# THE **POWER**
## OF THE
# **DOWNSTATE**

# THE **POWER**
## OF THE
# **DOWNSTATE**

Recharge Your Life
Using Your Body's Own
Restorative Systems

Sara C. Mednick, PhD

hachette
BOOKS

NEW YORK

Copyright © 2022 by Sara C. Mednick
Interior figures © 2022 by Emily Marshall Majer, MA
Cover design by Amanda Kain
Cover copyright © 2022 by Hachette Book Group, Inc.

Hachette Go, an imprint of Hachette Books
Hachette Book Group
1290 Avenue of the Americas
New York, NY 10104
HachetteGo.com
Facebook.com/HachetteGo
Instagram.com/HachetteGo

First Edition: April 2022
Hachette Books is a division of Hachette Book Group, Inc.

The Hachette Go and Hachette Books name and logos are trademarks of Hachette Book Group, Inc. The publisher is not responsible for websites (or their content) that are not owned by the publisher.

Editorial production by Christine Marra, *Marra*thon Production Services. www.marrathoneditorial.org
Print book interior design by Jane Raese.
Set in 11-point Chaparral Pro

Library of Congress Control Number: 2022931376

ISBNs: 978-0-306-92579-5 (hardcover); 978-0-306-92578-8 (ebook)

Printed in the United States of America
LSC-C
Printing 1, 2022

THIS BOOK IS DEDICATED TO

*Alpha, Captain, and Rebel Turkeys.*

*Glorious Turkey loves you.*

*There is only one holy book, the sacred manuscript of nature which truly enlightens all readers.*

**—One of the 10 Sufi Thoughts**

*What is essential in the existence of man is the fact that he has emerged from the animal kingdom, the instinctive adaptation, that he has transcended nature—although he never leaves it; he is a part of it—and yet once torn away from nature, he cannot return to it; once thrown out of paradise—a state of original oneness with nature— cherubim with flaming swords block his way, if he should try to return. Man can only go forward by developing his reason, by finding a new harmony, a human one, instead of the prehumen harmony which is irretrievably lost.*

**—From *The Art of Loving* by Erich Fromm**

*How long should I be working on this? At least till you die . . .*

**—From *The Places that Scare You* by Pema Chödrön**

# Contents

# Author's Note

All names and details have been changed or modified; some characters are composites.

# Introduction

This world is hard. Adulting is *hard*. It takes an extraordinary amount of time, energy, and other resources to respond to the pressures bearing down on you from work, finances, family, personal health, and other areas, not to mention the never-ending information barrage from the news and social media. And, in this dystopian new era of highly contagious viruses, planetary destruction, and all the other troubles of the world, you can easily find yourself living with heightened levels of anxiety, vulnerability, and hyperarousal that tax your ability to maintain any sense of balance.

Most of us live our lives as the human equivalent of smartphones running on 10 percent battery power. At any given time, you're just an hour or so away from shutting off, but you insist on eking out a few more minutes in Low Power mode. Which means you're slower than you need to be. Dimmer. You feel drained. Stressed out. Your processing time stinks.

The truth is that you have battery chargers everywhere, and I'm here to help you find them.

## Welcome to *The Power of the Downstate*

The Downstate is a comprehensive term that refers to the wide range of recovery systems you can tap into on a daily basis to restore your most vital functions at a cellular level, including giving your heart, brain, and metabolism a rest; repairing overtrained or inflamed tissue; and allowing time to process some of the more complicated business of being human—your memories, emotions, carefully made decisions, and Aha! moments. The Downstate is also the time for housecleaning the brain's toxic by-products of everyday living. It's your opportunity to plug yourself into a metaphorical outlet and power back up.

You won't find the Downstate I'm talking about in any self-help books, medical manuals, or laboratory studies because until now, there hasn't been a word for it. I developed the concept based on research insights discovered in my University of California lab. For the past decade, the scientific community has recognized that a type of Downstate happens every night, starting when your head sinks into your pillow, your eyes close, and your brain takes its delicious dive into sleep. As a professor of cognitive science at UC Irvine and world expert on sleep—specifically, the role that sleep plays in forming our long-term memories, regulating our emotions, keeping our cardiovascular system functioning properly, and helping older adults stay alert and agile—I have discovered just how important that nighttime Downstate is for our mental and physical health. Thanks to experimental findings from my sleep lab, along with other labs' findings, we now understand that in the depths of sleep, a healthy brain switches from On to Off mode in successive, one-second intervals, called Upstates (when brain activity is high) and Downstates (when brain activity is low). Together, the sleep science community has established that these Downstates are the driving force for all of sleep's restorative benefits. And most alarmingly, they are the very thing we're losing as we head into middle age.

But the story doesn't end with sleep. The Downstate is an integral part of all the physiological, cognitive, and emotional processes that allow us to stay resilient, yet it is often ignored by our go, go, go and do, do, do society. You can capture Downstate moments at any time of day by taking your fingers off the keyboard and sinking into a deep breath, taking yourself on a walk around the block with your furry friend, or mindfully preparing a meal that will do your body good. Downstate moments can also be harnessed by maintaining a regular schedule with your sleeping, eating, and exercise routines such that your mind and body synchronize to your own natural rhythm, rather than the rhythm imposed on you by society, your family, or your job. By honoring these Downstates, we tap into our personal renewable resources that help us live longer, wiser, and healthier lives.

I am a sleep researcher by trade. My lab showed that an hour-long nap rich in deep Downstate sleep can reverse the accumulation of fatigue that erodes our thinking during the day in ways that other interventions, such as caffeine, meditation, or even the promise of money, cannot.[1] These bite-size bits of daytime sleep not only increase alertness, they engage memory and emotional systems, restore tissues, enhance immune function, and provide a mini-cardiovascular holiday, making you smarter, more productive and creative, stronger, and healthier when you return to the daily grind. In fact, I showed that the magnitude of cognitive and restorative benefits from one daytime nap was equal to that of a whole night of sleep![2]

My first book, *Take a Nap! Change Your Life*, was written for the go-getter personality—Doozers, as I like to call them. Doozers are creatures who only know how to work.[3] They sport construction helmets, boots, and tool belts and build, build, build, or die. Doozers don't Downstate. They put their heads down and keep working. You're a Doozer when you eat lunch at your desk, forget to go outside all day, and get up at three a.m. to start prepping for that big presentation next week. *Take a Nap!* reinitiated the nap into Doozer culture as the best tool for increasing and igniting productivity, memory, and creativity, as well as the antidote for the epidemic of sleep deprivation that still shows no signs of abating.

After its publication, my attention turned to big picture questions about how all our rejuvenating subsystems—not just sleep, but cardiovascular, circadian, and metabolic—fit together. In particular, I wanted to figure out why these systems seem to simultaneously fall apart in older adults, and what these insights could tell us about the same, yet milder, cognitive changes that begin to appear in forty-somethings. Sure, there are some grandparents who are in tip-top shape, sleep well, and are cognitively sharp. But more fall into the middle of the spectrum: typical aging adults who struggle to sleep through the night, feel sluggish during the day, have trouble remembering words, and forget to take their medication. Moving to the far end, you find people with Alzheimer's or dementia who have completely fragmented, wholly non-restorative sleep, along with internal biological rhythms that are so discombobulated that they're awake all night and fall asleep involuntarily during the day. These problems don't just appear one day in the mail like the dreaded inaugural AARP magazine; anyone in their forties will tell you that these issues make themselves known much earlier. I thought that if I could understand the deeper reason for these differences between healthy and pathological aging, I might be able to catch the problem early, hopefully discovering the cause and, thereby, the solution to these problems.

One thing was certain: A fresh, holistic viewpoint was required that could bring together disparate scientific approaches, considering not just the basic neuroscience of the brain but the untapped secrets from the body as well.

The first inkling of that viewpoint came on a visit to colleagues at the University of Sydney, Australia, where I learned that the autonomic nervous system doesn't just maintain our most basic water and power functions, but that it also plays an important role in high-level information processing, with the two opposing autonomic branches, the sympathetic and parasympathetic systems, contributing independent parts. The sympathetic is known as the fight-or-flight response but actually encompasses all of the ways your body mobilizes its resources in response to new and exciting experiences, stress broadly defined, injury, or illness. The parasympathetic, also called the rest-and-digest branch, calms you down, decreases inflammation, rebuilds and replenishes your depleted resources, and supports your mental and emotional processing.

Parasympathetic activity is measured through heart rate and the calculation of heart rate variability (HRV), which reflects the amount of variation between heartbeats. I learned that HRV activity during waking hours was linked with cognitive ability, such that the higher the HRV—meaning the more milliseconds of variation between heartbeats—the better people performed in tests of attention, working memory, and self-control (a group of cognitive functions typically labeled *executive functions*).

This finding intrigued me because I also understood that the two branches of the autonomic system engaged in a little power play across the day and night, with the sympathetic system domineering the daylight hours, whereas parasympathetic activity reigned while we slept.[4] And my research had repeatedly shown that most of our cognitive improvement happened during sleep, not while awake. But, surprisingly, nobody had thought to consider how parasympathetic activity during *sleep* might be playing a role in cognition. I decided that my lab should be the first to investigate that question. That day I emailed my lab on the other side of the world and asked them to add a couple of new electrodes to our sleep recordings because we were going to start collecting information from the heart (in the form of an electrocardiogram [ECG]) along with the typical brain activity we get from electroencephalograms (EEGs). When I returned home, my then-graduate student, Dr. Lauren Whitehurst, dove into the new analysis of the ECG signals to determine whether they predicted any of the memory improvements we see in our research subjects.

I remember the first time we sat down together to review the results. Lauren came in and closed my office door so we could talk in private. She looked at me with a strange combination of intense excitement and deep concern, and said, "Sara, you are not going to believe these results." She proceeded to show me one of the most significant associations my lab had ever seen between sleep and cognitive improvement. By considering a combination of their brain (i.e., EEG) *and* heart (i.e., ECG) activity during sleep, we were able to account for 73 percent of participants' memory improvement after a nap.[5] These results showed plainly that there was more to understanding our mental processes than focusing solely on brain activity. In fact, neural activity was only part of the story; parasympathetic activity from the heart played the real starring role. And since parasympathetic activity reflected the REST (-and-digest) state of the autonomic system, this meant that just like those Off periods in the sleeping brain, the autonomic nervous system spent crucial time in the Downstate, too, and both of these restorative breaks contributed to making us smarter.

The question was rapidly forming in my head that if sleep and autonomic activity had a restorative Downstate, what other systems had one too? And was engaging these Downstate processes key to living a long and healthy life? I was taking my first bold glances into the eyes of the Downstate, and from that moment on, I have been continuously amazed by how clearly nature repeats itself when it has found a pattern that works. Using a broad scope of scientific approaches, I have shown that enhancing Downstate expression is the key to health, well-being, and longevity, and that is why I decided to write this book.

I compiled all these restorative processes into a single idea, the Downstate, an umbrella term coined from neuroscience, which can be defined as a noun or an adjective. As a noun, the Downstate is the time and space where restoration and recuperation from the rigamarole of living take place. As an adjective, it can describe all the activities that replenish and reenergize body and mind. What I've discovered is that the Downstate doesn't just happen at the neural level in the ups and downs of slow-wave sleep. The truth is, there is a whole lotta Downstate everywhere you look, especially when awake. You have it when you practice mindfulness and focus on your breathing. You have it when you take your dogs for a walk in the forest or when you hold hands with someone you love. You have it in the external glow delivered by an intense workout or an out-of-this-world orgasm and the internal glow that comes by eating whole grains, colorful fruit and veggies, fish and omega-3 fatty acids, and very little red meat. You have it when you confine eating times to a relatively short window, which gives your organs the break they need and deserve.

## What Goes Down, Must Come Up . . .

The Downstate is here for you whenever you need to recharge and restore so you can get back to the chaos of the day. I call this other half of life the Upstate (again borrowing from neuroscience), when all activities that require energy, focus, action, and the mobilization of mental and physiological forces happen. The Upstate is when you go to work, when you're industrious, when you kick ass and take names. It's when your body and mind naturally conspire together to make sure you have all the energy you need to climb a mountain, tackle a work assignment, or stand in front of a crowd and tell them what you know. It's when you're most resilient to stress and, not coincidently, it's when most stress happens. The Upstate is what makes living, living . . . but it's also what drains your batteries.

Whether your personal weakness is Lust, Gluttony, Greed, Sloth, Wrath, Envy, or Pride, the 24-hour Upstate Party is in permanent full swing, everywhere you go, luring you in with short-term rewards that offer up a million and one reasons to avoid nurturing/tending to your Downstate. Let's take a look at the usual suspects:

**Electronic Upstate Party:** There's a raucous Upstate Party happening on screens, social media, news, and work emails, none of which abides by day or night. We have all grown accustomed to letting our boundaries between home and work be crossed, especially in the wake of the pandemic when our bedrooms became our offices and our kitchens were piled high with the detritus of elementary school classrooms. Finding any semblance of a work/life balance has become nearly impossible, so much so that most of us couldn't name a single personal boundary if asked, especially around our electronic devices. We allow so many attentional traps to tear us away from the present moment: the zing of notifications that creates a dopamine/serotonin speedball and drives us to check our phones during conversations with partners and dinners with family and friends; the AutoPlay option on streaming apps that keeps us glued to the couch following up on some cliff hanger, instead of on some make-out time with the person sitting right next to us; social media or a favorite sex site that catapults us into a mental vortex of procrastination, even as the stress of our inaction drives up self-loathing.

**Convenience Food Upstate Party:** Whether you're cooking for one or for four, it's become easier to fill your grocery cart with insta-meals that come in pouches, boxes, and single-serve packets. We live in a just-add-water-for-dinner civilization. Fast food, convenience store munchies, and microwavable dinners are cheaper than vegetables and pumped full of preservatives so they can sit on a shelf or in a freezer for years without decaying. They are loaded with ultraprocessed ingredients that spike your blood sugar levels faster than you can throw the wrapper into the garbage.

**Social Pressure Upstate Party:** As a community, we lionize burning the candle at both ends and promote Upstate badges of honor, such as "I'm so busy," "I'm super stressed," and "I have so much work," which can be translated as "I'm not making Me Time," "I'm not feeling empowered at work," and "I have no time for giving and receiving love." Each of these statements pours acid on your ability to temper Upstate arousal. They also greatly increase your chances of burnout, which results in overwhelming exhaustion, feelings of cynicism and detachment from the job at hand, a sense of ineffectiveness and lack of accomplishment. And it's not just long hours of unrelenting paper pushing that can bring on burnout. Careers fueled by passion and purpose are the very ones driving people into the ground due to the expectation (implicit or explicit) that work should take priority over personal physical and mental health.[6] Compounding matters, technological advances promote the "always on" mentality. So, even loving what you do doesn't guarantee that you'll "never work a day in your life." Many of us are unable to find rest when our heads hit the pillow . . . or we wake up in a panic and can't get back to dreamland once our racing heart and churning thoughts take over.

**Self-Medication Upstate Party:** To get through the night, many of us rely on a slew of unhelpful coping mechanisms: late-night emotional eating, daily drinking, smoking or vaping tobacco or cannabis, consuming caffeine like it's your job, and using prescription stimulants, such as Adderall or amphetamines. Needless to say, all of these fallbacks are a gateway— actually, more like a luge race—to riskier behaviors. For many adults, the concept of relaxing and enjoying a moment without pharmacological assistance is a distant and unfamiliar concept. These coping mechanisms are closely linked with anxiety, depression, weight gain, and drug and alcohol abuse, not to mention they deflate your get-up-and-go, destroy your wellness routine, and share one guaranteed outcome: a jacked-up Upstate and a shut-down Downstate recovery system.

I want to emphasize a crucial point here: you can handle a significant amount of Upstate stress as long as you replenish yourself on a daily basis by engaging in Downstate activities that make you feel rested, full of energy, loved and cared for by others. The foundation of your mental and physical health is in the symbiotic relation between Upstates and Downstates, and this unifying theory is just as relevant to the smallest kernel of the neuron as it is to the cycles of day and night, the weekdays and weekend, seasons of the year, and even beyond that to a lifetime.

Think of the interplay between Upstates and Downstates as the ebb and flow of ocean waves eternally lapping against the shore. At the beginning of every wave cycle, the ocean draws the water and all its riches back into the cold, deep sea, pooling its resources and accumulating velocity, nutrients, mass, volume, and power in the process. This is the Downstate ebb of the wave, which is inevitably followed by the cresting, thunderous explosion of all that energy in the Upstate portion of the wave. The magnitude of drawing inward during the Downstate is directly proportional to the power of the outward Upstate blast; as long as there is a Moon and Earth to promote this rhythm it will always be there. All animals and plants are resource-limited, so they need to cycle between Downstates and Upstates to generate power and then release it. Whether your goal is to learn the ukulele; have more energy for your kids, grandkids, or garden; or to reach some work-related goal, playing at full capacity in the Upstate requires that your tanks get refilled to their maximum capacity as frequently as possible. The Downstate is where that happens.

*The Power of the Downstate* gives you a framework for understanding the synergy between Upstates and Downstates along with a comprehensive four-week Downstate RecoveryPlus Plan that provides the practical steps to achieve the harmony that nature intended. I will show you how to achieve the right Upstate/Downstate ratio every day by making specific changes to your life, including how you breathe, sleep, exercise, and eat.

For thousands of years, smart folks have lived by the simple, holistic principle that a system in harmony tends toward health, well-being, and sustainability, and a system in disharmony tends toward illness, disease, suffering, and collapse. If it sounds a bit unfamiliar, that's because modern health care has become reactive and silo-based, instead of preventative and holistic. You wait until you are already out of balance and in the ER before beginning treatment. You have one doctor for your heart and another for your kidney and another for your ears, nose, and throat. Appointments usually aren't made until a problem has already grown out of control, then you undergo tests and receive medicine *for that specific problem*: your heart, your kidneys, your ears, nose, or throat. You find yourself taking a mountain of pills with little oversight.

How often does your cardiologist ask about your sleep? When has your psychiatrist brought up potential links between what you eat and your depression symptoms? Where are the recommendations for young adults to maintain their working memory by ruthlessly guarding their good sleep far into the choppy waves of adulthood? What about nutrition, movement, sleep, breathing, and stress mitigation? Why have we been ignoring recommendations about balance and harmony from the smartest people throughout history?

And now we're in trouble. We relentlessly push ourselves to the brink of exhaustion and depletion, pushing ourselves to be stronger, faster, smarter, sexier, more productive and successful, and accepting invitations to each and every Upstate Party, which further drains our resources. Just like the ocean waves that can't keep crashing on the shore over and over without the critical preparatory phase, human beings are not designed to operate at maximum effort, hour after hour, day after day, without spending time in the Downstate.

Your day is literally filled with chances to de-stress at a physiological and emotional level, yet you don't snatch them up because you (a) don't know they exist, or (b) think that taking anything resembling a break will destroy your productivity. But they're there, like little $20 bills falling from the sky and landing on the seat next to you on the subway . . . tucked into the phone booth at your coworking space . . . stuck to the handle of your refrigerator. There's one sitting on your bike seat as you read this page. We'd never ignore free money, but we're blind to the Downstate opportunities and sooner or later, our health and happiness will pay the price.

*The Power of the Downstate* integrates *Upstate* and *Downstate* into the everyday lexicon, introduces them as a formal concept and a new way of framing all of your biological processes. This is not just a book about sleep, or an attempt to convince you that the answer lies in one health behavior. Think of the Downstate as the new way humans "take a break" that is based on principles as old as Earth itself, and which come in the most unexpected ways . . . a powerlifting session; a challenging mountain ascent; falling into a deep conversation with a friend; spending the last third of your day fasting; taking a walk in nature; making time for creative thinking; having a smoothie in the sun or pretzeled up with someone listening to the rain. (I know I said it can be a noun or an adjective, but it can even be a verb: *Come Downstating!*)

By following the guidance put forth in this book, you'll be living according to an instruction manual invented by Nature, designed to help humans get the most out of each day. Get ready to be more alert, productive, and cognitively sharp during the day, feel greater intimacy and affection, and enjoy consolidated, restorative sleep at night . . . not to mention expand your years of mental and physical vitality. Ready to get Down? Let's begin!

## The Desiderata of the Downstate

When I Downstate, I . . .

1. Give myself an almighty gift of harmony, love, and peace every day

2. Fill my tanks so that I can be of better service to those who depend on me

3. Am a better partner, friend, and family member with healthy boundaries who has energy, time, and space for intimacy and honest communication

4. Am a loving parent with self-mastery and compassion to guide and support my children with wisdom and patience

5. Embody an energetic, strong, and flexible body that is capable of protecting and caring for my physical needs and the needs of those around me

6. Harmonize with my internal rhythm and can choose to sync up with the rhythm of people around me and society at large when needed

7. Get deep rest by making space and time for the restorative power of sleep as it suits me

8. Blend my nutritional needs with my love of tasty foods and prepare each meal as an offering to the temple of my body

9. Bring awareness and connection to each moment through my full and steady breath

10. Meet my basic needs, heal my wounds, and replenish my resources on a daily basis so that I can answer the calling from my highest self for many years to come

# PART ONE

# Getting in the Right Ratio

Chapter 1 introduces you to the autonomic nervous system as the ultimate expression of the push-pull relationship that exists between your Upstate and Downstate. This system works in your favor when well tuned but can conspire against you when your response to stress creeps, unchecked, into your life. The best way to maintain a strong autonomic nervous system involves tapping into the natural rhythms that occur across the 24-hour day that give both the Upstate and Downstate their own special moment in the sun, or moon as the case may be. In Chapter 2, you will learn how, since the beginning of life on Earth, living plants and animals have survived best by relegating their Upstate sympathetic activities to daytime hours, and their Downstate parasympathetic processes to the night. Modern culture has steered you away from this simple truth, but Part 1 will explain the benefits to regaining alignment with these daily circadian rhythms, as well as the weekly, monthly, and annual rhythms of activity and rest that govern life.

# CHAPTER ONE

# Everything You Know About Balance Needs an Upgrade

I was a late bloomer when it came to learning how the brain works. As a young woman, I focused all my energies toward a future career on the stage and screen. It wasn't until my midtwenties when I leveled with myself concerning this childhood dream and realized that, after several hundred cattle call auditions, one too many unpaid East Village performance art pieces, and a series of casting couch invitations, I needed to find another way to "make it" in this life.

I accepted a job working in the psychiatry department at New York City's Bellevue Hospital, purely because it allowed me to take classes at New York University for free. Working with newly admitted psych ER patients opened my eyes to the fact that not all brains are wired the same—an experience so world-rocking and profound that I switched career paths from theater to psychology. After volunteering in several labs that gave me hands-on experience with experimental research and a chance to present my findings at a scientific conference, I applied to PhD programs and was thrilled to land at Harvard University's Psychology Department. During my first year, I was immersed in lectures about this strange organ called the brain, a complicated network of eighty-six billion or so densely packed cells, and practically overnight, the brain had become my new fascination.

It was during these first heady days of graduate training that I was introduced to a simple fact that would evolve into one of the foundational building blocks of *The Power of the Downstate*—to live your most satisfying, productive, enjoyable life, you need to replenish your resources regularly. And it all starts with the neuron.

## The World's Smallest Downstate

In my first neuroscience class, we received a big picture tour of the average brain cell, also known as a neuron. Neurons communicate through *action potentials*, blasts of information sent from one brain cell to the next. Picture it: Neuron A is buzzing with some juicy message—*"The light turned green; hit the gas"*; *"Dude, put away the bong, your mom is at the door"*—and tells her closest neighbor, Neuron B, by sending a prolonged and intense burst of chemical and electrical messengers his way. Once Neuron B grasps the full extent of that communication, he is ready to fire off a similarly bold message to his buddy, Neuron C. This train of action potentials between neurons resembles the human microphone of protest movements and is the basis for all thought, action, and reaction in any animal that trucks with anything resembling a brain.

This loud and persistent stream of A→B→C firing is called *long-term potentiation*, and every thought, feeling, and action—even you reading this sentence—is a result of your neurons communicating with each other in this manner. (As famed neuropsychologist Donald Hebb said (paraphrased by neurobiologist Carla Shatz): "Neurons that fire together, wire together.")[1]

This lightning-fast game of Operator is resource-depleting, and neurons need microdoses of rest between every action potential so as to successfully keep passing messages down the line. Contrary to the hopes of many computational modelers of the '80s and '90s, the human brain is not just a fancy circuit board of wires and resistors feeding off of a limitless electrical supply; it's a biological organ composed of billions of neurons, and as with every living thing, neurons are limited in resources. Because of this, each neuron requires programmed breaks that grant time to literally recharge and prepare for the next power punch. These rest states are called *refractory periods* and they represent our biological need for Downstates at the cellular level.[2]

As I learned more about the brain and body, I realized that not only has Nature, in its infinite wisdom, provided the refractory period to ensure your brain cells have the Downstate they need, but that this pattern of activation and recovery was a fundamental principle of every aspect of our

## REFRACTORY PERIODS REVEAL NATURE'S SECRET TO OUR SUCCESS

Neurons have two states: resting and firing. As the neuron moves between these two states, electrically charged ions flow between the inside and outside of the cell walls. At rest, there are far more negatively charged ions inside the cell than outside, with a resting membrane potential of −70mV. When Neuron A sends an action potential to Neuron B using chemical and electrical messengers called neurotransmitters, little doors on Neuron B open up, allowing positive ions into the cell. This sudden shift from negative to positive charge changes the membrane potential of the neuron to an all-time high of +33mV and sends a strong action potential toward Neuron C. Once Neuron B completes its burst of activity, it enters its refractory period, a time in which no amount of bribery, pleading, or seduction from Neuron A (or any neuron, for that matter) will make it react. Neuron B is engaged in a critical Downstate process of restoring its membrane potential one ion at a time until it can get back to its fighting weight—or charge, in this case. Nature has set up this mandatory work break, during which the neuron prepares for the next big communication by repositioning its ions in their rightful spots and reestablishing a resting membrane potential of −70mV, after which it's ready to fire off another action potential. In the time it takes you to read this sentence (five seconds), your neurons will have fired off anywhere from two hundred to four hundred action potentials and logged a corresponding number of refractory periods![2]

lives. Just as BIG YOU needs sleep, exercise, food, time in nature, warm touch, and more, in the right dose and at the right times, all the Little Yous—neurons, organs, muscles—need recharging too. And if you are wondering whether the refractory period that men experience after every ejaculation is another example of nature's built-in Downstates, you'd be right! That post-*YES!* full-body surrender and complete lack of say in the matter, evolutionarily speaking, "favours natural selection by maintaining sperm counts by limiting too-frequent ejaculation."[3] In other words, this particular Downstate is nature's way of preventing you from spilling the beans, so to speak.

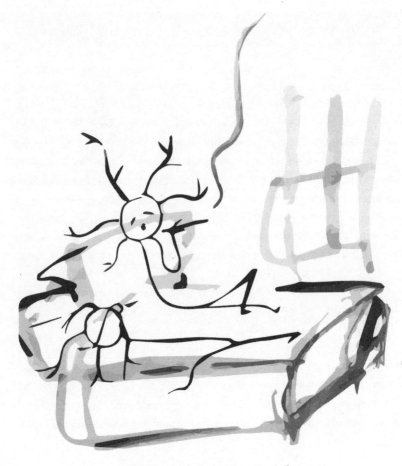

The Neuron's Refractory Period

## Homeostasis, Homeoshmaesis

Nature is abundant with evidence of two sides to every action—a preparatory buildup and an energetic release. Consider how the ocean wave inwardly draws up the power, motion, and intensity of the sea before the dramatic outward crash onto the beach. Think of the cold and dark of winter that produces strong crop yields in the summer, or the deep muscle exhaustion that comes after an athlete's long run or intense sprint that leads to muscle growth and facilitates fleeter feet later on. Borrowing from Newton's Third Law of Action and Reaction: *To every Upstate action, there is always an equal and opposite Downstate replenishment.*

Our health is maintained via the right amount of energy-consuming Upstates and energy-replenishing Downstates. Just as the neuron alternates action potentials with refractory periods to get its job done, Upstates and Downstates need to be in the right ratio so that you are ready for anything: the next physical challenge, big relationship talk, work presentation, night on the town, and so on. Digging deep into this phenomenon is critical to mastering "this thing called life."[4]

Throughout history, we've been told that survival depends on achieving balance in our basic physiological functions. This goal state, called *homeostasis* (*homo* meaning "same," *stasis* meaning "steady") was first coined by physiologist Walter Cannon, MD, in a wonderfully detailed 1932 treatise called *Wisdom of the Body*.[5] Consider a simple homeostat that you likely regularly use; the thermostat in your home. When set to 68°F, the heating/cooling system is constantly turning on and off to keep the area around the thermometer at that temperature. Cannon proposed that the same basic principle works for humans and described the exquisite sensitivity of our physiological functions to small perturbations in the environment that affect our *internal milieu*, the fluid that bathes every cell of the body transporting nutrient to cells (and waste away from cells). For example, our body temperature needs to be maintained at around 98.6°F (37°C) whether we are baking in the Palm Springs desert sun or sleeping in a Swedish ice hotel. To keep our internal milieu within a narrow homeostatic range, we sweat to cool down or shiver to heat up. Similarly, the cells in our bodies need to maintain a specific amount of glucose for energy. The pancreas releases insulin, which transports glucose into the cells as needed. If blood glucose levels drop too low, the liver steps in to maintain a specific level in the cells at all times. These are prime examples of how homeostasis— *same, steady*—works.

Cannon was not the first person to propose the need for balance. For thousands of years, Chinese medicine has based its practices on the simple principle that any system in harmony tends toward health, well-being, and sustainability, while a system in disharmony lists toward illness, disease, suffering, and collapse. Similarly, ancient Greek and pre-Socratic philosophers, such as Hippocrates, developed the humoral theory for human physiology, in which the human body consisted of four humors (blood, black bile, yellow bile, and phlegm) that continuously circulated through the organs and tissues.[6] When the humors were balanced and in harmony (*eucrasia* in Greek), a person enjoyed optimal health. When disequilibrium and disharmony (*dyscrasia* in Greek) erupted among those humors, disease occurred.

In fact, French physiologist Claude Bernard went so far as to say, "All the vital mechanisms, however varied they may be, have only one object, that of preserving constant the conditions of life in the internal environment."[7] In other words, we are searching for balance in all aspects of life.

But wait a second; let's think about this a little more carefully. Doesn't holding steady at one homeostatic set-point feel completely out of touch with every physical, intellectual, and psychological goal you've ever set? When is the last time you started eating better to stay on track toward heart disease, or embarked on a meditation training program because you wanted to maintain feeling strung-out and frazzled, or practiced an instrument so that you'd repeat the same mistakes? Progress, growth, and aiming high can't happen if your brain and body work like a homeostat. In reality, that concept only applies to a handful of physiological variables truly essential for life, like maintaining pH, body temperature, glucose, and oxygen levels. These functions have optimal set-points and only a narrow range of tolerable fluctuations, over or under which you're destined for rapid decline and even death.

## Introducing RecoveryPlus

From birth to death, humans want to become stronger, faster, smarter, sexier, and fitter. Whether you're seeking growth in an intellectual, emotional, physical, or spiritual domain, the way you get better isn't by looping around the same old circle trying to get back to your baseline. Let's engage with a more apt description of growth: an upward trajectory with a lot of zigzags along the way.

A great example of our bumpy progress toward goal achievement can been seen with exercise, which has the power to take you from couch potato to 5K-running gym nut within months. Balance? What balance? This transformation depends entirely on a call-and-response dialogue between your Upstate action and Downstate recovery that keeps ratcheting up your set-point to the next level.

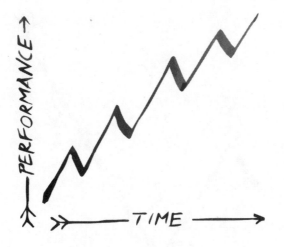

**Performance Improvement**

When you first begin (or return to) an exercise routine, you may only be able to withstand twenty minutes of cardio and fifteen minutes of strength training at the lowest weight before you feel that you're in cardiac arrest. After the first workout, you're exhausted.

But! That exhaustion sends a strong signal to jump-start your Downstate recovery process, such that you're better prepared for that hard workout next time. I call this process RecoveryPlus, with *Recovery* encompassing the necessary repairing and rebuilding of damaged muscles, replenishing of energy reserves, increasing in lung capacity, and bringing cardio functioning to a more nimble state, and *Plus* extending that recovery time just long enough to get you a little extra bump in resources, ensuring you'll have more juice the next time. (Think of it as your body's insurance policy against feeling as broken as you did after that first workout.) Your body interprets the inaugural workout as a major stressor—*"I'm moving fast! I'm lifting heavy things! Time to mobilize resources!"*—and that alone means you're already starting to nudge your set-point forward with that very first session. By sticking with your new regimen, your body learns how to use oxygen and glycogen (sugars) more efficiently, and your heart, lungs, and muscles grow stronger, bringing you to a new set-point for stamina and strength. You've recovered, but with a bonus, because instead of returning to the same old–same old, you have elevated yourself. With each bout of exercise followed by a sufficient recovery period, you can work out a little

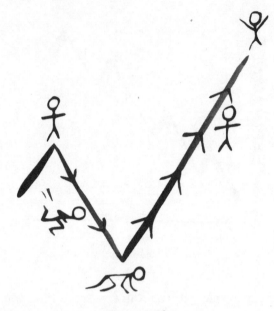

RecoveryPlus

longer, or lift slightly more weight. In time, the duration of your Downstate recovery grows shorter and shorter, and the next thing you know, you're someone who actually looks forward to going to the gym.

Exercise, therefore, is a prime example of one of the most important principles of this book: The Upstate action and Downstate RecoveryPlus pathway is THE mechanism by which you bounce your set-points—and with them, your potential—higher and higher.

The same RecoveryPlus trajectory can be applied to anything at which you would like to get better. Take the psychological process of learning. Your knowledge set-point is constantly changing as you absorb new facts, whether you're taking a class, tuning in to a podcast, learning Hungarian, or practicing the tuba. I recently boosted my own set-point by listening to psychologist Terry Real's audiobook on relationships, *Fierce Intimacy*.[8] I didn't know anything about his approach to working with couples, so my initial knowledge set-point was very low, as it is for every beginner learning about a new topic. As I listened, I found myself deep in Upstate *information-gathering* mode: taking voracious notes and noticing lightbulbs inside my head sparking up every few minutes as I began to understand myself and my experiences with love, starting with my most primary relationship—my parents. At times, I would turn off his voice and take a walk or run, have a deep conversation with my wife, Emily, or my bestie, Karen, or fall into a deep sleep. These intermittent periods of Downstate *information-processing* provided me with the time and space for consolidation and integration of these fierce new ideas with my prior life experiences, advancing my set-point for understanding myself as I relate to others.

Life throws at you a steady stream of challenging-in-a-good-way experiences, which I like to call "reasonable stressors"—things like buying a house at the upper limit of your bank account, taking a hard college course, training for a marathon, or falling in love (and the crimes and misdemeanors that often follow). These stressors are fundamental to the development of your own self-confidence and worldview, because they teach you that you can handle whatever comes your way. Sure, starting a new job, or a new grade in school, whether kindergarten or college, is hard, but great challenges wouldn't be great without a little agonizing strain and nauseating thrill, now would they?

When you're young and healthy, you are abundant in resources that allow you to handle these reasonable stressors. By that I mean you have ample neurotransmitters, hormones, nutrients, and robust physiological systems to efficiently pump these substances through your body, get rid of waste products, and make strong new mental and emotional connections. During these glory days, your Downstate support systems are optimized, making life's ups and downs manageable, allowing you to experience, recover, and grow. (As my wife likes to say: "Oh great, another f***ing growth opportunity.") Once you muster the courage and perseverance to scale that peak, the gift waiting on the other side is both a relief that the struggle has ceased and the confidence of "I did it myself!"

Similarly, as you develop and learn life lessons, your set-point for tolerating disappointment, regulating emotions, and expressing your needs adjusts to new levels. Difficult experiences that pepper your childhood, from being bullied to parental divorce, mold your views of the world and create set-points for how you will react to future difficult life experiences. At the time, it feels unsurvivable, but with support from family and friends and your own bootstraps, you make it through and bounce back stronger.

Psychological makeup also has a big influence on how you perceive yourself and your experiences. An adult with depression will experience a loss or disappointment very differently than someone without depression, and someone raised in a stable, loving household may be more resilient than someone who grew up in a dangerous or abusive home. Economic, racial, and gender privilege can enhance access to opportunities that help some people attain their goals more easily than others. Together, your individual personality, mental health, race, sex, ethnicity, sexual orientation, finances, and overall life history matter in how you adapt your set-points to daily life experiences.

All of which is to say, while Hippocrates, Cannon, and many other scientists throughout history were definitely onto something with their theories of balance and harmony, we need to reach for a new concept, one that encompasses the real biological, psychological, and emotional trajectory of progress.

As you move forward, keep the RecoveryPlus concept in mind: Intense experiences stretch you beyond your comfort zone and push you to reach for new set-points, physically, cognitively, and emotionally. As Jen Sincero writes, "If you want to live a life you've never lived, you have to do things you've never done."[9] Reaching each new set-point—achieving Recovery-Plus—can only be done by plunging deeply into the Downstate.

Now, let's meet the system that has evolved over billions of years to run the Downstate RecoveryPlus show . . .

## Meet the Two Sides of Your Autonomic Nervous System

The essence of your quest to elevate your set-points hinges on the actions of your autonomic nervous system, which, at a basic level, supports equilibrium of all your physiological functions, including maintaining the right levels of salt and electrolytes, controlling body temperature within a narrow range, keeping blood pressure high enough to circulate nutrients throughout the entire body, and managing waste disposal. On top of custodial care, the autonomic system also keeps you abreast of all new experiences, providing moment-to-moment support for every action and reaction you have to the world. It facilitates a little dopamine bump when you see something you like; mobilizes oxygenated blood to muscles at the gym (and then repairs those muscles during Downstate recovery to be even stronger tomorrow); and ushers you into the coveted flow state, when

RESTORE & REV

you become so deeply absorbed in an activity or task that you are indistractable and primed for creative insight.[10]

Along with these positive experiences, the autonomic system also monitors your darker moments, such as heartache during a difficult breakup, pressure from a toxic boss, or the constant rants and raves of social media. You process all these experiences by engaging and inhibiting both branches of the autonomic nervous system—the sympathetic and the parasympathetic—which are inextricably tied together and complementary, like yin and yang, inhalation and exhalation, day and night.

Think of the two branches of the autonomic nervous system as subsystems that have essential roles in the larger organism, YOU. They are two sides of the same coin with their own unique strengths; when they are working together in harmony, all is right with the world. One subsystem, I call it REV, is highly sensitive to incoming information; it is reactive and ready to expend energy quickly. REV is important for facing any challenge that might come your way and enables you to reach beyond the ho-hum of your comfort zone, giving you the gusto to elevate set-points and grow. REV is critical for tough situations but, without careful monitoring, becomes an out-of-control bull in the china shop. You've probably already guessed that REV represents your sympathetic nervous system.

RESTORE, on the other hand, is a force of calm and level-headedness, providing space for thinking through problems, and feeling through emotions, without reacting to them. RESTORE is in charge of all parasympathetic responsibilities, including RecoveryPlus. RESTORE needs adequate time for stocking resources, healing tissues, connecting ideas, and teeing you up for the next challenge.

Each of us relies on both subsystems, but some of us might have a strong tendency to REV, making them a little heavy on the reactive, assertive, and even hypertensive side, whereas others might find themselves leaning toward RESTORE, which keeps them wading in the calm pool so long that they don't always have the drive to make sh*t happen. This is because RESTORE reigns when you need to draw inward, nurture a creative idea, heal your wounds, and replenish your resources, whereas REV evinces the muscular release of energy and the git-er-done pursuit of goals. As such, RESTORE and REV are equally matched and rely on each other. When both sides are synced up in a good ratio your autonomic nervous system works in your favor and you are at your best. But, when Upstate stress responses start to outnumber your Downstate cool-down sessions, REV can become overbearing.

REV supports all Upstate functions, such as novelty-seeking (e.g., our attraction for bright shiny new things like sports cars; exhilarating experiences like jumping out of planes racing high over the earth's crust; mingling professionally with people above your current station) and information-gathering (e.g., engaging in an exciting conversation; taking in a lecture, book, or podcast filled with knowledge that intrigues you; exploring and navigating a complex landscape like a forest or new city). It also revs up the body's readiness response so that you can assume a defensive or offensive stance, get your energy stores ready, mobilize your body for action, and focus your mind on the target. This burst of activity also tags exciting experiences as important and worthy of further processing by your cognitive and emotional brain after the immediate fires have been put out.

Evolutionarily speaking, REV is charged with keeping you safe from harm, whether that harm is presented in the form of a saber-toothed tiger 500,000 years ago or the driver who nearly mowed you down last week as you crossed the intersection. The millisecond you perceive trouble, your brain sounds an alarm triggering a cascade of events designed to propel you out of danger so you can fight, flee, freeze, protect, or do whatever you need to do to keep you and your charges safe. This massive mobilization response is generally referred to as the *fight-or-flight* response, but there is evidence that we can generate less aggressive responses to stress as well, including freezing in fear, or emotionally joining hands to protect the group, termed *tend-and-befriend*.[11] All of this happens instantaneously and unconsciously, and all under the direction of REV.

Your body isn't designed to have adrenaline coursing through your veins 24/7 and your heart rate doesn't like being elevated all the time. In fact, these stress responses can be downright corrosive to your brain and body. So, once it's saved your butt, REV falls back and its calmer, gentler half, RESTORE, takes center stage, undoing all that physiologic wear and tear that came from successfully avoiding the tiger or stopping in your tracks mid-intersection to avoid being hit by that careless driver. RESTORE's job is to inhibit and reverse your stress response and help you recover such precious physiological resources such as glycogen, body fluids, and blood flow. If you ever wonder how some people can maintain a sense of calm alertness even in the most high-tension-wire moments, that self-regulation is due to RESTORE working right alongside REV.

This same call-and-response exchange occurs following less lethal, yet still stressful experiences, such as being asked to introduce yourself in a meeting full of strangers. Now, let me remind you that not many people enjoy speaking in front of large groups. In fact, some rate public speaking as scarier than death itself.[12] So, if this is you, the moment you get called on to speak, the gaggle of seemingly innocent people sitting around a table will seem to transform into a deadly horde of terrifying goblins who are judging you, eye-rolling like they invented it, and texting under the conference table about what an idiot you are. At this particular moment, you'd rather a meteor hit this meeting than survive the next thirty seconds of abject humiliation. Chances are your fear response rivals any tiger-in-the-jungle scenario your forebears faced, which means REV is in full offense mode and RESTORE is preparing for damage control.

Inside your internal milieu, your brain and body are flooded with "stress hormones," such as cortisol and adrenaline, and all liquid and blood are shunted away from your digestive tract and erogenous zones (Who can think about sex when you're about to die from mortification?) toward your hands, arms, and legs to prepare for a swift escape or mortal combat. Your palms slicken, your mouth dries up, and your heart pounds in your chest like the drum of an 808 sound system. At this moment, even though you may not be in real danger, you are in the throes of REV's fight-or-flight response.

After you haltingly say your name and what department you are from, the bull's-eye shifts to the victim seated to your right, allowing you to grok that you didn't actually die, at least not this time. Now, the trusted, stabilizing force of RESTORE will make rapid work of pulling you back from the cliff of hyperarousal. First, as the need to mobilize your extremities for either a rapid sprint for the door or a battle-to-the-death has subsided, your heart rate slows, drawing back the blood and sweat from your hands, arms, and legs. Simultaneously, salivary liquids are replenished in your mouth and digestive tract, in case you want to go back to working on that oatmeal cookie, and your brain goes into Monday Morning Quarterback mode on whether you stuck the landing. All of these functions inform your concept of public speaking so when the next opportunity to speak in front of an audience arises, you might engage a little more *suave* (and a little less mortal combat) response. Welcome to the rapid response team of the autonomic nervous system, with its subsystems REV and RESTORE, who constantly trade insider information on all your internal workings to keep your Upstates and Downstates optimized.

But RESTORE does so much more than take over the nonessential mind-body functions put on hold during REV's domineering act (e.g., digestion, urination, sexual arousal, heart rate relaxation, and general lubrication of the eyes, mouth, and erogenous zones). While crusading and conquering occur in the realm of Upstate, our restorative, creative processes—all under RESTORE's purview—flourish in Downstate Land, including the transformation of recent experiences into long-term memories, engagement in complex thinking, creativity, and regulation of emotions. It provides a safe space for your mind to wander, dream, and create. All the things that were shunted to the back burner under stress come alive like a desert superbloom in the springtime.

In a nutshell, your RESTORE system gets elevated whenever you enter the Downstate. And the Downstate, which I have mentioned (and will continue to throughout the book), is the key to health, well-being, and longevity. Most important, it's your ticket to RecoveryPlus.

## Running on Empty:
## The Scourge of Autonomic Imbalance

When confronted with reasonable stressors, REV pumps your arousal up to the proper level and you feel excited to go explore the world and seek out novel experiences. (This sort of positive stress is technically called *eustress*, the prefix *eu* meaning "good, easy, normal." In contrast, negative stress is called *distress*, with *dis* meaning "unpleasant.") That first day of school, board exam, or long day of travel don't feel as intimidating. In fact, they seem downright exciting, and you feel ready, because a little bit of excitement mobilizes REV's forces (e.g., the stress hormones cortisol and adrenaline) in just the right amount to light a motivational match and help you zero in on the task at hand.

And because these hormones, in appropriate quantities, improve memory, they leave a lasting "Yes, we can!" imprint for the next time a similarly challenging situation arises. As long as REV is appropriately reigned in, things that put you right at the edge of stress get your blood pumping in an empowering, but not panicky, way. As Susan David, PhD, author of *Emotional Agility: Get Unstuck, Embrace Change and Thrive in Work and Life*, writes, "Courage is not an absence of fear; courage is fear walking."[13]

Oh, that life were but a basket of reasonable stressors! Instead, so many of us live under a 500-pound weighted blanket of chronic distress, held down by career pressure, financial worries both personal and global, relationship drama or abuse, the chaos of caretaking both aging parents and kids, the fear of the next pandemic, and the general grind of life that seems to grow more precarious and uncertain by the day. The nervous system interprets each of these troublesome situations as unsafe. And when you are consumed by them around the clock, which is the case with so many of us, your brain and body start to view everything, even not-so-dangerous situations, through the filter of "Yikes!"—galvanizing REV's army far more often than Mother Nature ever intended, but without the much-needed RESTORE follow-up to help replenish your resources and get you ready and able to handle the next attack.

With prolonged distress, you can end up in a state of *autonomic imbalance* that debilitates the entire system, causing the stress response to essentially become stuck in the On position. People spend weeks, months, even years submerged in toxic work environments or relationships that are spiraling down the drain. They feel plagued by financial worries or bear the burden of caring for kids and/or ailing parents, duties that call for the prioritization of others' needs above your own. In all these situations, built-in Downstate RecoveryPlus systems, such as sleep and exercise, are the first things to go. When this happens, the amount of time you spend in recovery mode doesn't match how long you spent swimming in the distress pool. This creates a serious challenge to your optimal REV/RESTORE ratio.

During the COVID-19 pandemic, stress levels were over the top. "There is a price tag to be paid individually and societally from the cumulative stress we have experienced from the pandemic," says Christine Runyan, PhD, cofounder of Tend Health, a program to protect the mental health of health-care professionals.[14] "It's not just about the mental health crisis. In the next two to five years, it's going to show up in medical conditions with the stress response at their core, including diseases of the cardiovascular and inflammatory systems, even cancer."

Mercedes, a mother, wife, and corporate lawyer, leaned into her career. Between the late work nights, school events, and pro bono work, life was demanding, but Mercedes found ways to make time for exercise, dinners with friends, quality time with her husband, and at least one free weekend day with her kids. Then, in 2020, *la merde* hit the proverbial fan. Her children's school closed, forcing her and her husband to work from home while assuming the job of homeschool teachers. Gone were any opportunities to exercise or spend time with friends, and because her days were filled with reading and writing lessons, her nights were spent working on the couch. Six months into the pandemic, she started to feel bad. She used to love her job, but began to dread every approaching Zoom meeting and saw every project as a waste of time. Lying awake wondering what happened to her once-robust sleep patterns and worrying about how she was going to get through the next day's to-do list, Mercedes began avoiding bedtime and started experiencing nighttime panic attacks, a hallmark sign of sympathetic overarousal.

So, how did a young, healthy, and capable person like Mercedes go from having it all to curling up in a ball and wanting it all to go away? And how do so many otherwise indomitably successful adults go from kinda stressed to a state of complete mental, physical, and emotional burnout?

It happens when that daily ratio of Upstate stress response and Downstate RecoveryPlus is ignored, or the magnitude of Upstate needs outpaces the hours left in the day for Downstating. When that happens repeatedly, you can find yourself in a state of autonomic imbalance and chronic stress. This is the way Mercedes, and millions just like her, live life: REV rages unbridled, while RESTORE is silenced.

Living too long in this mode can wear down the very resources that keep you Teflon-resilient, and can cause irreversible damage to organs, leaving you at a heightened risk for a litany of health issues. Here's what chronic stress looks like:

**Your memory and cognition suffer.** When a stressful event is repeated over many weeks, your brain cells, or neurons, change in supremely unconstructive ways. Lab studies have shown that neurons inside the hippocampus (the memory brain) atrophy, leading to memory failure. Other neurons in the amygdala (the fear/anger brain) grow and fearful-rageful responses become enhanced.[15]

**You age prematurely.** A dominant REV hastens aging, from the skin on in. Autonomic imbalance predisposes you to wrinkles as levels of the stress hormone cortisol ramp up the aging process. Think of before-and-after pictures of US presidents—the enormous stress of their job often speeds up admittance to the Cotton Top Club.

Stress is associated with less activity and more sedentary behavior. Without moving around, your muscles and bones weaken, and your hippocampus diminishes in size. A weaker hippocampus means less brain power and fewer reserves for problem-solving, creative thinking, or learning new skills. This is one reason older adults tend to be more rigid in their thoughts and behaviors—a weaker hippocampus forces them to rely on alternate brain regions that prefer the easier route of deferring to old habits.

**Your immune system weakens.** Like exposure to the flu virus, a short burst of acute stress directs immune cells to quickly move to places they are most needed to fight infection and disease. But with chronic stress comes excessive inflammatory responses that *suppress* immune function and *increase* susceptibility to infection.[16] And the damage to your body caused by stress can linger even when the specific stressor, an angry boss for example, isn't even in the room.[17]

**You're more apt to develop various long-term diseases.** Your cardio-vascular system regulates the rise and fall of blood pressure during the day to ensure that you have enough blood supply for any number of daily activities, from getting out of bed in the morning to accelerating your heart rate so you can run to catch the bus. But when your blood pressure goes up and stays up, as it does with chronic stress, it promotes atherosclerotic plaques, which narrow the blood vessels, making it harder for blood to flow through. Inflammation is so common with increasing age that research-ers have coined a portmanteau, *inflammaging*, which is associated with increased rigidity of the arterial walls, making cardiovascular disease one of the main causes of death for men and women.[18]

Chronic stress metes out similar punishment on your metabolism, the system that keeps us physically fit. The rapid and short-term conversion of food to sugar by the stress hormone cortisol is important if there actu-ally were a tiger from which to get the hell away, as this process provides a fast track to energy by increasing locomotor activity, appetite, and food-seeking behavior.[19] However, many of today's tigers appear when you're tied to your desk next to a grouchy coworker; subjected to slights, unfair treatment, or harassment at work; stuck in the car filled with murderous road rage; terrified on a couch watching the nightly news; or lying in bed with someone you don't like—all situations in which you don't actually need highly sweetened blood. The combination of low physical activity, ele-vated cortisol levels, and high blood sugars can shut down your whole met-abolic system, leading to such conditions as *insulin resistance*, in which the cells of your muscles and organs get so overwhelmed that they stop being able to use insulin to get the glucose they need, all of which increases your risk of obesity and type two diabetes.[20,21,22]

---

**AUTONOMIC IMBALANCE CAN BUMP UP YOUR EXPIRATION DATE**

Many roads lead to death, but chronic diseases like cardiovascular disease, type 2 diabetes, and cancer all share a common path—autonomic imbalance, characterized by high blood pressure, high fasting glucose, high lipids, and elevated resting heart rate. This last one is particularly important—when your body is stressed, tired, and unfit, the heart is forced to work harder to keep blood circulating. As a result, resting heart rate increases. Study after study has linked elevations in resting heart rate not only with a heightened risk of all the aforementioned diseases, but also with the chance of dying early.[21] One study found that every ten beats-per-minute increase in resting heart rate increased people's risk for death by about 20 percent.[22]

This mountain of medical data draws a straight line from autonomic imbalance to an elevated, inflexible heart rate to chronic disease. BUT this is actually great news because both a healthy autonomic ratio and a strong, resilient heart rate are two things that you can control. Just by reading this book and letting the knowledge impact your daily behaviors, you are already on your way to a healthier you. Working your way through the Downstate RecoveryPlus Plan and letting these good habits become second nature will reduce your risks for chronic disease and keep you healthier, longer.

---

## The Stress of Social Dominance

Along with your psychological makeup and personal life experiences, the world at large and the cultural norms into which you were born can wield a mighty influence on your well-being and Upstate/Downstate ratios. Our world today is shaped in part by a history of dominance of certain individuals and groups over others. Generally speaking, the political and financial power is concentrated in the domain of wealthy, White, Christian, heterosexual males, and the extent to which you were born with one or more of those characteristics can influence your access to a healthy, safe, and opportunity-rich life. Inequality gaps in health care, wages, education, justice, incarceration, and housing are ever widening, with more and more people living in the underserved end of the spectrum. Living in these compromised circumstances makes the crisis of chronic stress and auto-nomic imbalance even more dangerous, and the goal of healthy Upstate/Downstate ratios even more challenging.

Consider that living in the upper strata translates into living in larger, less dense, higher-quality housing (e.g., away from trains, planes, and auto-mobiles, with better windows blocking noise and offering improved aller-gen control); higher quality health care (e.g., treatment for asthma, sleep, and cardiovascular and metabolic disorders); and access to health education (e.g., knowledge of sleep hygiene, nutrition, stress-reduction techniques, and exercise). Living in the upper strata also relieves you of the pressure of needing to make difficult decisions, such as whether to put dinner on the table or replace your child's worn-out shoes; or how to make time for any restorative practice when you are parenting and working multiple jobs. Day-to-day living in the underserved end of the spectrum creates physi-cal and mental health holes for people to fall into due in part to a danger-ous combination of stress-induced autonomic imbalance and limited time for Downstate recovery. For these reasons, living in poverty is associated with all the telltale precursors to chronic disease: high blood pressure, low heart rate variability, elevated REV (i.e., high sympathetic nervous system arousal), and autonomic imbalance, as well as being one of the strongest predictors of early mortality.[23] But recent studies have shown that it's not just the deprivation of poverty, but also the experience of discrimination due to one's poverty, that contributes to poor levels of mental and physical health, with lack of respect and social exclusion correlated with elevated blood pressure, high cortisol, and high body mass index (BMI).[24]

Although there are individual differences in the lived experience of dis-crimination, studies have shown that these experiences share similar out-comes. Discrimination due to poverty, race, ethnicity, sexual orientation, sex, physical ability, or religion all cause the same stress response on the brain and body as physical threat or injury.[25] The most commonly used measure of discrimination is the Everyday Discrimination Scale, which asks people how often they have experienced events that were disrespectful, discourteous, insulting, fearful, threatening, or invalidating.[26] Everyday discrimination is often expressed subtly through microaggressions, defined as "brief and com-monplace daily verbal, behavioral, or environmental indignities, whether intentional or unintentional, that communicate hostile, derogatory, or negative . . . slights and insults," and widely referred to as "death by a thousand cuts."[27] High ratings on Everyday Discrimination have been linked with several precursors to chronic disease including hypertension, arterial stiffness, high oxidative stress, systemic inflammation, and depression.[28]

Being part of a group that is marginalized due to sexual orientation, as is the case for lesbians, gays, and bisexuals, is fraught due to a long history of discrimination, including criminalization, classifications as mentally ill, attempted forced conversion, hate crimes and violence, and exclusion from employment, housing, public spaces, and social institutions.[29] Along with these structural inequities, the stigma of homosexuality can create internalized negative feelings and a lifetime of hiding one's true self in the closet. All of this has been linked to poor health behaviors, such as tobacco use, heavy drinking, eating disorders, and physical inactivity, as well as depression in lesbian, gay, and bisexual individuals.[30] Importantly, everyday discrimination experienced by people who are marginalized due to sexual orientation is linked with cardiovascular profiles associated with greater REV in these groups.[31]

In late 2020, the American Medical Association officially and explicitly recognized racism as a "serious threat to public health," one that "negatively impacts and exacerbates health inequities among historically marginalized communities."[32] Studies across different countries and populations report similar findings—that racial discrimination is associated with poor self-reported physical health, obesity, blood pressure, and cardiovascular disease, with chronic cardiovascular, inflammatory, and metabolic risk factors elevated in Black and Hispanic Americans even after controlling for such health behaviors as smoking, physical exercise, or dietary variables.[33] Due to a lifetime burden of discrimination, harassment, and/or assault, Black people have the highest prevalence of hypertension worldwide, developing it at an earlier age than their non-Black American peers and experiencing more hypertension-related chronic diseases, with REV overdrive identified as a major cause for hypertension and cardiovascular dysfunction in this group.[34] Greater everyday discrimination is associated with lower heart rate variability (HRV) in Black Americans.[35]

Racial discrimination is also a sleep saboteur, with groups as varied as Asian American and Latino adolescents, middle-aged Black adults, and Asian and Pacific Islanders showing correlations between high levels of discrimination and poor sleep quality, suggesting that prejudice and bigotry are infringing on the most fundamental Downstate recovery resources.[36]

My colleague, one of the few women of color in her field of neuroscience, says that she experiences hurtful or awkward race-based slights on a daily basis from her White colleagues. (She has given me permission to share her story.) She comes home every night to her partner exhausted and spends so much time activating Downstate RESTORE systems to heal from these microaggressions and insensitive remarks that she has lost out on precious hours that could have been spent enjoying her favorite hobbies or exercising, not to mention devising new experiments, writing papers for scientific journals, or developing her theoretical models. Think about this in person-hours—compared with her colleagues, how much Downstate time has she and other people of color lost to processing trauma? How many hours have been spent tolerating and even apologizing for other people's microaggressions? These are hours that could have been used to further her career and make the world a better place.

## Onward! Let's Do New Things . . .

At this point, given the mountain of evidence about the dangers of autonomic imbalance, you're probably wondering if there's any good news. *Of course, there is!* Otherwise, I wouldn't be writing this book. As I've been driving home in this chapter, life experiences change your set-points either in a positive or negative direction depending on your ability to intentionally prioritize Downstate RESTORE processes. The simple and exciting act of reading *The Power of the Downstate*, followed by the not as simple but far more important act of embarking on the Downstate RecoveryPlus Plan, are exactly the type of novel life experiences that can shape the trajectory of your life.

There are many ways to intentionally enhance your Downstate recovery periods so as to reap the benefits of RecoveryPlus and start your next day as a better/stronger/smarter/happier version of yourself. In the next chapter, you'll learn about how the rhythms of day and night promote built-in periods for Upstate and Downstate functions, and how harmonizing with this universal rhythm can move the stress needle into the positive green zone of *eustress* and away from the anxious red zone of maladaptive *distress*. It's time to change some set-points.

# CHAPTER TWO

# Get in Sync with
# Your Inherent Rhythm

O n the heels of World War II, Eleanor Roosevelt famously chaired the United Nations committee that adopted and ratified the Universal Declaration of Human Rights. These thirty principles were created in recognition and preservation of the inherent dignity of human life and are considered inalienable. Some of them are fairly obvious: Article 3 states that "Everyone has the right to life, liberty, and security of person."[1] Article 4 prohibits slavery in all forms. Article 18 guarantees freedom of thought and religion.[2] A key element of all of these rights, whether they're political, civil, social, cultural, or economic in nature, is that they are each equal in importance and interdependent; none can be fully enjoyed without the others. Together, they lay the foundation of freedom, justice, and peace in the world.

Nevertheless, there's one article that's never discussed at any human rights convention and is often maligned as being unworthy of inclusion with the others. Article 24 of the Universal Declaration of Human Rights is the right to Rest and Leisure.[3] With all due respect to the important work of human rights advocates around the world, I strongly believe that our modern culture's denial of rest as an essential human right is the main reason for the mounting psychological and health problems we face today.

Nature gets the supreme importance of rest and has, over many billions of years, worked out a system of indomitable rhythms that ensure you get the downtime you need. All living things are controlled by these natural rhythms: the daily rhythm of the sun and moon; the yearly cycle of seasons; the monthly rhythm of sex hormones in females; and the

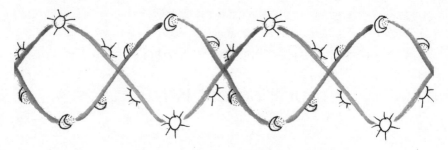

The Sun Moon Cycle

minute oscillations of inhibition and excitation among brain cells. The list goes on . . .

Rhythms provide humankind with a specific framework to take care of every task at hand in every aspect of life. They set aside time to achieve equity between the forces of creation, or Upstate Doozery (exploring, advancing, taking on, building, all of which require energy and lead to the depletion of resources), and the forces of Downstate RecoveryPlus (whereby those resources are restored so as to maintain and promote vitality). They're the *when* in everything we talked about in Chapter 1—the key to optimizing health, well-being, and cognition, guiding and actively supporting both sides of the activation/restoration seesaw.

On top of this durable, collective foundation of universal rhythms is You, a unique combination of genes, personal experiences, social and cultural backgrounds, which has been stirred up in a pitcher of water with a twist of lemon or lime (your preference). The secret to a long, happy life is discovering how to incorporate the you-ness of you with the universal principles that govern life on Earth.

## Walking on Sunshine (whoa)

The most irrefutable and recognizable universal rhythm happens when you wake up and rub the sleep from your eyes each morning. By starting your day as the sun rises in the east, you're participating in an Upstate ritual that's been practiced by animals for 4.5 billion years, and by your fellow humans for a few million.[4] Before the technological trappings of the modern world, we didn't have to consciously make time for recovery systems because the Upstate/Downstate processes of all plants and animals were adapted to follow the sun, and the sun told us what to do. We diurnal creatures slept when it was dark and woke when it was light. We were in perfect sync with nature's rhythm because we hadn't invented ways to dominate and control it just yet. The planet spun on its axis approximately every 24 hours, giving us day and night, and we followed this natural rhythm without thinking, much like birds that automatically fly north each spring without consulting a map, or bears that store weight for winter hibernation without so much as a second thought.

The daily ritual of opening and closing our eyes to the sun and moon for 1.65 trillion mornings has set up a strong rhythm that regulates the biological and psychological processes of all living things. Scientists refer to this daily rhythm as *circadian*, from the Latin *circa* meaning around, and *dia* meaning a day. This chain of action governs the sleep/wake cycle of every human, animal, plant, and even bacterium on the planet, and countless processes depend on the circadian rhythm to time-manage their Upstates and Downstates. Since the beginning of time, daylight has been the period where plants voraciously invest in photosynthesis, opening their petals early in the day to drink in the sunlight, and all of us diurnal animals are safe to hunt and gather, *veni-vidi-vici* à la Julius Caesar, or explore the outermost banks beyond which there be dragons. In contrast, nighttime has long been the right time for decreasing energy expenditure by closing up petals, or for critters great and small to nestle into the darkness of the burrow or cave, avoiding the many predators that seem to prefer night to day.[5]

So, how do we know when to do what? It all comes back to Sol Invictus and the specific types of light it shines morning till night. Light is your circadian rhythm's strongest signal, but not all light is created equal. It comes in many different colors, determined by the frequency of the light's wavelengths. Within visible light, we can see wavelengths between 400 and 700 nanometers, the shorter wavelengths being cooler colors (purple and blue) and the longer wavelengths appearing as warmer colors (red and orange), with yellow and green in the middle.

As the sun begins to rise, the bluish light of dawn enters the retina and is detected by three different types of retinal cells. Two of these, rods and cones, are used for processing visual perceptions; the third, the retinal ganglion cells (RGCs), specifically process information for the circadian system. Whereas rods and cones can process a broad spectrum of wavelengths, RGCs pick up only blue light, as this particular wavelength is the semaphore that signals the brain what time it is and when to release either melatonin, the circadian rhythm's main Downstate hormone, or cortisol, your trusty Upstate go-juice. Like a rooster, RGCs excitedly send this color information to your brain—the hypothalamus, specifically—which starts to get very, very excited that daytime's a-comin'. In particular, a cluster of about twenty thousand neurons called the *suprachiasmatic nucleus* (SCN) becomes extremely pumped, triggering a cascade of events designed to get you going so you can kick your day's ass in the best possible way.[6] This includes, but is certainly not limited to, cueing the pineal gland to stop producing sleepy melatonin; the adrenal glands to ramp up production of energizing hormones, such as cortisol and epinephrine; and your metabolic system to start heating up your body temperature.

As the sun sets in a westerly bath of fiery red and orange, the Downstate Show begins. Your eyes look out into the night and sense impending darkness. The absence of blue light alerts the suprachiasmatic nucleus to stimulate the pineal gland, so you get your melatonin fix for the night, sending the whole system down a gradual descent toward wind-down mode again. The brain orchestrates the release of melatonin, which keeps pumping in large quantities until early morning, while cortisol, which has already been experiencing a slow decline all day, dips low. You feel sleepy . . . veryyy sleeeepy.[7]

Many of your most critical biological processes rely on this millennia-old structure of day and night. Classic examples include your body temperature heating up in the morning, preparing for daytime action, then cooling down at night, conserving energy and signaling to your brain that it's time for sleep. As I previously explained, the stress hormone cortisol bursts from the adrenal glands (small glands that rest above the kidneys, like little top hats) in the early morning hours, helping rouse you from deep to light sleep, and preparing you for several daytime to-dos—from revving up your metabolism to allowing you to make quick assessments of friend or foe. In a healthy body, cortisol decreases at night and its antidote, growth hormone, is released to repair the damage from all that

**MELATONIN IS THE DOWNSTATE HORMONE**

Most of us think of melatonin as a supplement taken at night for help drifting off, but it's anything but a one-hit wonder. A powerful antioxidant in its own right, melatonin also reduces free radical burden and diminishes system-wide inflammation, improves heart health, and is responsible for shifting the balance between the two branches of the autonomic nervous system in favor of RESTORE across the night. In fact, given its role in decreasing blood pressure in animals and humans, its reduction in REV and enhancement of RESTORE, and its relative safety for long-term use, it is being investigated as a possible treatment for hypertension.[7]

Upstate overwork, emotional toil, and general Winnie-the-Pooh feeling of "too much day for me." Produced only during deep sleep, growth hormone increases cell reproduction and regeneration and benefits a range of restorative processes, including stimulating height in children, increasing muscle mass, and fostering the growth of every organ, including the brain. It's a RESTORE wonder hormone.

## The Rhythm Is Gonna Getcha

Every cell in your body is equipped with a tiny metronome, tick-tocking away but in need of a main conductor. The suprachiasmatic nucleus (that cluster of neurons in your hypothalamus) is that conductor, synchronizing all the cells and organs of the body to the tolling of day and night and orchestrating the rhythms for glucose and fat metabolism, energy expenditure, recruitment of nutrient-rich blood, and appetite stimulation. In plain speak: The suprachiasmatic nucleus ensures that the right hormones and right behaviors are in the right place at the right time of day.

Each of your different subengines—your guts, heart, autonomic and central nervous systems—has a rhythm, with the common theme being that they collectively maximize efficiency by positioning your resources to be most available during the Upstate day and least available during the Downstate night. Take a look at a few . . .

## CIRCADIAN RHYTHM OF EATING AND METABOLISM

Your guts live and breathe by your biological clock, with Upstate daytime (morning to midday) the clear favorite in terms of optimal eating times. Think of the hunger signals you feel at least 30 minutes before your typical lunch time, reminding you to shove a BLT down your piehole. These pangs are relayed by appetite hormones that tell you when to start eating and when you are full: ghrelin and leptin, respectively. Both hormones rise across the day, peaking between one p.m. and three p.m., then start to fall, indicating it's time to slow your roll with the face-stuffing.

Eating activates REV, which provides a quick burst of energy to support ingestion, digestion, and absorption of nutrients, as well as to transport the resulting nutrient-rich blood to your organs. Processing food in the body produces heat and burns calories via diet-induced thermogenesis, which peaks in the morning. In one study, it was 2.5 times higher in the early hours than at night—an impressive difference that has prompted nutrition experts to recommend frontloading calories (i.e., making breakfast the biggest meal of the day) as a strategy for reducing risk of obesity and preventing metabolic diseases.[8] A hearty brunch, therefore, takes advantage of a natural Upstate swing in metabolism.

Glucose, which provides the body and brain with energy to take action and think, is highest in the morning, and your body's ability to process glucose from meals is also faster early in the day, rendering nighttime glucose utilization nearly 20 percent less efficient.[9] Insulin is needed to transport glucose from the bloodstream into your organs; this is how you get energy. In the morning, the pancreatic cells that produce insulin are very sensitive to glucose, but they tire out by the end of the day, becoming less sensitive to glucose. This leaves more glucose in the bloodstream, which ultimately gets stored as fat. Basically, when you're lounging on the couch snacking at nine p.m., your whole metabolic system is saying, "I'm exhausted. Take me home."

Are you sensing a theme here? Your nutritional rhythm is set up to eat a horse in the early part of the day, and twigs and nuts in the evening.

These aren't just cool medical facts to impress your spouse on her midnight run to the freezer for a bowl of Peanut Butter Pandemonium. Results from several studies support the benefits of shifting eating times to earlier hours, with a 10 percent decrease in body mass index; double the reduction in waist circumference; and a 25 percent greater weight loss in groups who ate earlier but had the same caloric intake and physical activity.[10] Compared with late eaters, early eaters show greater reductions in total cholesterol; better insulin and glucose metabolism; and a greater increase in HDL, the "good" cholesterol.[11]

Beyond physical fitness, earlier mealtimes are also associated with higher melatonin levels. In a study of medical students, half were advised to skip breakfast and consume 50 percent of their daily food intake in the night, while the other half ate three even meals a day. After three weeks, levels of melatonin and leptin were suppressed in the night eaters.[12] These findings demonstrate the important fact that all of your biological subengines are interdependent; eating patterns affect sleeping patterns, sleeping and exercise patterns affect fitness and metabolic health, and so on. By honoring the universal Upstate/Downstate rhythms, you bring all these subengines into alignment.

## CIRCADIAN RHYTHM OF EMOTIONS, AND COGNITION

It's not just your biology that likes to stay in sync with the sun and moon. The brain uses 20 percent of all glucose created or consumed, and since glucose is more readily available earlier in the day, you are cognitively sharper at that time too. In healthy adults, executive functions, including working memory and attention, give premium performance between sunrise and high noon.[13]

Emotions, mood, and clinical levels of anxiety and depression are influenced by circadian rhythm. Things that go bump in the Upstate day are far less disturbing than if they go bump in the Downstate night, as fear and anger emotions are reined in during daylight hours.[14] For example, being held up at gunpoint in a sunny park is frightening, but it typically results in a smaller emotional reaction than if it were to happen in a deserted, shadowy corner of that same park at night. This is because the brain areas that regulate and control emotions are at their peak functioning capacity in the day, helping keep a lid on emotional reactions.[15] And even though REV dominates during the day, these brain areas are even stronger and able to rein in your stress response. At night, on the other hand, these brain areas

## FECAL TRANSPLANT, ANYONE?

Studying bacteria found in poop samples is one of the primary methods scientists use to determine which flora and fauna live in the gastrointestinal tract, otherwise known as the gut microbiome. Your microbiome is home to trillions of bacteria and it's vitally important for keeping you alive and healthy. (You're actually half microbe, as these microbes equal your human cells one to one!)[16] The majority of these bacteria are good-for-you bugs, helping with digestion and immunity; protecting you from disease-causing bacteria; and producing many essential vitamins.[17]

Sometimes, however, the ratio of good to bad bacteria gets thrown out of whack, resulting in *dysbiosis*, a.k.a. a messed-up microbiome. This condition can increase disease risk, including diabetes, obesity . . . even mental disorders, such as schizophrenia.[18] Since the large intestine is both home to the microbiome and the place where poop is made and ejected, scientists had the crazy thought that sending a "poop present" from a healthy host (human or animal) into a sick host via colonoscopy could allow the healthy microbes to invade and flourish in the guts of the sick host, facilitating healing. (This treatment route actually originated in ancient Chinese medicine more than 1,700 years ago, when doctors would advise sick patients to tuck into a bowl of "yellow soup,"[19] a broth made with dried or fermented stool from a healthy person.) This procedure is called a fecal transplantation, a term you may have heard thrown around in the news and wondered whether it really means what it sounds like it means. In fact, it does!

And by golly, those ancient and contemporary scientists were right. Fecal transplants have been helpful in treating fatal bacterial infections, such as *C. difficile*; colitis, constipation, and irritable bowel syndrome; and there is hope that

are done for the day, so not only do you have less control over your emotions, but you're also waking up REV from deep slumber, and you know what they say: Don't wake the bear! It's, therefore, always better to have that difficult talk with your partner in the middle of the day when you have your wits about you, than during the wee hours of the night when REV is cranky. It can wait till morning . . .[16,17,18,19,20,21]

Having control over your emotions—letting them happen, observing them, and not letting them run you—ensures that negative experiences they may be useful in treating many more diseases not traditionally thought to be gut-related, such as depression, arthritis, and fibromyalgia.

So, why am telling you all this? Two reasons: Number one, I have the humor of a six-year-old and it delights me when I find study titles like "Stool Substitute Transplant Therapy for the Eradication of Clostridium difficile Infection: 'RePOOPulating' the gut."[20] Reason number two ( . . . "number two") is because it's recently been discovered that the microbiome has a strict circadian rhythm!

When scientists analyzed the activity pattern of bacteria in mice poop, they showed that the bacteria that were active during the Upstate day were in charge of energy metabolism, while the ones partying during the Downstate night were poised for detoxification of harmful substances from the brain and body.[21] This means that even your guts are conspiring to keep you raring to go during the day and in healing and cleaning mode at night.

Interestingly, these scientists were also able to induce dysbiosis in these animals by experimentally shifting the mice's feeding times by twelve hours, essentially creating a state of rodent jet lag. The connection between jet lag and dysbiosis may not be surprising, as you just learned that when you disrupt one circadian subsystem (in this case, eating), you upset others as well (in this case, metabolism). Well, here's the amazing part: When they transplanted the dysbiotic poop into the guts of healthy, non-jet-lagged animals, guess what happened? The healthy mice not only became dysbiotic, they developed glucose intolerance and obesity—results strongly indicating that when you don't honor the universal and natural pattern of your Upstate/Downstate circadian rhythm, your guts get angry. Even more reason to save that cupcake till breakfast and go to bed!

are less likely to harden into long-term traumas. Studies have shown that losing control of REV (e.g., experiencing faster heart rate and shallower respiration) during a frightening experience increases the likelihood that an individual will suffer from post-traumatic stress disorder (PTSD) (intense, disturbing thoughts and feelings related to a traumatic experience that last long after the event has ended).[22] Think of the mental health disasters that could be avoided if people encountered potentially PTSD-inducing situations preloaded with interventions that helped them remain in the calm hands of RESTORE and able to regulate REV even in the most difficult moment of their lives. This kind of forward-thinking approach could protect everyone from soldiers headed into warfare to emergency medical personnel during a natural disaster or pandemic crisis. Instead, we are more likely to wait for the problem to happen and then rely on the pharmaceutical industry for treatment options.

Preventative strategies that help people enhance RESTORE and down-regulate REV is an approach that Dr. Runyan of Tend Health describes as "vastly underutilized in our healthcare system." Stay tuned for Chapter 8 and the Downstate RecoveryPlus Plan, where you will be introduced to such methods as heart rate variability (HRV) biofeedback training, which have been scientifically demonstrated to keep people cool as cucumbers under stress.

Beyond feelings, memories of emotional experiences are processed better during daylight hours. Returning to that park incident, if it happened during the day, you would be more likely to put together an accurate picture of the circumstances leading up to the event and then avoid those conditions in the future, such as choosing a different route home or not walking alone through that park again. A person held up in a sunny park at noon will also more readily understand it was just that one specific park where the scary incident happened, but if that same incident happened in a dark park at night, the victim is more likely to view *all* dark parks as dangerous. This type of overgeneralization can fester into persistent anxiety and even PTSD, whereby even small reminders of dark parks will prompt you to relive the full terror of the experience no matter how long ago it happened.

This all means that your cognitive processes have a circadian preference; preferring daytime for attentionally and emotionally demanding processes. And when you don't honor this preference, you might have a rockier time regulating your emotions. Having a personal preferred time (e.g., early morning or late at night) for such Upstate functions as being alert and productive and getting exercise is called *chronotype*. There are five, which I have done you the favor of renaming because scientific labels tend to suck (except for the *sonic hedgehog* protein, of course): Roosters (definite morning types), Morning Glories (moderate morning type), 9-to-5ers (neither morning nor evening), Sunsetters (moderate evening), or Owls

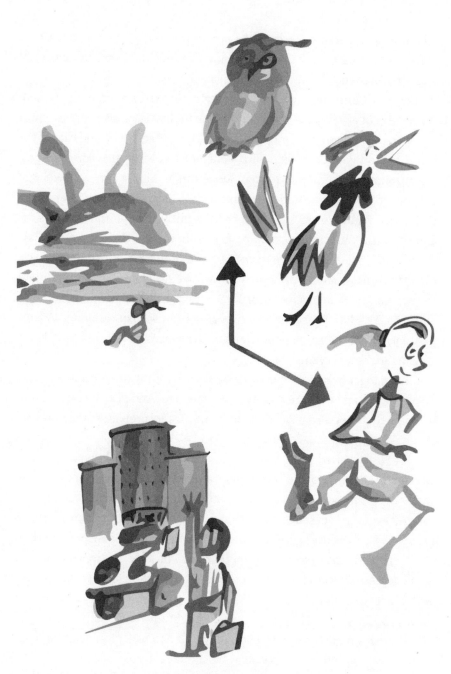

The Five Chronotypes:
the Rooster, the Morning Glory, the 9-to-5er, the Sunsetter, the Owl

(definite evening type). Chronotype can be assessed via a questionnaire or it can be measured in the lab by checking timing and levels of melatonin and cortisol in the blood, urine, or saliva.

Being a Sunsetter or Owl—moderate to extreme evening chronotypes—is not always to your advantage due to the disconnect between your own personal preference for the timing of Upstate activities and that of the world around you. Compared with Roosters and Morning Glories (morning chronotypes), Owls and some Sunsetters exhibit more symptoms of depression, take more antidepressant medications, and have poorer access to emotion regulation strategies, such as cognitive reappraisal, which is the ability to use your head to reframe experiences. In addition, people diagnosed with major depressive disorder commonly have dysregulated circadian rhythms. This has prompted innovative developments in treatment for depression that involve incorporating bright light in the morning to shift the circadian phase, hoping to coax a sunnier disposition.[23] Not surprisingly, bright morning light is one of the suggested Action Items in my Downstate RecoveryPlus Plan.

I have to stop for a moment and apologize for my description of Owls. So far, I have said they are moody and depressed. And I can go on . . . studies show that they also have more drug and alcohol problems and increased suicidal behaviors too.[24] Does this mean that people who love to stay up late are just screwed, end of story? Of course not! We all know plenty of wonderful night owls . . . you might be one yourself or in a relationship with one. It's important to remember that the differences between morning and evening types are based on averages with a lot of variance in each group. Even if the average of all the evening types is more depressed than the average for the morning group, there will be a lot of happy Owls (and some depressed Roosters) in the bunch. Some studies suggest that people who burn the midnight oil just for fun may not experience some of the darker aspects of #OwlLife. For example, one study found that in a group of people with a nighttime preference, only half had biological delays in melatonin onset, and these people also had significantly worse depression.[25]

Presently, we don't have enough data to understand what, exactly, is going on with Sunsetters and Owls. One possibility is that the increased rates of emotional problems stem from a biological shift in their circadian rhythms. Some Owls have a delayed onset of melatonin, the hormone driving the shift into Downstate nighttime mode, so they really *can't* get to sleep until the wee hours. In this case, living in a morning-happy world leaves them constantly sleep-deprived, tired, and moody . . . and thus more vulnerable to depression or likely to self-medicate with booze or drugs. On the other hand, for people who are Owls-by-choice, melatonin onset is not delayed, instead personal preference drives them to be awake when the rest of the world sleeps. There are many reasons why you might prefer the quiet and solitary night to the day: you might have mild anxiety or hyperarousal that keep you ruminating in the dark; or maybe you like the way your brain thinks when the rest of the world has stopped making so much noise; or maybe it's the only opportunity you have to control your own time. Creative people tend to be Owls.[26] My musician/poet sister, Lisa Mednick, remembers feeling a kinship with the night from early on:

> As a kid, I stayed up past bedtime, reading by flashlight and later on listening to music . . . I also remember waking up before it got light out and coloring with crayons before I could see the colors . . . all of that time I was alone and not afraid of the dark. I was too young to realize it of course, but I was taking advantage of the solitude and the rare chance to control my own time. For an artist, that is crucial—to be able to have control over how you spend your hours. Even at the age of six, believe it or not, I think I knew that. I am sure that is one reason why creative people train themselves (or maybe they're wired) to be awake and alive while the world—the authorities!—sleep. I mean, you can work sort of "outside the radar" I suppose. Otherwise everyone else is directing your thoughts and activities . . . at least that is how it can feel if you'd rather be left alone with your dreams and actually create something worth having spent your time on![27]

Regardless of the source of your circadian misalignment, the urge to stay awake is in conflict with society's rhythm, and problems can ensue. It's a real chicken-vs-egg debate, only in this case, the chicken is an Owl and the egg is depression. Generally speaking, if you are a Sunsetter or Owl who has made this schedule work for you, stay with it. But if you feel significantly stressed and unhappy and wonder whether your circadian

## ARE CHRONOTYPES A MODERN INVENTION?

Like many chronic diseases, night preference may be a recent development caused by modern society. Toba (a.k.a. Qom) is a culture in Argentina that has not been exposed to electricity, and researchers have recently discovered that they show pretty uniform bedtimes, with the majority of people within the same age range going to sleep two hours after the sun sets (around ten p.m.). But, when people from this culture move to more industrialized areas and transition to using electricity (e.g., lightbulbs), they start having shorter sleep, later bedtimes, and delayed melatonin onset.[28]

But the good news is that circadian preference is malleable and can be pushed back to its original factory settings by reducing your light exposure, such as by going camping. Circadian researchers measured circadian preference and melatonin onset before and after a six-day camping trip in the Rocky Mountains where experimental subjects were exposed to only natural light (i.e., sunlight, moonlight, and campfires; no flashlights, no personal electronic devices, etc.). Compared to the subjects' normal lives under modern electrical lighting, sleep start times moved up 2.5 hours earlier, and sleep duration increased by similar amounts, but with no change to wake time. In addition, melatonin onset began 2.6 hours earlier.[29] Together, these findings show that your circadian preference might not be set in stone; rather, it is determined by your exposure to light at night (LAN) as described on page 53.

rhythm is to blame, be sure to visit a sleep clinic to learn about possible treatment strategies.[28,29]

Discovering your chronotype—your preferred peak period for engaging in Upstate tasks—hinges on having the freedom and time to self-determine your optimal Upstate/Downstate schedule. This would require a sufficiently long experimental period that would allow you to judge for yourself the costs and benefits of shifting your times for workouts, meals, work, sleep, and socializing. You would then measure your productivity, mood, health, mental and emotional sharpness, and quality of life under many different schedules and lighting conditions to see which gets you the best results. If you work remotely and your job offers ample flexibility, this is a real possibility. Many people took advantage of this personal autonomy during the pandemic with fantastic results for their sleep.[30] But if you do not have the freedom to choose your work/life schedule, figuring out your personal chronotype may be harder. As we will read about later in the chapter, many people's work schedule goes against their own internal rhythm, and the cost to their health and well-being is definitely something to lose sleep over.

## CIRCADIAN RHYTHM OF ILLNESS

Illnesses also observe a circadian rhythm, with some flaring up in the morning hours during the switch from sleep to wake and from RESTORE to REV, such as migraines; allergy symptoms such as sneezing, runny, and stuffy noses; and chest pain, heart attacks, and strokes.[31] Meanwhile, evening tends to bring on ulcer symptoms and epileptic seizures.[32] This is because the organs and hormones involved in each disease have internal clocks of their own. For instance, the body produces a substance that facilitates blood clotting that peaks in the morning, then slowly wanes throughout the day, whereas cardioprotective melatonin is low in the morning. It's likely no coincidence that heart attacks, which can occur when blood flow to the heart is cut off or severely restricted by one or more blood clots, are two to three times more likely to strike in the morning.[33]

A new movement in disease management involves incorporating circadian rhythms during treatment, an approach called *chronotherapy*. A single daily five thirty p.m. dose of inhaled corticosteroids is as effective at treating asthma as four doses spread throughout the day.[34] Cancer cells are more active during the day, meaning evening chemotherapy may have the advantage of sneak-attacking malignant cells when they least expect it, nearly doubling their tumor-shrinking capability.[35] Circadian clocks in the skin are more active during daylight hours—burns heal nearly 60 percent faster when the injury occurs during the day than at night—and while you can't exactly plan when to accidentally singe your wrist on the stove, patients with in-the-know doctors may one day be advised to have surgery at a specific time, once chronoresearchers are able to pinpoint the precise time when fibroblasts (wound-healing skin cells) are working at their max.[36]

**GET THE LED OUT**

Before the advent of electricity and artificial light, the world was bathed in the sun during the day and fire or candles at night. Flames emit long, red wavelengths, so even if every candle in the world were burning at the same time, your circadian rhythm would still recognize it was nighttime and let the melatonin's powers take over. Edison's incandescent lightbulb mirrored the warmer tones of candlelight as well.

In the 21st century, though, we rely heavily on light-emitting diode (LED) products that are far more energy-efficient than the lightbulbs of yore. Computer screens, tablets, and phones are all made with LEDs, as are industrial lights in parking lots and gigantic wholesale stores.

I'll give you one guess as to what kind of light LEDs emit. If you said blue, you'd be right.

Unfortunately, your circadian rhythm is so sensitive to blue light that even short exposures can shut down melatonin production and prolong Upstate processing. By exposing yourself to blue light after six p.m.—whether that's watching a TV show with your family, scrolling through social media after dinner, or wandering down the ice cream aisle at the grocery store for a late-night fix—you're basically sending an unwanted wake-up call to your suprachiasmatic nucleus. Not to be mean, but your circadian rhythm is not exactly a subtle thinker. It's not paying attention to context; it sees light, it blocks melatonin, and then you're up for a couple more hours whether you like it or not. (This is why even just a quick peek at your smartphone at two a.m. when you get up to pee should be avoided.)

The potential benefits of chronotherapy are vast in terms of disease progression, not to mention the potential cost-savings that could come from reduced medication needs. However, widespread adoption of chronotherapy by medical professionals has been unsuccessful due to a general lack of knowledge about circadian rhythms and, somewhat ironically, the lack of time needed to study it.

To summarize, circadian rhythms serve to automate Upstates and Downstates, giving you times to reap and times to sow, times to push the oars and times to pull them back, times to activate and times to recover. As these examples so clearly demonstrate, the success of countless processes depends on these rhythms functioning properly. Your clocks are ticking . . . and that's a great thing!

## BURNING THE MIDNIGHT OIL

Over the past century or so, a shockingly large percentage of the population has decided to give the middle finger to the sun and the moon. Edison's lightbulb paved the way to 24-hour Target stores blazing with blue light. The average American spends more than ten hours a day staring into a screen of some sort.[37] We caffeinate all day long, snack after dark when our digestive tract is begging for a break, binge-watch mindless TV, pop an Ambien at midnight and pass out with our windows lined with blackout curtains and a sound machine app serenading us with faux rainfall. Sound familiar?

The long-term consequences of betraying nature's rhythms are abysmal. Living life out of sync increases the risk of heart disease, high blood pressure, diabetes, cancer, depression, obesity, Alzheimer's disease, and more. Shift workers are especially at risk, facing abnormally high rates of these conditions as they ask their bodies and brains to constantly battle Nature's will.

Lifestyles that reverse or oppose your natural rhythm—high-stress jobs; evening screen use and abuse; nightshift work; subpar eating and exercise—prolong Upstate levels of cortisol; prevent the nightly RESTORE downshift; dampen growth hormone and melatonin; and turn sleep into a fragmented and relatively futile mess. Dysregulated rhythms are powerless when it comes to putting the indomitable REV in its place, leading to autonomic imbalance, plus a host of short-term health risks, including insomnia, gastrointestinal upset, increased risk of injuries and accidents, decreased quality of life, and a general feeling of blah.

One of the primary culprits that has spun our circadian world out of control is overexposure to light at night (LAN). More than 99 percent of individuals living in the United States and Europe experience LAN.[38] The world is illuminated by parking lots aglow around the clock; streetlights penetrate bedroom windows; the blue light of screens pulls you away from your soft pillow; work and social media make demands on the job and off. These intrusions are known to contribute to rising levels of depression and poor sleep.[39,40,41]

## THE DRAG OF SOCIAL JET LAG

Living in a daily state of misalignment between your personal preference and public timetables can put you in a permanent state of jet lag, something researchers call *social jet lag*, measured in the difference in sleep-wake times between work and free days. Say you have children or a job that gets you up before dawn Monday through Friday. But, like many, you enjoy decompressing at night with one too many episodes of *Top Boy*, shortening your sleep on "school nights." Then, when you're at liberty to sleep in on the almighty weekend, you jump at the chance, skipping breakfast and maybe even passing on lunch to catch up on some winks. If this sounds familiar, you are one of approximately 70 percent of people living with social jet lag.[40] This carries with it the same health risks as sleep deprivation, including depression, cognitive impairment, metabolic syndrome, and every hour of social jet lag is associated with an 11 percent increase in heart disease risk.[41] So, whether you have a constitutional make-up that positions your most productive hours to coincide with the darkest hours of the night, or a boss assigning you the graveyard shift at work, if you notice a big difference between the times you get out of bed on weekend and weekday mornings, you are probably social jet-lagged. Finding ways to reduce this gap is critical for helping Upstate REV stay in its own lane and reestablishing your Downstate RESTORE system to its rightful place and time.

## She Works Hard for the Money

For some, LAN is unavoidably and inextricably tied to keeping food on the table and a roof overhead. Shift workers make up 20 to 30 percent of the industrial world population, including medical staff, factory workers, airline employees, truck drivers, performers, and others, all of whom require light at night to do their jobs.[42] Among many scary health statistics, working the nightshift is associated with poorer fitness; increased cholesterol, hypertension and obesity; and more diagnoses of metabolic syndrome, a cluster of conditions including elevated blood pressure, blood sugar, cholesterol, and triglycerides, as well as excess belly fat.[43] Long-term shift work is tied to depression, but even young nurses during their first three months of this trial-by-fire work schedule report feelings of helplessness, loss of control, apathy, and low social support, all of which predispose one to depression. The level of emotional and physical toil that goes with these jobs has prompted the World Health Organization (WHO) to cite shift work as a probable carcinogen, and wonderful Denmark started compensating women who develop breast cancer after spending their lives working at night.[44]

Hospital staff are exposed to LAN regularly, but so are the patients they treat, with one study reporting that lights are switched on at least thirty minutes every hour throughout the night, a practice linked to increased inflammation and pain in these patients.[45] Think about it—your built-in Downstate recovery and healing systems are being screwed over by the very institutions endeavoring to fix you—and those systems are also screwing over the healers! So much is wrong with this picture.

Though it's hard to imagine, there are modern day cultures who have successfully eschewed the temptations of LAN, along with a whole lotta other Upstate Parties, and they're healthier for it. The Old Order Amish is a large rural group descended from the Amish Mennonites who self-impose severe restrictions on dress and use of modern technology. As such, they are not exposed to light from televisions or computers. This lack of LAN may help explain why the Amish have greatly reduced rates of cancer, depression, and other psychiatric disorders compared with the general population.[46]

Bottom line: If you can, turn off your screens at night, or get yourself some jazzy, 1980s Blublocker glasses from the erstwhile SkyMall catalog or invest in a pair of blue light filter Swanwick glasses (I have no financial interest). Swanwicks have actually been scientifically tested in two applied settings (managers and call center representatives) with positive results reported for sleep measures, as well as next-day benefits including increased employee engagement and performance (measured in client-rated interactions).[47] You can also try to romance-up your evenings with candlelight teeth-brushing and add an adjustable, circadian lightbulb to your bedside table lamp. Rather than doomscroll in bed, read from a hefty historic tome that will knock you out halfway through the first paragraph. (Kate Pierson of the B-52s says, "*Wolf Hall* is like a sleeping pill.")[48]

## When It's Been a Really, Really Long Night

There are natural cases of circadian gut punches to be found if you venture to the extreme latitudes of Earth, some of which experience sunlight or complete darkness almost 24 hours each day during certain times of the year. In Tromsø, Norway, about 200 miles north of the Arctic Circle, the sun refuses to rise from November to January, enveloping the city in what's known as Polar Night. Then, from May to July, they experience the Midnight Sun (the sun never sets), meaning it's daytime 24/7.

Given everything I've told you about the premier importance of the sun rising in the morning and its sleep-inducing descent into the horizon at night, you'd probably imagine these Tromsønians are up poop's creek in a major way. And in some respects, this has proven to be the case. When researchers looked at the seasonal variation of suicides in Greenland, a country that experiences the same extremes in annual light, between 1968 and 2002, they detected a cluster of suicides in the summer months that was particularly pronounced in the country's northern region, which also experiences several months of constant daytime.[49]

But it's not all circadian doom and gloom. Surprisingly, Tromsø residents actually have lower rates of depression than those seen in other cities with traditional cycles of day and night. Despite the circadian misalignment, these people move through life with a pervasively positive mindset and residents seem to actually look forward to the Polar Night, "full of snow, skiing, the northern lights, and all things *koselig*, the Norwegian word for 'cozy,'" according to Stanford health psychology graduate student Kari Leibowitz, PhD, who spent a year living in Tromsø studying psychology and mental health.[50] Instead of feeling suffocated by darkness, residents relish the time to snuggle up with loved ones or a good book; enjoy the great outdoors; and take in the stunning midnight blue hue that cloaks Tromsø during the Polar Dark, which many insiders have rebranded "the Blue Time."

Given the small and isolated nature of the population, it's possible that there is a protective genetic mechanism at play in which only the happy survive these extreme circumstances. Research out of the University of Tromsø has shown that Arctic reindeer adapt to the extreme light and dark seasons by essentially turning off their circadian clocks and relying on an independently regulated cycle of melatonin release.[51] Humans are not reindeer, of course, but one can speculate that a similar phenomenon is at play with Tromsø's human inhabitants, as genetic variation has been tied to differences in human sleep durations.[52] Over hundreds of years, the *koselig*-or-bust types lived longer with more opportunities to procreate, while the "normal" people removed themselves from the gene pool.

There are two main takeaways here: First, unless you enjoy a long Tromsø lineage, you need to heed your body's natural circadian rhythm. Second, Midnight Artic Reindeer would be a killer band name.

## The September of My Years

Circadian rhythms change with age. Though your brain and body are still yoked to the sun and the moon, the connection to these signals weakens, and melatonin and growth hormones' levels decrease dramatically. These shifts in rhythms are pathologized by modern medicine with doctors usually throwing drugs at the "problem" starting with your first Ambien prescription in your thirties. But in reality these changes are normal and natural and simply require a doubling down on your part to support your naturally restorative Downstates on a daily basis.

Adult sleep periods usually start between ten p.m. and midnight and end between six and eight a.m. Toward middle age, your circadian rhythm shifts toward what scientists call a *phase advance*, meaning that you start to get sleepy earlier in the evening. Gone are the days when working at night was a viable option; now, all you're good for is a British crime show and light pillow talk. As the years accumulate, these small shifts become ever more dominant, to the point where you can go to sleep as early as eight or nine p.m. (but few of us do), then inevitably wake up at four or five a.m., leaving you sleep deprived. For most people, aging is met with a gradual dampening of circadian rhythms, but for some, the decline is more sudden and severe. For these individuals, weaker rhythms (e.g., having lower melatonin levels; falling asleep involuntarily during the day, and not sleeping through the night) are linked to poorer cognition, especially executive function, as well as later risk of mild cognitive impairment and dementia.[53]

When I give talks, I usually ask the audience how many people experience middle-of-the-night waking. Half of the room (and most people

### GO THE F**K TO SLEEP

If you've spent any time with adolescents, you have noticed that starting around age twelve or thirteen, something changes. Your once-obedient sleeper now seems to have added the phrase "Time for bed" to their ever-growing list of sentences for which they have selective hearing loss. (Not even your best Samuel Jackson impersonation urging them to put down the phone and "Go the f**k to sleep" will work.)[54] Although this might seem like direct evidence of their willful rebellion, it actually has a biological origin in what scientists call *circadian phase delay*. Although we don't know why exactly, adolescents experience a shift in their evening melatonin release that can stretch to hours beyond their preadolescent timetable. This means that no matter how hard they try, they cannot fall asleep at what their parents consider a "normal" bedtime. Some kids can lose up to three hours of sleep every night due to this phase delay, because they fall asleep at one or two a.m. but they have to still wake up at six a.m. to get to school on time. No wonder these kids don't leave their rooms until two p.m. on Saturdays and Sundays . . . they are sleep deprived!

The traditional mentality around school schedules has been that as kids get older, their classes should start earlier and earlier. I know some middle

over age forty) raise their hand.[54] This is another phenomenon that is pathologized in modern society (doctors call it "maintenance insomnia") but appears to have roots in early human history, suggesting it's not a disorder, but simply a natural shift in your rhythms that you might do better to embrace than freak out about. Consider that people in the pre-industrial, pre-electric lightbulb, Western society used to divide the night into "first sleep" and "second sleep," and spent the intermission sweeping the floor, having a smoke with the neighbors, or getting down with their bed partner.[55] This wasn't diagnosed as "maintenance insomnia" as it would be today; it was an accepted part of the daily rhythm, along with a daily nap, of course. In fact, some researchers explain these variations in our nightly patterns as evolutionary adaptations to ensure safety of the tribe.[56,57,58] school kids who have to leave home by six fifty a.m. to catch the bus. Moreover, adult teachers slate difficult classes like math, science, and English in the morning, operating under the belief that cognitive abilities are at their sharpest at that time (which they are for many adults). Many studies have shown that this approach to pedagogy has set a lot of students up to fail academically.[56] Under these schedules, kids are more likely to fall asleep during class and perform poorly on tests because they (1) slept through the lesson, and (2) are so tired that their focus is shot and their emotions are stuck on irritable, impatient, and hopeless. Several studies have shown that experimentally increasing kids' sleep by even thirty minutes shows marked improvements to cognitive/academic abilities.[57] In contrast, restricting sleep in kids intensified behaviors associated with attention deficit/hyperactivity disorder (ADHD), including impulsive and aggressive behavior, depression and anxiety symptoms, and impaired quality of life.

My advice: Let them sleep! Some forward-thinking Parent Teacher Organizations have started petitioning their schools to allow later start times, which has benefited students by decreasing sleepiness and increasing attention and school performance for many.[58] This real-world example demonstrates the power and benefit of aligning your personal schedule with your nature-given rhythms.

## Beyond a Day, a Time to Every Purpose . . .

Now, let's consider the universal rhythms that govern different aspects of life, each operating on massively different time scales: a lifetime, a year, a week, and a night. For the individual person, the rhythm of the life cycle begins with walking on four legs in the morning . . . two legs by midday . . . and three legs (with a cane or walker) in the evening, as per the Riddle of the Sphinx. Whether you believe that you will reincarnate into your favorite furry friend, hope to spend eternity with some chubby winged cherub, or are just content with the idea that your lifeless body will become food for worms and trees and that's enough, the first law of thermodynamics says that energy cannot be created or destroyed. This means that the energy your life holds contributes to a larger cycle of life on the planet.

These renewable cycles of life are also captured in how the four seasons of a year contribute to life on the farm. Planting and seed germination take place in spring, followed by the ripening of life energy in summer, the harvesting of the fruits of our labor and the turning of beds in the fall, followed by a period of winter dormancy that sets the groundwork for the next cycle.

Winter on a farm may look like an uninviting, cold waste of time, but plants need this Downstate period of shorter days and lower temperatures to bloom and blossom in the subsequent Upstate summer. Under these "chilling hours," plants enter a period of "deep, almost anesthetized sleep" when energy reserves are built up for the taxing process of sending out new growth.[59] Without sufficient chilling time, a fruit tree will generate fewer, weaker buds, limiting fruit production before spring has even had a chance to start. Just like for humans, Downstate time for plants directly predicts Upstate riches. This continuous loop of active growth and restorative repose is critical for nature to provide a healthy yield at harvest time, year after year.

Distilled down even further, humans have organized every week into seven days. For every five days of work, we have two days of rest. If you think about it, our weeks have been organized into a 1-to-2 ratio, one part rest for two parts work, which happens to resemble the proportion of sleep to wake within a single day. Under ideal conditions, a third of our lives is supposed to be taken up by Downstate rest (sleep or the weekend break) and then the other two-thirds, we work our tushies off. The beloved weekend was formalized by workers' unions, but has been an integral part of creation myths, holy sabbaths, and educational systems since the inception of these social structures. Yet, compared to other industrialized nations, such as those in western Europe, US workers are the least likely to avail themselves of this rejuvenating break from the rat race, and they, not surprisingly, suffer from the highest amount of stress-related disorders and burnout.[60]

**FOR PEOPLE WHO DON'T LIKE BEING TOLD WHAT TO DO . . .**

When I was learning how to act in college, I got the part of Miranda in Shakespeare's *The Tempest*. Shakespeare wrote in verse, a very specific cadence called iambic pentameter, which meant that all my lines sounded something like this: da-DUM da-DUM da-DUM da-DUM da-DUM. When I first learned that I had to speak on stage in this stupid, sing-songy way, I was horrified. Where was the art? Where was the self-expression? Where was my individuality and imagination? But, in time I saw things differently. I saw that instead of choosing between ten million different ways of saying one line, there were just a few ways that worked with the emotions and motivations of the character actually written into the verse. By getting in sync with the rhythm, I would naturally fall into the deeper meaning that Shakespeare intended. Instead of golden bars, I found freedom.

If you're anything like me, the idea of fitting your life into a specific temporal structure may seem confining, an affront to the American spirit of "Don't fence me in." So, you might get slightly triggered by my asking you to follow a pattern set up for you by something other than your own design. It helps me to think of these rhythms not as human rules, but as laws of nature. In general, we humans treat Earth like we own it, instead of being one of its creatures, and this thinking led us to where we are now, at the brink of losing it all. You have the opportunity to shift this relation by thinking of yourself as a subcomponent of a larger system guided by the time-honored wisdom of nature. Taking away some of the responsibility of deciding when you should be doing each task can eliminate the stress of choice overload, the phenomenon where you have too many choices. Leave it to the expert: Nature.

## WWED? (What Would Eleanor Do?)

So, how do we find balance? By demanding and honoring the human right to rest and leisure that Eleanor Roosevelt and the United Nations delegation enshrined. Nature has provided optimal times of day for your get-up-and-go Upstate, and times when it's right for getting down. Harmonizing to these inherent rhythms can keep you aligned with some seriously powerful regulatory systems that sustain health and well-being.

# PART TWO

# Activating the Downstate

N ow it's time to turn your focus to the Downstate and learn the ins and outs of this bastion of calm and recovery . . . and how you can get even more of that good, restorative stuff. The next four chapters will get into the nitty-gritty details about the four main ways that the Downstate flourishes. I call these the *Domains of Action*, so named because they are actions that are under your control and just waiting to be given their marching orders. Part 2 will start with a master class in how the RESTORE system works and how you can hone its regenerative chops. Next, we will check in on sleep, exercise, and nutrition, each of which need to be brought into line when one is becoming a Downstate Maven. The last chapter of Part 2 will look at how the strength of and access to the Downstate erodes across the decades like a sandcastle carried off by the ocean waves . . . and how it's in your hands to build and maintain a resilient long-term home while you're on this planet.

# CHAPTER THREE

# Replenish, Revitalize, Rebuild, RESTORE!

—————————— • ——————————

To fully understand the magnitude and prowess of the RESTORE system, you'll first need a quickie neuroscience primer to get you caught up on how the different parts of the brain and body communicate and function. Let's start at the very beginning, with the lightning-fast sequence of events that takes place when new information first enters your brain through your five senses. Light hits the eyes, sound waves enter the ears, smell molecules waft into the nose, substances wash over taste pores in the mouth, and touch sensors respond to changes on the surface or inside the body. These stimuli are turned into electrical transmissions (the action potentials we learned about in Chapter 1) that the sensory areas of the brain assemble into perceptions: the familiar smell of tomato soup; the dramatic hues of the sun setting over the ocean; a muddy dog excitedly heading your way.

These perceptions now need to be interpreted, so the second step involves further processing by various brain areas that control fear and anger (amygdala); memories (hippocampus); value judgments (orbitofrontal cortex); empathy for and awareness of ourselves and others (insula); detecting when reality doesn't match our expectation, and assessing how much you have to lose or gain by each course of action (anterior cingulate); and many other processes and brain areas.

Say you're at a fancy dress party, wearing new white pants, when that muddy dog starts trotting in your direction. As the perception of the pooch looms larger and larger on your retina, your brain divides its processing power between the polite party chatter and a whirlwind of lightning-quick thinking happening inside your head. First, the visual brain area tags

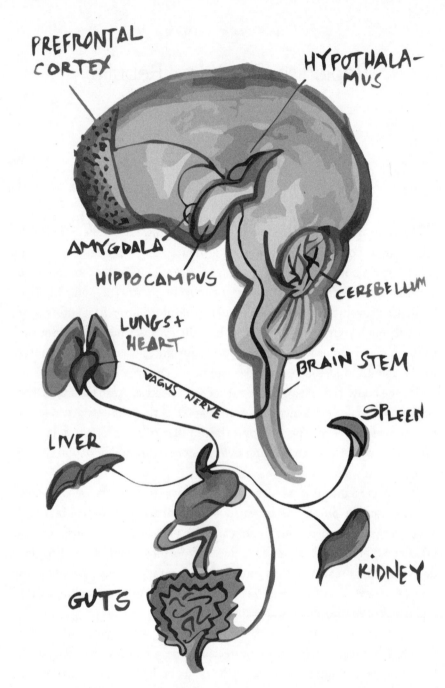

The Brain Network of Central Command and the Vagus Nerve

the image as a four-legged creature, and your hippocampus reminds you "That's a dog" and "Dogs jump on people." Those familiar concepts are filtered through the amygdala, which floods your mind with fears of a doggy onslaught on your new white pants. Your orbitofrontal cortex makes a judgment call about whether the price tag on the pants is worth the social embarrassment of screaming and running away, and your anterior cingulate assesses the various outcomes of each of your possible reactions.

The last stop on this 500-millisecond thought train is the prefrontal cortex, which weighs all the information coming from each brain area and decides on the best course of action.

I like to call the prefrontal cortex "Central Command," as it controls all of the so-called executive functions, such as working memory (which, in the case of the fancy dress party, motivates you to remember people's names while also engaging in clever banter); selective attention (which helps you focus on your cocktail conversation even as multiple other conversations take place around you, and then there's that approaching dog to consider); and goal-driven attentional shifting (being able to make the split-second decision to remain stoically calm about the dog so as to prioritize your too-cool-for-school reputation over the purity of your new white pants).

As the most recent brain structure to develop in the course of evolution, the prefrontal cortex, or Central Command, is the structure that separates us highly intelligent, social animals from the beasts.[1] Animals in the wild have no delay between the moment they sense danger and their physical reactions; when their peripheral vision picks up movement in a nearby bush, they fear a predator is nearby and hightail it out of there. In the same vein, animals also instinctively go after desirable stimuli without a second thought, such as the squirrel that dashes across a road for a fallen nut even though there's a high chance of being hit by a car.

But we primates have evolved to depend on Central Command's exquisite control over base survival-mode reactions, as it's a huge waste of energy to react to every small motion or sound, and besides, nobody wants to look like a moron running in terror at the slightest noise or startle. Central Command has the big picture in mind and isn't afraid to put the kibosh on any derailing thoughts and actions your reptilian brain might be up to.

## What Happens in Vagus

For a long time, scientists believed the brain reigned supreme and that it alone made decisions without input from the body (a.k.a. the autonomic nervous system). But more and more research points to an important role for REV and RESTORE at each stage of processing, even in the early stages as we formulate our initial perceptions and assessments. In fact, we now know that many brain areas, including the amygdala, prefrontal cortex, and others, are highly connected with both REV and RESTORE systems, meaning that your big decision-maker at the front office integrates information from perceptual, reward, emotional, and memory areas along with data from both branches of the autonomic nervous system to shape your thoughts, feelings, and responses to the world. For example, it's Central Command's job to gauge the accuracy and importance of whatever factor is causing REV to fire up the body (e.g., racing heart, sweaty palms, knocking knees) and make the decision that a tiger is in fact a tiger and let's run like hell, or that sometimes a tiger is just a neighborhood cat and let's all take a chill pill.

The main artery of influence transmitting RESTORE information to and from Central Command is the vagus nerve.[2] Stretching from the colon to the brainstem, it is the longest cranial nerve in the body, conveying 80 to 90 percent of information about the state of the body's organs to the brain.[3] Heart rate, breathing, pain, alertness, hunger, thirst, and consciousness . . . all of these must-have functions are transmitted via the vagus nerve, which carries them to the brain stem, the On/Off switch for most of your basic functions, as well as the bottleneck for all brain-body communication. The brainstem directs all vagal information to the brain areas responsible for complex cognitive processing, such as memory, emotions, and decision-making.

On top of these more cognitively driven responses, you also rely on the vagus for your gut instincts and intuition-driven responses. Think of the butterflies in your stomach you feel for that special someone, or how an upcoming job interview sends you to the toilet. These are all messages from your guts transmitted via the vagus nerve to the brain telling you that something has definitely piqued your interest. The vagus is announcing: *Achtung*, Baby!

When you realize the scope of brain areas touched by the vagus nerve (*vagus* means "wandering" in Latin, which makes sense because like a *vagabond*, it wanders around . . . in this case, from organ to organ), you understand why vagal activity, and RESTORE functions in general, have such a profound impact on thinking, feeling, and doing.[4]

Importantly, however, the vagus nerve is not solely running the RESTORE show. Central Command has the final say over how much influence any single brain area has over what we think and do by applying "top-down" inhibition on everything, including the vagus nerve.[5] In moments of danger or stress, Central Command holds back the vagus, thereby dampening RESTORE processes and releasing REV activity (e.g., it jacks up your heart rate and shunts blood to your extremities so you can prepare yourself for real or perceived danger), whereas when Central Command gives the all-clear signal, it releases the brakes on the vagus nerve, and RESTORE activity can resume. Hello, Downstate!

Generally speaking, holding down the brakes, or inhibition, affords the brain efficient, detailed, dynamic control of all its subsystems. Think of the Central Command as an automobile driver with REV and RESTORE as the car's two pedals: Different than normal cars, in this car, REV is the gas pedal glued to the metal and RESTORE is the brake pedal with complete authority over the car's speed. The brake pedal needs to move up and down in a tightly controlled manner to manage all that energy in a purposeful way. The benefit of having this type of operating system is that it affords very quick reflexes when you need them. So, the nanomoment you get the Spidey sense that there is a bug crawling through your hair, you can go from calm, cool, and collected (brake pedal down) to a complete and total flailing freak-a-zoid (brake pedal released) before you have time to remember that you are at a somber funeral.

Oops.

Central Command uses this inhibitory brake pedal to assess and respond to all incoming messages, keeping excitation in check and allowing for very complex neural networks to work together, thinking through complicated problems and dreaming up brilliant solutions.[6]

Central Command is not born into its role; it has to earn its inhibitory chops through real life experiences, ripening with age and experience. (Nice to know that getting older has some advantages!) When you are young,

Central Command is thin and not well connected to other brain areas, so its inhibitory sway is understandably poor; this immaturity means you are fairly incapable of discerning safe from dangerous conditions or good from bad decisions. You are more wild animal than domesticated human, and your responses are poised to react with hair-trigger velocity. (Think of the cute little pygmy jerboa in the desert making quick getaways from owls and snakes.) This is the reason toddlers don't always look both ways before running across the street, and teenagers can have a hard time sticking to the speed limit, just saying no to drugs, or turning the other cheek when their feelings get hurt. In those cases, when an experience excites a teenager, even if some part of her brain can hear her mother's voice telling her to stop and think, she usually does not have the Central Command muscle or maturity to stop her reactions to emotional situations or stupid dares (see #TidePodChallenge). In fact, this brain area does not reach full thickness and commandeering potency until the end of adolescence, which occurs in the early twenties for girls and midtwenties for boys.

With every passing year you accumulate challenging life experiences ("growth opportunities," as I mentioned my wife euphemistically calls them) and Central Command toughens up, allowing you to learn about cause and effect, action and consequences. You learn that, to a certain extent, you can call the shots by controlling your own actions and reactions, by weighing pros and cons, by making wiser decisions, by focusing on long-term goals, and by tearing yourself away from momentary temptations. Your ever-strengthening Central Command sends a robust signal to the vagus nerve to restrain the fearful, worried, or aggressive posturing of REV defense mode and turn on the relaxed, "I got this" RESTORE system. As such, your ability to control REV's fear and anxiety responses beefs up with age.

### Gimme an H, Gimme an R, Gimme a V! What Does That Spell?

We know so much about the vagus nerve and the RESTORE system because researchers have found a way to quantify them using a variable called heart rate variability (HRV; remember my Aha! moment in Australia?). HRV assesses rhythmic patterns that naturally occur in the heart rate. Autonomic nervous system scientist Fred Shaffer, PhD, captured the essence of these rhythms when he wrote, "A healthy heart is not a metronome," meaning it doesn't have a standard, consistent amount of time between heartbeats.[7] Instead, the interbeat intervals can vary by hundreds of milliseconds. This cadence is a symphony of rhythms that tells the secrets of how well your internal regulatory systems are working together, including your REV/RESTORE ratio, blood pressure, gas exchange, and gut and heart activity.

Analyzing HRV is like looking under the hood of a car to view the engine and being able to account for the individual dynamics of each different part (e.g., the pistons, the crankshaft, the spark plugs), as well as how they work together. As our brains and bodies rapidly adjust to sudden physical and psychological challenges, these complex and ever-changing rhythms reflect our heart's difficult task of responding to stress and then recovering its resting state once the thrill or fear is gone. The superstars among us who boast RESTORE, or parasympathetic, mastery have high HRV, meaning there's a bigger variation in the time between heartbeats reflecting the ability to solidly handle the slings and arrows of life. But chronically stressed-out individuals have low HRV, meaning the variation between heartbeats is low. This represents a system stuck on overdrive and unable to flexibly respond to life's demands and then appropriately calm the system down.

## When the Heart and Lungs Resonate

Just like all biological systems, the heart has a rhythm with an Upstate and Downstate; the interbeat intervals speed up, then slow down rhythmically. One of the heart's most important jobs is to grab oxygen from the lungs as they fill up on the inhale. For this to happen most optimally, the heart's Upstate needs to be perfectly timed to coincide with lungs' Upstate, the intake of breath, and then the slowdown of the heart needs to happen as the lungs start to empty. This coordinated cardiorespiratory interaction is thought to improve efficiency, in that the heart is only pumping fast when there is oxygen-rich air in the lungs, then slows down to almost nothing when the air quality in the lungs tips toward greater $CO_2$ during the exhale.

This interaction between respiratory rate and heart rate has a fancy name, respiratory sinus arrhythmia (RSA), which quantifies the degree to which the rhythms of the lungs (the *respiratory* in RSA) and heart (the *sinus* in RSA) are in sync. Through its inhibitory command on the heart, REV and RESTORE play important roles in the tempo of the RSA tango, whereby REV increases the heart rate, and this faster heart rate signals the vagus nerve to slow down the heart rate. Remember, REV and RESTORE are matching subsystems; when one gets excited, the other immediately senses it and wants in on the action.

The average person breathing at a normal rate takes around ten to twenty breaths per minute.[8] At this respiration rate, the heart rate peak is at the midpoint of the inhalation and the heart rate nadir is at the midpoint of the exhalation. This is fine—it will keep you alive and let you tackle your daily to-do list—but it rarely results in your heart and respiration rhythms syncing up. By slowing your breathing rate to about six breaths per minute, however, you can harmonize the Upstates and Downstates of both systems. When you do this, the heart and lungs find their *resonant frequency*, the point at which there is the most efficient uptake of oxygen into the blood and a huge amplification of HRV.[9] It's pretty amazing to see resonance in action. In one moment the HRV is rolling at a low hum, then the moment resonant frequency is achieved, RESTORE is singing its best aria to the cheap seats.

Yoga, tai chi, and many other ancient contemplative practices embraced and utilized resonant breathing techniques long before modern science was in diapers. The tradition of breath regulation, or *pranayama*, includes paced breathing, manipulating the nostrils, chanting or humming, retaining the breath, and other techniques. As ancient Indian yogic texts describe, "As the breath moves, so does the mind, and mind ceases to move as the breath is stopped," which is a pretty good description of the RSA.[10] For people plugged into the spiritual aspect of the mind-body connection, mystics have long believed that the basic principle of resonance stretches beyond the individual, suggesting that aligning your own personal rhythm or frequency with that of the universe amplifies your spiritual energy and brings you closer to a perfect state of consciousness and oneness with everything.[11] For the purposes of this book, all you really need to know is that six breaths per minute will increase your HRV, and that is good.[12,13]

**SIX! IT'S THE MAGIC NUMBUH...**

Six breaths per minute is the universal resonant frequency. But, thanks to slight deviations in anatomy and cardiovascular fitness, everyone has their own unique resonant frequency breathing rate, which can range anywhere between 4.5 to 7 breaths per minute, with the most common being 5.5 breaths per minute.[12] To find your own resonance, you'll need a device or an app that uses pulse oximeter technology to measure your pulse. Once you're set up, you will take turns breathing at 4.5, 5, 5.5, 6, 6.5, and 7 breaths per minute for two minutes each (Hint: It's easier to start with the fastest rate and progress to the slowest).[13] Afterward, you can review your results and find the breathing rate that produced the largest changes in HRV. You will see that as you slow your breathing down and approach your own personal resonant frequency, HRV amplitude will increase significantly. If it feels too tricky and hyperspecific to try to stick to, say, 5.5 or 6.5 breaths per minute, don't worry; overall, resonant frequency is pretty forgiving and the universal six breaths per minute rule gives you what you came for. Just do your best and breathe on.

Try it now and see how it feels. Take ten seconds per full breath (five seconds for the inhale and five seconds for the exhale). After practicing it for a few days, try to make a habit of slowing your breathing as often as you possibly can. Do it while driving, while cooking, while knitting and watching a show. Do it while sitting down to work at the computer (*email apnea* is a thing; people stop breathing when they start working) or Zoom meeting, standing in the elevator, bored on a long flight, or strolling down the street. Use it whenever you want to gain control of your fired-up amygdala—in the middle of a heated argument or just before giving a presentation. Do it while you think to yourself, "I never have time to meditate." (Don't worry about it—this breathing technique delivers the same HRV results.) Chapter 8 will revisit deep breathing in one of the Domains of Action.[14,15,16,17]

## THE HIGHER THE HRV, THE HEALTHIER AND SMARTER YOU ARE

Findings from large, epidemiological studies provide strong evidence that higher HRV predicts a range of sought-after outcomes. Remember "The

## DO IT THROUGH YOUR NOSE

Your mouth excels at many tasks: eating, drinking, talking, laughing, kissing, and other sensual pleasures, as well as dropping the occasional F bomb when your computer crashes. But guess what it's *not* so great at?

Breathing.

Chronic mouth breathing can make your upper cleft smaller and your jowls sag. This reduction in airspace lowers oxygen intake and increases the risk for breathing-related sleep disorders, such as sleep apnea. People who breathe through their mouth show lower memory performance, meaning it compromises your intelligence, putting you in the same company as other figurative and literal mouth-breathers like Napoleon Dynamite and Biff from *Back to the Future*.[14] It also causes bad breath, tooth decay, and gum disease.[15]

Luckily, you've got two perfect little holes just an inch above your mouth that do an outstanding job when it comes to breathing. Your nose is your body's natural filtration system, warming, cleaning, and detoxifying air as it comes in. Nasal breathing also organically slows your inhale and exhale significantly compared with mouth breathing. This slowing is better for your lungs, as it gives them more time to suck up oxygen from the circulating air, thereby increasing oxygen capacity and energy levels. (Mouth breathing is inherently faster and shallower, which affords less opportunity to extract oxygen from the air.)

Somewhat related, nasal breathing is calming at a cellular level. If you've ever experienced anything resembling a panic attack, you will remember that horrible feeling of not being able to breathe as your inhalations quicken. That scary sensation is actually your brain alerting you of a carbon dioxide–oxygen

Scourge of Autonomic Imbalance" from Chapter 1? Having a system where the balance is tipped toward REV compromises your emotional and cognitive processing and puts you on the path toward a range of chronic diseases, system-wide inflammation, and all sorts of other conditions that will bump up your expiration date. High HRV, which reflects increased RESTORE activity, reverses this downward spiral. Here are some key takeaways . . .

**General health:** Like eating whole, healthy foods or getting regular exercise, high HRV is just plain good for you. It favorably predicts lower rates imbalance caused by not enough time between inhales for your lungs to extract oxygen from the air. Nasal breathing optimizes oxygen consumption by increasing levels of both oxygen and carbon dioxide.

The nasal cavity is also in direct communication with your autonomic system, and there are some data to suggest that alternating breathing through the left and right nostrils may differentially access REV and RESTORE. Studies have shown that right nostril breathing can activate REV by speeding up heart rate and blood flow and increasing blood pressure. On the other hand, breathing through your left nostril appears to galvanize RESTORE by lowering blood pressure, exerting a calming effect. A slew of breathing techniques play with shifting the dominance between the autonomic branches by flipping back and forth between nostril channels, either heating you up and getting you excited (via right nostril breathing, which involves pressing the left nostril shut), or bringing you into a state of rest (via left nostril breathing).

Nasal breathing is not new, dating back some five thousand years to highly developed cultures of ancient India.[16] But as James Nestor points out in his fabulous book *Breath*, the nose has become "more or less an ancillary organ."[17] Nestor and a friend of his bravely guinea-pigged themselves for the sake of rhinoscience by plugging up their noses for ten days to see what would happen. Short answer: it sucked. Nestor developed raging sinus headaches and sleep apnea; he felt dumb; and he was completely destroyed by even short bouts of exercise. In contrast, when he switched back to nose breathing, his blood pressure dropped, his HRV increased by 150 percent, and the apnea completely disappeared. Read *Breath* for a deeper nosedive into this honker of a topic!

of diabetes, cardiovascular disease (heart disease), and even mortality, in high-risk as well as low-risk populations.

**Cardiovascular health:** You don't need a cup of tea leaves to predict your future heart health; just look at your HRV. In one longitudinal study, lower HRV predicted hypertension (high blood pressure) three years ahead of the diagnosis, as well as the chances of dying from a heart attack.[18] People with hypertension have significantly lower HRV compared to normotensive people, even after adjusting for age, race, gender, smoking, diabetes, and education.[19]

**Form and fitness:** Being fit affords you a healthier heart, a.k.a. higher HRV. As body mass index or waist circumference go up, HRV goes down.[20] Studies have found that not just adults, but adolescents with unhealthy weight are more likely to have lower HRV.[21] The relation between fitness and HRV is a two-way street, as studies show that becoming fitter ramps up your HRV, and the opposite direction has also been reported.[22]

**Healthy blood sugars:** People with higher HRV are nearly one and a half times less likely to develop type 2 diabetes, as well as cardiovascular disease.[23] Among those with type 1 diabetes, specific unfavorable changes in HRV can foreshadow a hypoglycemic episode that, untreated, can result in seizures, loss of consciousness, and possibly death.[24] Nondiabetics show higher vagal activity than do diabetics after adjustment for age, race, and gender.[25]

**Sharper cognition and better emotion regulation:** Along with the benefits to health, research in cognitive performance and HRV shows a strong bidirectional relation between a healthy heart and a smart, happy brain.[26]

*Cognition:* As I stated at the beginning of this chapter, the vagus nerve's far and wide connections in the brain make it an important influencer of how you think, learn, and react to life experiences. Each of these areas use vagal input to discern which information is salient, personally relevant, and in need of deeper processing, with Central Command having the final say on all your thoughts and feelings and modulating REV/RESTORE ratios as it sees fit. Therefore, your HRV is an index of how well Central Command is able to regulate and control all these emotions and cognitive processes.[27]

Having a strong Central Command is associated with both higher HRV and better working memory and inhibitory functioning.[28] The brain training apps you've heard about that claim to help you stave off your dotage actually strengthen Central Command by training executive functions. You can also achieve the same endgame by enhancing your HRV. Since your HRV levels are thought to reflect the potency of Central Command, researchers have gone so far as to say that HRV is a marker of self-regulation.[29] Studies show that improving HRV sharpens executive function by way of a stronger Central Command and improves your ability to manage your emotions and thoughts, especially under stressful situations.[30] All of which gives you plenty of reasons to take this improving-your-HRV business seriously!

*Emotions:* Individuals with high HRV have better management of undesirable emotions. They're also better able to maintain an upbeat attitude by turning to self-soothing strategies, such as reappraisal ("Maybe she was wrong for me after all") and suppression (pushing aside pessimistic thoughts). In contrast, people with lower HRV are vulnerable to extreme swings in emotional states and have a general tendency to focus on gloomy feelings and perseverate on unhelpful thoughts.[31] People with diagnosed mood disorders, such as major depressive disorder, anxiety, and post-traumatic stress disorder, exhibit lower HRV.[32] These individuals are thought to have less flexibility in how they adapt to changes in their environments.[33] So, when life throws them a curve ball, such as the loss of a job or a romantic breakup, REV's panic button gets glued to the On position and it's an uphill battle for RESTORE to reverse the physical and emotional spirals that ensue.

Thus, the higher functioning your Central Command, the more robust your RESTORE system and hence your HRV, and the better you are at controlling your emotions, which is key to staying on the sunny side of life. This three-part circuit is illustrated in one study where college students' brains were scanned by functional magnetic resonance imaging (fMRI) while they viewed neutral or emotional pictures and were asked to intensify or reduce their emotion state, or to simply passively view the pictures.[34] Subjects with high HRV were better able to explicitly control their emotions and had higher activity in their frontal lobe, as such they were able to flexibly bring on the waterworks or push blue feelings away. In other words, the HRV superstars among us put the "Command" in Central Command.

## Got GUTS?

One of my favorite living scientists, Julian Thayer, PhD, and his colleagues have a theory that the human stress response doesn't come from stressors out there in the world. Rather, humans ARE stress! The Generalized Unsafety Theory of Stress (GUTS) proposes that the fundamental state of every animal (including you) is the equivalent of that pedal-to-the-metal engine I wrote about before, but without the brake pedal: fearful, reactionary, and defensive, basically all REV, no RESTORE.[35] Consider that babies are born into this world screaming and wailing as a survival mechanism. Those screams signify the stress of not knowing friend from foe, where food and warmth will come from, and a general feeling of unsafety. The GUTS model interprets the bloodcurdling screams of babies to mean that they are naturally in a state of REV overdrive.

But, by living through those reasonable stressors, you learn that your parents got you, that your community got you, and, eventually, that you got you. Each moment teaches you that you *are* safe and that you *can* handle life's ups and downs, and this growing understanding helps develop the branches of your Central Command along with its ability to use the brake pedal to inhibit REV's stress response, and to self-regulate; temper emotions; and make solid, long-term, goal-oriented decisions. This is how you mature from a college sophomore who funnels beer on a Tuesday night instead of studying for tomorrow's exam to a thirty-four-year-old with the wisdom to walk away from that second glass of wine at the end of a long day because you know you'll be a worthless lump of cells at that job interview tomorrow.

A key to the GUTS model is that when you perceive yourself to be vulnerable and unsafe, which can happen at any age and in a wide range of situations that may be emotionally or physically dangerous, Central Command may not develop properly and, therefore, loses its inhibitory control of the rest of the brain including the amygdala, leaving REV on at full blast 24/7. This explains why people who live with a long-term illness, the frailty of aging, a physical disability, or who are part of a marginalized community have heart rates stuck at an elevated level (i.e., low HRV), high blood pressure, and all the other problems associated with autonomic imbalance. Kids experiencing the stress of parental neglect or resource scarcity due to poverty can be deprived of the safety signals that help them grow a stable and strong Central Command, and therefore may tend to become adults with low HRV, smaller brain volumes, and poorer self-control.[36] This underscores why early childhood experiences of stability and safety are so crucial.

A generalized feeling of unsafety can also arise when we can't predict what the future holds, such as the uncertainty of every aspect of life during the COVID crisis. And because we're pack animals by nature, spending more time alone can also be stressful. It causes wear and tear on your physiology, with brain activity profiles looking more stressed than they do when people are nearby.[37] Isolated animals have cortisol and heart rate levels as high as those being purposefully stressed under laboratory conditions.[38] Scientists believe this stress response to being alone comes from a very basic survival instinct that make you feel safer in a pack and more defenseless on your own.

Whether you're isolated or not, you can feel lonely, an emotion that serves as an ever-increasing threat to your well-being. It's that disconnected feeling that can happen when you don't see people regularly, as is the case with so many seniors living longer and outlasting their friends. But it can also manifest when you are with people, but disconnected—in a marriage, a family, a friendship, even in a big group. Loneliness can also be due to more time spent on social media, as those online "friends" are about as comforting as a hill of beans when it comes to reducing the stress of life and may even exacerbate the feeling of loneliness.[39] Unsurprisingly, the lonelier you are, the lower your HRV, the higher your cortisol and the worse your immunity.[40] It even increases your chances of early death.[41]

When you're feeling isolated, lonely, or stressed, you're lacking something that makes you feel safe, warm, supported; something that, when you have it, makes your vagus nerve take hold of the wheel. As Thayer and his GUTS colleagues write, you're missing "something which is so important for social animals such as humans; call it love for a better word."[42] Scientists don't often use the word *love*, so I thought I would quote them directly to show how powerful and meaningful this idea actually is. Love = Downstate. Boom. Done.

## PUTTING IT INTO PRACTICE

You can improve your HRV and a wide range of benefits will follow. In this section, you will learn techniques that have been scientifically demonstrated to increase RESTORE vagal activity and, as a result, boost vitality in many areas of your life. These proven methods will appear again in Chapter 8 as the possible Action Items you'll choose from for your Downstate RecoveryPlus Plan. They're the verbs, the deeds, the Dos that I talked about in the Introduction.

## Slow, Deep Breathing

Breath is the game changer at the base of every RESTORE-boosting Action Item you'll learn about in this book. Slow deep breathing, defined as around ten to twelve seconds per breath, five to six breaths per minute, is not only relaxing, but serves as the direct switch from REV to RESTORE dominance. Remember to do it through your nose only. Slowing your breath brings your respiration into alignment with your heart rhythm, so you go from respiratory sinus *arrhythmia* to respiratory sinus *harmonia*.* As I detailed in the section on RSA, when you sync up your heart and lungs, you increase the heart's chance of gobbling up all that fresh oxygen, thereby making the entire cardiovascular system more efficient, and recruit Central Command to take the reins.

Scores of meditation and mindfulness practices incorporate breathing exercises that feature a slowing and holding of the breath followed by an extended exhalation. Everyone from the Dalai Lama to legendary NBA coach Phil Jackson has sung deep breathing's praises, and it's among the most heavily researched health practices out there, promoting REV decreases (reductions in blood pressure and heart rate) and RESTORE increases (improved HRV).[43] Once you become accustomed to the slow, deep breathing practice, you may eventually want to try experimenting with the wide range of breathing rhythms available. A good place to start is in a yoga class or online videos that engage pranayama. Check out techniques from Wim Hof, and/or read Nestor's book *Breath*.[44]

## HRV Biofeedback

In the freezing cold foothills of the Himalayas live a group of Tibetan Buddhist monks who practice a form of mind-body mastery called *g-tummo* yoga. Living in chilly, uninsulated stone huts with earthen floors and flattened tin cans for roofs may have necessitated the invention of their astonishing ability to shift their body temperature by at least 14°F (8.3°C).[45] Researchers have documented an overnight competition in which monks draped in icy towels engage in specific breathing and visual-

---

*Dumb science joke.

ization techniques. The winner is the one who can dry the most towels off his back! This Iron Monk endurance practice helped inspire researchers at the Mind/Body Medical Institute at Beth Israel Deaconess Medical Center to train the minds of regular folks to regulate and control blood pressure, breathing, metabolism, and heart rate through a practice called the *relaxation response*, with the goal of benefiting a wide range of stress-related problems.[46]

Using biofeedback training, your mind can learn how to self-regulate and gain control over your seemingly uncontrollable autonomic functions. With practice, you can use biofeedback to direct blood flow to different areas of the body (helpful if you suffer from poor circulation–related conditions, such as Raynaud's disease or swings in sexual function); reduce pain and tension (it can be as effective at easing headaches as medication); and more.[47]

HRV biofeedback involves intentionally aligning your breath and heart rate while hooked up to a sensor that measures heart activity, which can be done using visual cues for guidance, such as rolling waves or, for kids, video game characters. HRV biofeedback can be viewed as a form of concentrative meditation with a focus on observing and attempting to control the breath and has been shown to increase HRV as well as grease the wheels on all Central Command processes.[48]

HRV biofeedback was first shown to help restore autonomic balance in patients with hypertension and other cardiovascular problems, as well as in patients with depression or anxiety, chronic fatigue, and post-traumatic stress disorder.[49] In more recent years, though, studies report that HRV biofeedback has stress-busting benefits in healthy people too. In one study, experimental subjects were assigned to thirty-minute HRV biofeedback training (or a control task) once a week for five weeks, with their autonomic function and emotional reaction to a stress test measured at the beginning and end of the intervention.[50] At the end of the training, subjects in the biofeedback group had significantly lower depression and anxiety scores, lower blood pressure, and higher HRV. The researchers noted that the decreased blood pressure during the stress induction was due to the subjects using the slow, deep breathing they had learned during the study. This shows that HRV training can make even the most difficult moments a little easier.

HRV biofeedback's antistress benefits have been tested in competitive sports. In a trial of young male athletes, researchers measured REV and RESTORE activity, anxiety, and self-esteem levels, as well as brain activity using EEG.[51] Half of them received ten HRV biofeedback training sessions over the course of three weeks; the other half did not. HRV went up and anxiety and stress went down in one of these groups—I'll let you guess which one. In addition, the biofeedback group showed amplified brain activity associated with more robust self-regulation, attention, and control of emotions. On the court or field, these kinds of improvements translate into keeping your head about you when focusing during high-stakes free throws, handling defeats with grace, and playing the long game by avoiding momentary scuffles with opponents.

As with so many things in life, there's an app for measuring HRV. Several, actually.

Some apps come with separate devices that measure heartbeats, whereas others use the phone's camera, which employs light to measure blood volume changes when the finger is placed over the lens. Heart activity is turned into a visual signal on the screen to illustrate how well you are modulating your HRV. So, in addition to snapping selfies, serving as alarm clocks, and chronicling your meals on social media, today's smartphones can also be used as "gamified" instruments for heart rate assessment and analysis that give you fun, real-time visual feedback of the synchrony between your heart and breathing rates. The gamified aspect makes these biofeedback apps good for kids too.

## Yoga . . . Especially Inversion Poses

*Yoga* can mean many things to many people: a path, a divine union, a sequence of exercises performed in expensive, stretchy pants. But one thing we can all agree on is that it's old, dating back to the pre-Vedic age in India around 3000 BCE.[52] Yet it's still one of the most popular forms of exercise in the world today. That's some impressive staying power.

In yoga, every movement has a breath. Imagine standing in *tadasana* (Mountain Pose), ready for your first *surya namaskar* (Sun Salutation). Your first movement is to lift your arms up and out to the sides, fingers meeting above your head in *urdhva hastasana* (Upward Salute). Whether you're practicing in New Delhi or New York City, this movement occurs with a deep inhale. In fact, yoga instructors usually start the Sun Salutation sequence by saying, simply, "Inhale." Next, you bend at the waist into *uttanasana* (Standing Forward Bend), exhaling as your arms swan dive toward your feet. And so on and so on, each movement taking about four seconds to complete and accompanied by slow, coordinated inhales and exhales. This combination of slow, deep breathing with stretching and gentle movement has been shown to deliver a wide range of health benefits, including the usual RESTORE suspects of boosted heart rate variability; decreased heart rate; improved cognitive performance, blood glucose, and blood lipids; reduced cortisol levels; decreased pain; and enhanced sleep.[53]

Regular yoga practice has been associated with increased Central Command brain volume—the longer the practice, the greater the volume—as well as higher levels of circulating brain-derived neurotrophic factor (BDNF), which scientists often call "fertilizer for the brain" for its ability help grow new brain cells.[54] In one study, healthy, physically active male volunteers were divided into three different age decades: the twenties, thirties, and forties.[55] Everyone practiced an hour of yoga a day, six days a week, for three months. Yes, I know that's a lot, but check out the results: at baseline, the researchers had found, as expected, the beginning tremblings of autonomic imbalance in the thirty- and forty-year-olds, including increases in heart rate and blood pressure. But after three months of regular yoga, these REV indicators decreased significantly, as HRV simultaneously rose. Other studies involving less rigorous yoga routines have yielded similarly promising results. In a recent German study, for instance, a group of high school students was asked to engage in either ninety minutes of yoga once a week for ten weeks, or the equivalent amount of conventional school sports (basketball, volleyball, etc.).[56] The young yogis experienced a more pronounced increase in HRV at the end of study than did the sports group.

Inversions,* yoga postures where the head is at or below the level of the heart, will help you Downward Dog your way toward healthy HRV. These poses are less taxing on the heart, as it takes less effort to pump blood to the

---

*If you have high blood pressure, check with your doctor before attempting inversion poses.

brain when you're horizontal or upside down. Swedish researchers recruited healthy men and women for an eight-week yoga program (60 minutes of yoga, once a week that included a series of inverted and semi-inverted postures, including Downward Dog (*adho mukha svanasana*), Waterfall Pose (you lie down with your legs straight up in the air, hips propped up on a yoga block), and a shoulder stand variation.[57] As the weeks went on, subjects spent increasing amounts of time in these inverted poses, and by the last month of the study, everyone was hanging out upside down or semi–upside down for fifteen to twenty minutes per session. Researchers measured subjects' blood pressure and HRV at the beginning of the study, then again eight weeks later. In the end, they found a significant improvement in HRV among participants, indicating greater RESTORE activity.

You don't even technically have to do anything to reap the benefits. Daily practice of *savasana* (Corpse Pose), which involves lying flat on your back and breathing mindfully, can lead to significant reductions in blood pressure, implicating Corpse Pose as an easy, effective tool for hypertension management.[58] (Have you read my nap book?)

## Intimacy

Sex is complicated for many reasons. I'm just going to focus on the autonomic one. It involves an intricate interaction of both REV and RESTORE systems, from arousal to postorgasm euphoria. During the initial stages of getting turned on, the RESTORE system warms up the body and mind for sex, as any fight or flight–type thoughts or feelings can be a real buzzkill. But while RESTORE is critical for arousal mechanisms like erections and clitoral engorgement, REV takes over as things heat up, increasing heart rate, blood pressure, sweat production, and pupil dilation . . . this last sign being a universal signal for "Come and get it."[59] REV also handles the swelling of breasts, vaginal walls, and testicles; tightens the scrotum; and lubricates the tip of the penis. These actions all continue through REV's final push toward the Big O.

The massive RESTORE rebound following all that exertion makes orgasms your gateway drug to deep Downstate bliss. Post-*YES!*, RESTORE covers your entire body in calm.[60] Central Command, which made a big push during the lead-up to the fireworks show, takes five, and the brain is soaked in a warm bath of attachment-facilitating oxytocin and feel-good serotonin. And to all you insomniacs out there, to the anxiety-prone people who spend hours ruminating, to anyone who feels exhausted all the time, whether or not they get good sleep: sex is the answer. Curiously, vaginal orgasms may beat clitoral ones when it comes to RESTORative gains, due to stronger connections between the vagus nerve and the vagina (as opposed to the clitoris).[61] Less is known about whether anal sex might lead to the same RESTORE perks, but intriguingly, vagal connections do reach the anus, suggesting that it's possible.[62] Along with improved REV/RESTORE ratios, orgasms give your cardiovascular system a run for its money; help combat restless sleep; and just make you happy. And happy mood is associated with higher HRV.[63]

Good sex and HRV are a two-way street, with a healthy REV/RESTORE ratio crucial for a good sex life. Becoming aroused requires just the right amount of REV; too little or too much and you'll experience trouble becoming and staying aroused.[64] High HRV is associated with better overall sexual function, and people with higher HRV tend to be the ones having more sex.[65]

On the other hand, sex or touch that doesn't feel right is the exact opposite of Downstate comfort, making you feel unsafe, on your guard, and everything BUT relaxed. Even slight touches, such as a stranger placing a hand on your back, or a colleague or boss giving you a too-often pat, can make you feel vulnerable and can even send you into a full-blown stress response due to the casualness with which they cross your physical boundary without consent. It's up to you to decide the whos, whens, hows, and wheres of physical touch and intimacy. Understanding and training yourself to embody the rules of consent can be helpful for self-empowerment.[66] Say yes only when it is a real yes. Say no when it is a maybe or no. Change your mind at any time; that is, you might be a yes, and then start feeling weird and switch to a no. When you take responsibility for setting the boundaries in a clear and honest way, physical touch can be a pleasurable way to welcome the Downstate.

You don't need to be sexually active to receive the warm, fuzzy Downstate effects of feeling close. Remember, we are pack animals, so having supportive relationships, including nonromantic ones, is hugely important for maintaining autonomic balance, a strong immune system, and a long, healthy life.[67] Friends, family, mentors, your book club buddies—anyone who makes up your village has the power to help spark these benefits. There are also many ways to satisfy your *skin hunger* needs, a recognized human need for affection that provides general well-being, mental health, and physical health.[68] My friend Susan gets regular massages to satisfy her skin fix. When I was in a long-distance relationship during grad school, I went salsa dancing six nights a week; this afforded me one hundred two-minute sweaty romps with everyone in the club, no strings attached.

The type of affectionate touch found in supportive relationships (defined as touch intended by the toucher to demonstrate love, care, fondness, or appreciation, such as hugging, kissing, caressing, hand-holding, hair stroking, and other nonsexual physical contact) is a way of conveying comfort and safety.[69] Even imagining loving touch can be a stress buffer, and simple hand-holding is da' balm in the face of impending threat.[70] In studies that induce stress by having subjects give a public speech, holding hands with one's romantic partner prespeech decreased cortisol, heart rate, and blood pressure during the actual talk.[71] Preemies who experienced skin-to-skin contact from their caregivers at birth showed decreased cortisol levels up to ten years later, compared with the kids who received no skin-to-skin immediately after being shot from the womb.[72] Adults who are huggers and touchers have higher HRV, lower blood pressure, and fewer physical ailments (e.g., aches, rashes, insomnia, upset stomach).[73] So, whether you're sitting side-by-side on the couch watching your favorite rom-com with your BFF, scheduling a weekly Sexy Sunday date with your spouse, or enjoying your morning warm beverage beside your favorite furred or feathered friend, you've got a golden ticket to the Downstate.

## Nature

While visiting a safari park with her children, Glennon Doyle, author of the book *Untamed*, watched a cheetah chasing a pink stuffed animal in return for a piece of frozen steak. Doyle opens her book by recounting the scene:

Day after day this wild animal chases dirty pink bunnies down the well-worn, narrow path they cleared for her. Never looking left or right. Never catching that damn bunny, settling instead for

a store-bought steak and the distracted approval of sweaty strangers. Obeying the zookeeper's every command . . . Unaware that if
she remembered her wildness—just for a moment—she could tear
those zookeepers to shreds.[74]

Doyle goes on to turn the cheetah into a metaphor for the way so many
women allow themselves to be "tamed" by society. But her words also perfectly capture the conflict between our civilized, electrified, urbanized,
industrialized, computerized selves and our suppressed wild animal selves,
who yearn to reconnect with nature.

Over the last two hundred years, people have gradually shifted from
working outside in fields and farms toward a more sedentary life in facto-
ries and offices. Good-bye, wild cheetah; hello, buildings, indoor plumbing,
and convenience stores. The average American spends over 90 percent of
his or her time indoors, and by 2050, more than 60 percent of the world's
population is projected to live in cities.[75] Emerging research investigating
the impact of this fluorescent-lit, cement-coated migration on our health
has determined that our inner cheetah is not happy. We do better when we
do what we do outside, regardless of sex, age, or fitness level.[76]

Time spent outdoors improves your REV/RESTORE ratio. A recent
study estimated that nearly 10 percent of people with high blood pressure
could get their levels under control if they spent at least thirty minutes in
a park each week, partly because of the heart-related benefits of getting
fresh air and reducing stress hormones.[77] Being outside boosts immune
function, improving chances of fighting off infection, inflammation, and
even cancer, by increasing humans' intake of aromatic plant compounds
called phytoncides that trigger natural killer cells, a type of white blood
cell that supports the immune system and is linked with a lower risk of
cancer.[78] In one study, researchers found that people who took a long walk
through a forest for two days in a row increased the number and activity
of natural killer cells by 50 percent.[79] Those activity levels also remained
a good deal higher than usual for the month following those walks. That's
just two walks!

Exercising in nature, or green exercise, is a smart move too. There are
rocks and branches to look out for, animals to observe, and different directions to decide between, all of which is far more mind-activating than the

ever-spinning hamster wheel of the gym treadmill. This excitement and fun sparks up endorphin- and serotonin-related mood enhancement; outdoor exercisers report feeling more revitalized, happier, engaged, and energized, and experience less tension, anger, and depression than do those who sweat indoors.[80] All of which keeps people coming back for more. In fact, when older people are active outdoors, they do at least thirty minutes more moderate-to-vigorous physical activity per week, and they feel healthier.[81]

Beyond HRV, being outdoors enhances another Downstate domain: sleep, which benefits in both duration and quality.[82] In one study, people either took a mile-long green walk through grassland, wooded areas, and a small lake, or a mile-long urban walk through city streets.[83] During that night of sleep, the forest and field walkers showed greater RESTORE activity, with higher HRV, compared with the cement pounders.

This growing fresh air fascination has created a wave of approaches that all share the goal of moving you back outside, including *shinrin-yoku* ("forest bathing" in Japanese) and horticultural therapy.

Developed in Japan during the 1980s and now widely employed there as a preventive healing modality, forest bathing refers to immersing oneself in nature and experiencing a forest's atmosphere with all five senses.[84] If savasana is a souped-up version of vegging on the couch, shinrin-yoku is an enhanced version of a walk in the forest. And it needn't be an actual forest; fields, nature preserves, and hiking trails can do the trick too. The benefits: heightened mood; decreased depression and anxiety; lower stress, heart rate, and blood pressure; and a greater immune system.[85]

Using plants and gardening to improve mental and physical health—horticulture therapy—has been used with a wide range of people, including the elderly, children, veterans, and people dealing with mental health and addiction problems. Beyond the simple goal of experiencing nature in forest bathing, this technique offers an active role in plant caretaking, as well as learning about the natural rhythm of nature and the cycle of the seasons. Working with plants instills patience, confidence, and courage to work on a long-term goal, as well as the calmness afforded by observing and physically working in a garden. Depending on the need, you can visit healing gardens, rehabilitation gardens, and restorative gardens. These usually feature accessible entrances and paths, raised planting beds and containers, and a sensory-oriented plant selection focused on color, texture, and fragrance. Reported outcomes are just what you would expect: RESTORE is blooming, and REV is in energy-saving mode. Gardening is also a great way to make friends with your green neighbors; you might even hold a progressive garden party where a flock of gardeners tour one another's oases. Personally, gardening is my refuge, one activity that helps me turn off my analytical mind and get creative, dirty, and sweaty all at the same time, and the friends I made gardening became a lifeline for me during the pandemic.

## Self-Hypnosis to Feel Warm and Calm

Autogenic training is a relaxation tool with origins in self-hypnosis commonly taught to clients undergoing therapy to help them find the power in themselves to produce a state of calm throughout the body and mind.[86] *Autogenic* means "self-generating" or "produced from within," and after a few sessions, you'll understand why. It's like a Jedi mind trick you play on your own autonomic system, training it to relax at will and steering it toward healthy physical and emotional responses to stress. Users are taught to think standard phrases several times in a row, with those phrases centering on specific physical sensations (e.g., warmth and heaviness) in six bodily systems, processes, or parts: the musculoskeletal system, circulatory system, heartbeat, breath, abdomen, and forehead. Examples include: "My right arm is warm," "My heartbeat is calm and regular," and "My forehead is cool." Studies show elevations in HRV after just one session, with improvements in headaches, asthma, heart disease, hypertension, irritable bowel syndrome, mild and moderate depression, anxiety, and sleep disorders.[87]

This relaxation modality may also be specifically helpful in bringing you back to YES in the sex department. We've all been there, mind racing with thoughts that take you so far from the warm-body comfort that can come from intimacy with a partner. Autogenic training can help here because even though it is not specifically targeting your erogenous zones, diving into your sensual body and away from your busy thoughts warms up your RESTORE system, which, as you read earlier, can get you in the mood.[88]

In this chapter, you have learned about the many $20 Downstate bills that are floating around you all day ready for you to then slip into your pocket for an immediate payoff in the RESTORE department, including more relaxation and energy, lower blood pressure, peace of mind, better emotion regulation, and sharper thinking. But this Downstate train never stops—it's heading into twilight, ready to show you all the hidden rejuvenating powers that reside in the dark, behind closed eyelids. Let the Downstate Sleep Show begin . . .

# CHAPTER FOUR

# Join the Rest-o-lution, Deepen Your Sleep

—————— • ——————

Whenever I'm asked what type of research I do, when people hear the word "sleep" in my response, their reactions tell me what age decade they are in. The twenties and younger are always excited to tell me about their dreams. The thirties are a toss-up, with the parents grumbling some discontent and the kidless half wanting to share a recent podcast they heard about nap optimization.

But once I'm talking with people in their forties and up, I'm treated to audible groans followed by an unbidden launch into their personal problems of either too little sleep or too many memory problems, which they are beginning to suspect may have something to do with their poor sleep.

Um, YES!

And I totally get it. I've always been a light sleeper, but now that I'm in my forties, I have trouble getting into the deepest slow-wave sleep (SWS), a problem that so many middle-aged adults experience. I get tired at ten p.m., spend a little too much time watching a show, working on the computer, or having fun with my wife, Emily, and then, when I turn out the lights by eleven thirty p.m., I've somehow missed my *sleeportunity*. I then spend hours with one eye open, aware of the moments ticking by as Emily gently snores beside me. It's such a drag.

Fractured sleep is a hallmark of getting older, and through my experience in the sleep lab, I have come to see it as entirely due to the slow wearing away of the Downstate.

Sleep is the ultimate Downstate . . . and so much more than just the absence of wakefulness. It's a meticulously orchestrated voyage during which your brain leaves structured thought behind and endeavors to sort through the clutter of the day, consolidate memories, regulate hormone levels, replenish energy stores, open the RESTORE floodgates, and just generally repair all the cellular damage incurred during your typical sixteen or so hours of Doozering.

In an ideal world, after spending seven to eight hours in this dreamy Downstate, you would open your eyes with the rising of the sun, ready to greet another day. Your mind would be in that coveted state of Inbox Zero: cleaned out, replenished, and ready to work.

Our ancestors understood this, relying on sleep as their main resource for Downstate restoration. But today, precious few of us get to bed early enough to log seven to eight hours of sleep. More likely, you're lucky if you get six hours, punctuated by a blaring smartphone alarm. That phone probably slept on your nightstand, bathing you in the type of blue light, buzzes, and *pings* designed specifically to keep consumers awake and alert.

You can reap a lot of Downstate benefits by revamping your nighttime rituals. But I don't just want you to revamp—my goal is to convince you to burn your old view of bedtime to the ground and learn how to capitalize on the inherently restorative, explicitly kick-ass benefits sleep has to offer.

### *Sleep that knits up the raveled sleave of care*[1]

Along with clean air and water, nutrient-rich food, and shelter, sleep is an essential need for human survival. Although medical science can explain everything related to those first four must-haves and how they impact our well-being, sleep has, until very recently, been almost completely disregarded. It's hard to explain exactly why this centuries-old blind spot developed around something that every living being does for one third of their lives, but it's dangerous and potentially lethal.

Between most people not knowing what a sleep specialist is and doctors frequently failing to ask their patients about sleep issues, many people have spent years enduring sleep problems that are entirely treatable (seventy million Americans currently have chronic sleep issues).[2] Faced with the sheer numbers, you would think that medical schools would wise up to this gaping educational hole and start developing curriculums on the topic of sleep. Yet, the average medical student only receives a total of two to three hours of sleep medicine education.[3] The majority of doctors don't ask about their patients' sleep; instead the pharmaceutical industry dominates treatment of sleep problems with pricey pills rather than cheaper yet equally effective therapies, such as cognitive behavioral therapy for insomnia, that help clients make long-term improvements.[4]

Sleep disturbance is one of the first signs that something isn't right with your body and/or mind, and chronically poor sleep is strongly associated with anxiety and depression; attention and memory deficits; hypertension and cardiovascular disease; diabetes and obesity; dementia and Alzheimer's disease; and all-cause mortality.

All this to say, sleep needs our attention. And once you start sleeping properly, gentle reader, you're in luck, because sleep is your direct line to all the rejuvenating perks of the Downstate on your RecoveryPlus journey.

## Stage by Stage

When we talk about sleep, we're not talking about just one monolithic Downstate experience. Science has divided sleep into four stages based on specific, consistent, and recognizable brain and body activity patterns, and the Downstate ebbs and flows depending on what state you're in.

Understanding what happens from waking throughout the four stages of sleep requires a quick primer on the measurements used to describe brain activity in each stage. Using electroencephalograms (EEG), researchers can measure the dominant electrical neural activity in the brain, which manifests in the form of brain waves of varying amplitude (or height) and frequency (cycles per second). Using this data, human brain waves are then typically divided into five principal bands, identified by Greek letters: gamma (25+ Hz), beta (13 to 24 Hz), alpha (8 to 12 Hz), theta (4 to 7 Hz), and delta (under 4 Hz, including slow-wave activity [0 to 1 Hz]). The insight here is that each brain region oscillates at a certain frequency, with a specific EEG signature associated with an individual brain area. Much like an orchestra that has high-frequency sounds coming from the woodwinds and deeper notes produced by the double bass section, EEG signatures from each brain area emerge at different periods in your night's symphony. By reading the EEG traces, cognitive neuroscientists can tell that sleep onset has occurred by a reduction in alpha waves at the back of the brain, or that the sleeper has entered slow-wave sleep, a.k.a. the Downstate Jackpot, by slow waves in the front of the cortex.

When the brain is actively awake, it is controlled by attentional and executive function networks that focus your perception on the most exciting or interesting feature in the environment and govern your responses accordingly. Waking EEG reflects the multitasking mayhem that is your day-to-day existence, characterized by a wide range of gamma and beta activity. Every brain area is talking at once and rather independently of its neighbor, which makes for low-amplitude, high-frequency EEG signals.

Occasionally, your attention transitions away from the external environment to a quiet, inner awareness, and a network of brain areas called the *default mode network* takes over. Default mode is the place you go when your mind is between moments of goal-oriented Doozering—a place where you can think about what you'll eat for dinner; contemplate your social interactions; daydream; or listen to a story without the pressure of formulating a response, like your favorite true crime podcast. It's also where you go during some forms of meditation, or as you begin to fall asleep and the executive at the head of the car sits down and stops ordering everybody around. These relaxed states feature larger amounts of alpha waves. As you fall asleep, brain activity moves into lower frequencies and larger amplitudes, with brain areas of the default mode network nodding off as you lose self-awareness and head into deep sleep.

**Stage 1:** The first few minutes of sleep, called Stage 1, are characterized by a shift in brain activity from alpha to theta, along with slow rolling eye movements from left to right and generalized involuntary muscle contractions called hypnogogic jerks (or Hypnic Jerks, which sounds like the name of a skateboarding band of hooligans from Glendale, California) that are usually accompanied by short-lived dreams of losing control, such as falling off a curb. This layover in Stage 1 sleep lasts for only a few minutes as the brain works diligently to quiet and synchronize activity across the entire brain in an effort to keep you asleep. Think of Stage 1 as your friendly Walmart greeter, welcoming you into Stage 2.

**Stage 2:** As I wrote in my nap book, "If sleep is a soup, then Stage 2 is its stock. Not only does it provide the medium in which all the other stages 'float,' but it's pretty nutritious all by itself."[5] We spend about 60 percent of our total sleep time in Stage 2 sleep, and it serves as the transition stage between deep slow-wave sleep (SWS) and active rapid eye movement (REM) sleep, such that you are always passing through Stage 2 on your way to SWS or REM. Stage 2 is chock-full of brain activity patterns that signal heavy CPU processing, including short bursts of brain activity from the thalamus called *sleep spindles* (12 to 15 Hz), and large, slow EEG waves from the cortex called *K-complexes*. K-complexes are precursors to the slow waves—the most fundamental Downstate source—that emerge in SWS. (More on that in just a bit.)

**Slow-wave sleep (SWS):** The longer you stay in Stage 2 sleep, the greater your chances are of transitioning into the molten core of your Downstate: SWS, which is basically all-slow-waves-all-the-time, including delta (1 to 4 Hz) and slow waves (0 to 1 Hz). SWS is comprised of Stages 3 and 4 (see the progression of sleep stages across the night on page 103), and should be called the Fountain of Youth for its regenerative powers. During this brain state, and ONLY this state, all systems enter a state of deep winter characterized by relaxation of muscle and vasculature, reduced brain activity and body temperature, decreased renal function, and slower intestinal motility. In addition, sympathetic stress-related chemicals take a nap while growth hormone, aldosterone, testosterone, insulin, glycogen, and prolactin—all critical for tissue repair, immune and metabolic function, and inflammation control—are released. (Growth hormone keeps you strong, youthful, and able to leap tall buildings in a single bound, and it's the antidote to cortisol's corrosive effects. Prolactin helps with milk production in lactating moms and supports immune function.) Just as with the seasons, where the deeper Downstate winter produces a more fruitful spring, the same goes for SWS; the deepest, slowest sleep is associated with the greatest metabolic rest (e.g., oxygen consumption decreases by 25 percent and glucose by over 40 percent), creating optimal conditions for the Downstate processes that build organs and tissues, and enhancing protein synthesis for the restoration of cell structure and function.[6] Additionally, the mounting electrical potential that builds during a long day of neural communication needs to be downscaled, or else the neurons will get overstimulated and oversaturated, rendering them incapable of functioning. Sleep, SWS in particular, promotes the downscaling and renormalization of neurons that help maintain a flexible and ready-to-learn brain upon waking.[7] In terms of RecoveryPlus, SWS is the time when your brain and body are replenishing resources in greater quantities than you had yesterday (remember that insurance policy I mentioned in Chapter 1?), preparing you to reach beyond your last set-point.

The most important thing to know about SWS is that the list of physiological changes associated with it are completely unique to SWS; they don't happen during wake or even lighter stages of sleep. This is because the acceleration of protein synthesis in the brain requires the deceleration of energy metabolism below the level attainable in wake or lighter stages of sleep. In fact, Upstate hormones, such as cortisol and catecholamines, block protein synthesis, whereas Downstate hormones, such as growth hormone, stimulate the synthesis of proteins and amino acid uptake, the fuel for the brain and body.[8] A profound quiet is also necessary for downscaling the potentiation of the neural network, something that can only happen during deep sleep. Thus, SWS is ground zero for all RESTORE recovery processes in the nervous system, and that is why I believe that the loss of SWS and its many benefits is one of the main reasons aging happens.

Understanding why SWS is the most profound opportunity for Downstate repair and recovery is one of my personal favorite contributions that my lab has made to sleep science (with reinventing the nap coming in as a close second). My lab discovered that the cognitive benefits of SWS are made possible by the combined action of slow waves in the brain and RESTORE activity in the autonomic nervous system.[9]

To get the full picture, shift your gaze below the neck and consider what the autonomic nervous system is up to once you fall asleep. When you are young and healthy, waking hours are dominated by an energetic REV, whereas from sleep onset to deep sleep, you experience a dramatic shift from REV to RESTORE with the slowing of heart rate and a large boost in heart rate variability (HRV). These influences are bidirectional, meaning the brain and heart are talking to one another such that changes in autonomic activity trigger sleep onset and the transition between sleep stages further enhances RESTORE.[10] Slow-wave sleep takes the brain and body on the deepest dive into the Downstate lagoon by letting REV go dark and RESTORE to flourish, even more than during other stages of sleep or when awake.[11] Healthy Upstate/Downstate ratios derived from the long RESTORE soak during SWS reduce risk for cardiovascular disease, diabetes, and all-cause mortality, leading some researchers to describe sleep as a "cardiovascular holiday."[12] Thus, if the circadian night is when Downstate recovery is optimized, SWS is the bullet train that transports the body and mind from depleted and drained to replenished and ready for the morning.

The rough part is that this natural rejuvenating bath is wasted on the young. As you get older, you lose precious minutes in SWS, with RESTORE essentially banished from your sleep kingdom. In fact, in my way of thinking, aging is defined by the loss of these restorative functions, a concept you will learn more about in Chapter 7. The good news is that by fully embracing the power of the Downstate, you will learn the whens and hows of these changes and what you can do to counteract them as soon as they start to rear their run-down, strung-out heads.

**Rapid eye movement (REM):** The first three stages, Stages 1, 2, and SWS, show a progressive slowing in brain electrical activity and heart rate, as well as a decrease in blood flow and metabolism. RESTORE is having a field day. All of which is completely reversed when you enter the final sleep stage, REM sleep, a veritable Upstate carnival of activity in the amygdala, anterior cingulate, and thalamus, with marked inhibition in the executive function and logical thinking areas of the prefrontal region. This pattern of brain activity is why REM dreams are characterized by heightened motivation, gripping emotions, and crazy, illogical structure. REM sleep is also marked by almost full-body paralysis of skeletal muscles, also called *atonia*, which prevents you from acting out your dream about showing up to work naked.

At the end of your first bout of REM sleep, you have traveled through a ninety-minute sleep cycle featuring all four sleep stages, taking you from the depths of restorative SWS to the dizzying heights of REM. After that, everything starts over again, minus the unnecessary introductions by Stage 1. Very quickly, your sleep stages recognize each other like old friends and settle into a long night of rhythmic cycling through Stage 2, SWS, Stage 2, and REM, Stage 2, SWS, Stage 2, REM, etc. . . .

### YOU ARE WHAT YOU SLEEP

Two of the main functions of Downstate sleep are the integration of the day's experiences into your knowledge, memory, and emotional networks and brain cleaning. Let's start with the cognitive benefits of sleep: memory and emotional well-being.

*Memory is not an abstraction. It is solid or it is smoke.*[13]

Every day, you process around thirty-four gigabytes of information.[14] The dilemma is that you need to store much of this information so you don't lose it or overwrite it with similar incoming data. This important task is one of the primary functions of sleep. During sleep, while you're cozily wrapped around your body pillow, Sylvia, your brain is hard at work, transforming your new experiences into long-term memories and integrating these new memories with all the other knowledge you have accumulated over the course of your life. During sleep, you update what you know about your friends and family; how you feel about romance and whether it's worth another try; or maybe even discover an innovation that will make or break your career. Such complicated tasks could never be carried out during the confusion of the Upstate, when you are exploring, hunting, and learning. So, Nature, in her ancient wisdom, decided to relegate the conservation and reassessment of your life to sleep, a quiet time for consolidating and reframing your experiences.

Your memories are important; they make you who you are. Babies are learning machines, from language development to figuring out how to crawl, cruise, and canter. They take in so much new information every day that they need frequent offline periods of consolidation (i.e., naps) to commit it all to memory. In adulthood, sleep helps you learn how to play a new musical instrument, remember the route to a new job, or understand how to incorporate remote technology for every aspect of your life in your late forties.

In the animated movie *Inside Out*, a poetic rendering of how early life experiences help construct a person's identity, long-term memories are symbolized as translucent glass orbs that glow with different colors depending on the dominant emotion at the time.[15] When the main character, eleven-year-old Riley, sleeps, her emotions and memories from the day are packed into a vacuum tube and shuttled to a library-esque space called Long Term Memory. Just as for Riley, your memories are inextricably linked with your identity and how you live your life. They make up the painted brush strokes of your self-portrait. Memories build identity (a carpenter, a scientist, a writer, a parent, a bus driver); habits and hobbies (snowboarding, knitting, a five p.m. glass of pinot; reading bedtime stories to kids or mystery novels to yourself); pet peeves and triggers (chaos, neediness, abandonment, messiness, tardiness). All of these aspects of your personality come from early life experiences that formed long-term memories and were integrated into your own personal knowledge-feeling-motivation network.

We use the term *memory* to represent all the information we hold on to for a long time, which can come from any cognitive domain, including perception, verbal and autobiographical memory, spatial navigation, motor skills, the learning of rote behaviors and habits, and many others. If any of your experiences are tinged with heightened arousal, either negative or positive, your brain will recruit the amygdala along with a little dash of REV substances, such as cortisol and epinephrine, to tag a new memory as extra important and prioritize processing during your next bout of sleep.

In cognitive science speak, memories can be explicit (or declarative, as in you can declare you know them) when you consciously decide to memorize and recall them, as with a phone number; where you parked your car; or who attended your last birthday. Or memories can be implicit (or nondeclarative) because access to this information is unconscious and automatic. Implicit memories include complicated motor sequences, such as those involved in riding a bike, forming habits from sheer repetition, increasing sensitivity to the sounds of individual musical instruments, or encoding subliminal messages. Or memories can have both explicit and implicit aspects. For example, a professional basketball player has explicit knowledge of what she should be doing with her body to shoot a basket from the free throw line, but because she has done it so many times those sequences of movements have now jelled into an implicit skill, such that if you ask her to use her explicit memory to perform a free throw, she would likely miss the shot. This is because you have different brain areas controlling your explicit and implicit memories, such as the hippocampus, which reigns over your explicit memories but has little access to your implicit memories. Consider the difference between driving to a new destination and your regular drive home from work. The new destination engages the hippocampus to help you learn all the explicit, step-by-step instructions to get you where you need to go, whereas the familiar drive home is so locked up in your implicit memory that you could zone out listening to your podcast and be home before you know it.

Explicit and implicit memories are processed differently. On the one hand, for explicit memories, your recall begins to worsen the moment after you experience each event, so the goal of your explicit memory network is to prevent further forgetting of the details by stabilizing the memory in long-term storage areas in the cortex, ensuring conscious access to everything from your first kiss to your most recent Zoom gaffe. On the other hand, implicit memories don't involve the hippocampus, rendering them less vulnerable to forgetting. Rather, they grow stronger, faster, and more accurate via the striatum (the brain's habit center) and cortex. With implicit memories, the end goal is enhancement by sharpening and speeding up of processing. You might lose explicit memory of your fifth birthday party, but you'll never forget the implicit skill of swimming the breaststroke.

One of the most exciting breakthroughs in memory research over the past twenty years is the discovery that sleep plays a large role in the formation of your long-term memories. Results from the sleep lab typically show that subjects have more detailed and resilient memories after sleep (whether it's a nap or a night) than after an equal period of wakefulness. But the most intriguing result is that the type of sleep matters. Sleep scientists have discovered that SWS helps people hold on to explicit memories, whereas REM sleep is better for improving implicit memories. Furthermore, Stage 2 supports motor learning, verbal memory, and general perkiness, whereas SWS is important for clearing away the information buildup that happens across a normal day (clearing the desktop, so to speak), as well as deep memorization of all explicit material and navigating through new spatial maps. REM is key for implicit cognitive processes, including perceptual learning, unconscious associations, as well as soldering creative links between ideas and memories in your head and processing emotions.

## EMOTIONAL WELLNESS

REM is critical for emotional well-being. Think about the last emotional experience you had—a bad breakup, a job loss, or the death of a loved one.

**GET PAID TO NAP!**

In my Sleep and Cognition Lab, our goal is to discover all the secrets of the brain during sleep that lead to better performance during waking hours. We do this by experimenting on individuals who agree to get paid to take naps (or sleep overnight) in my lab. Participants arrive in the morning and sit in front of a computer screen where they interact with information to be tested on later. This could involve memorizing a list of words or a set of emotional pictures; learning a motor or perceptual skill; or even finding and memorizing the location of buried treasure in the video game platform *Minecraft*. After lunch, participants nap while several physiological monitors, including electroencephalography (EEG) and electrocardiogram (ECG), read out activity in the central (EEG) and autonomic (ECG) nervous systems. Then, sleep technicians (i.e., trained graduate students) count the minutes in each sleep stage (Stages 1, 2, SWS, and REM), as well as the number of sleep events (slow waves, sleep spindles, and more). After a nap of anywhere between thirty and ninety minutes, we wake them, give them a moment to wipe the sleep from their eyes, then test them on the information they learned that morning. We also test a group of people who didn't nap, to quantify memory improvement across a period of wake instead of sleep. The same basic procedures work for nighttime sleep studies, but subjects get their first test in the evening, sleep overnight, and leave the lab after their morning test.

Now remember the timeline of your pain and how you processed the event from the very first moment that it happened, to the next day, to a week later, up until now. Did it go from the worst ache imaginable to a gradual contraction of the emotional pain as your understanding of what happened expanded? If you answered yes, you experienced the trajectory of a healthy emotional response.

Research has shown that REM sleep plays a protective role in helping people adjust to emotional events by helping move processing of the event from your amygdala-centered emotional brain to your Central Command's rational brain (the prefrontal cortex). REM sleep right after an emotional event can help predict the intensity of your feelings in the coming days and weeks ahead. Let's think back to that emotionally traumatic experience of getting attacked in a dark park at night. You want to learn from this experience so that you avoid similar situations in the future, so the brain makes sure that you don't forget this experience by tagging it with a strong amygdala response and an uptick in REV substances during the event, followed by an increase in REM sleep that night, all of which boosts your emotional response to the event. REM sleep right after the event helps gradually decrease your amygdala-centered emotional response. This means you might be very emotionally raw in the few days after the event, but eventually your emotional response becomes weaker (e.g., fewer sparks of rage or uncontrollable tears). Meanwhile, cognitive reappraisal of the experience allows you to objectively think through what happened and what you can do to avoid the situation in the future.

It is possible to have too much of a good thing, as is the case with people who live with periods of deep emotional distress due to depression or anxiety. They often have more REM sleep than nondepressed people and as such are more prone to perseverate on negative experiences, burdening them with darker moods. A recent cutting-edge therapeutic approach for depression called triple chronotherapy curtails REM sleep by waking people up early and exposing them to bright light, resulting in positive benefits for mood.[16]

Notably, the cognitive benefits of each sleep stage are just as true for naps as they are for nighttime sleep. We study naps because they make it easier to tease apart the separate contributions of each sleep stage by just waking people up before they head into deeper SWS or wacky REM, giving us the ability to measure the effect of a nap containing only Stage 2, or only Stage 2 and SWS, or all three stages. Ultimately, the results from nap experiments show the same outcomes as those from nighttime sleep experiments.

## This Is the Rhythm of the Night . . .

As you follow along with this book, you might start to see the Downstate/ Upstate pattern everywhere you look. If so, you'll pick up on the same ocean wave–like pattern in the drawing-in of SWS (Downstate), followed by the blast of energy in REM (Upstate). Each time you pass through SWS and REM, you complete one sleep cycle, which lasts about ninety minutes.

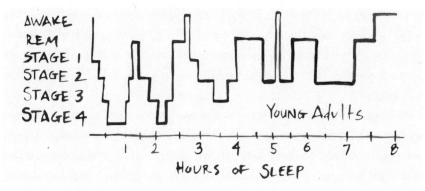

A Typical Progression of Sleep Stages Across the Night in Young Adults

A full night of sleep may contain four to five cycles before the rooster crows, but all sleep cycles are not made equally. The proportion of SWS and REM varies greatly depending on whether you are starting your first sleep cycle of the night (a concentrated bolus of Stage 2 and SWS [Stages 3 and 4], with very little REM sleep), or finishing up your last one in the early morning (mostly Stage 2 and REM sleep).

The transition across the night from SWS-dominant to REM-dominant is driven by a range of factors, some of which are in your control, some of which are not. This means if you consistently push bedtime back to eleven p.m. or later, you will miss out on that very important, highly Downstatey first sleep cycle, which is naturally programmed to occur a couple of hours after sunset. The brain has a stopwatch and it knows how long you've been awake, and what time you're popping in your night guard. You can't trick it by going to bed at midnight, saying, "No biggie, I'll still get my first SWS-heavy sleep cycle. I'm just starting a bit late." Nope. The two sleep rhythms you will now learn about have their own periods of the night devoted to them, and they don't like to get pushed around.

Many of us spend our lives going to sleep late and sleeping too long in the morning. By doing so, we miss out on the built-in Downstate opportunities ($20 bills) and only hasten the forces of decay that are coming for us, rain or shine. Understanding the inner workings of our nocturnal rhythm will help us determine when we should be getting to sleep and waking up for maintaining optimal health and cognitive sharpness.

Using its trusty stopwatch, the brain regulates two vital processes that together determine the proportion of SWS and REM in each sleep cycle. The first dictates when and how much SWS you get and is called Process S, for Sleep. The second regulates REM sleep and is called Process C, for Circadian.

Think back to the concept of homeostasis from Chapter 1, when I explained that only your most critical functions are maintained at a strict set-point, including water, salt, pH, and temperature. Well, now you can add sleep. Because sleep is so crucial for survival, Process S homeostatically balances your wake and sleep each day, paying specific, stalkerlike attention to SWS. This is due to all the RESTORE benefits that can only happen during SWS; to maintain a balance between the Upstate forces that empty your tank and the Downstate forces that fill it up, your body keeps score of the minutes you've been awake and measures out a precise amount of SWS to compensate for all that wear and tear.

Process S wakes up the moment you open your eyes to the day, launching a phenomenon called sleep pressure, which tracks how long you've been awake, essentially counting down the moments until you go back to sleep. Sleep pressure is low in the morning and starts climbing with each additional minute of Doozering. With increasing sleep pressure, your brain produces neurochemicals that mark the time awake. Think back to your biology class: Remember the Krebs cycle and ATP, the energy currency of every cell in the body? Absolutely anything your cells need to do (e.g., moving a muscle, having a thought) requires the small amount of energy that gets released when you turn ATP into ADP by pooping out a phosphate. A demanding Upstate life uses A LOT of ATP and therefore creates A LOT of ADP, otherwise known as adenosine. The amount of adenosine in your brain is a strong indicator of how long you've been Doozering and determines how sleepy you feel and how much SWS you need. In fact, when the buildup of adenosine reaches a fever pitch, this natural compound signals to your autonomic nervous system that it's time to transition from REV to RESTORE dominance and tells your central nervous system that it's time for SWS, ushering you into the greatest place on earth, the Downstate.

As I mentioned earlier, under normal sleep conditions, the first cycles of your night are rich in SWS followed by REM-heavy cycles in the early morning. We know that Process S works like a homeostat because when you stay up extra late or skip a whole night of sleep, your wake counter keeps ticking away, pushing up your sleep pressure to higher and higher levels. This happens for many people on a weekly basis when you stay up late Monday through Friday and then try to "catch up" by sleeping in on the weekends (social jet lag). The homeostat of Process S will try to make up this SWS debt as soon as it can, such that the next sleep opportunity will be even heavier than usual on the slow waves.

But one day of good behavior doesn't make up for several bad ones. Trying to pay back your entire sleep debt on the weekend is a false economy because the Upstate wear and tear that happens on a daily basis becomes impossible to balance out by sleeping in on Sunday morning. The buildup of brain toxins even after one night of sleep deprivation isn't cleared out after multiple nights of subsequent good sleep.[17] Several nights in a row of suboptimal sleep throws your eating hormones out of whack, making you hungrier than usual and driving your appetite for high-fat and sugary foods, sending your metabolic system into a prediabetic state.[18]

Beyond sleep, this false economy can be found in every Upstate/Downstate balancing act. One healthy meal a week can't make up for six days of fast food; one vacation won't balance out a year of late nights and no weekends; one long walk isn't enough to stave off the negative consequences of sitting at the computer fifty hours a week. The fact is you can only maintain a healthy Upstate/Downstate ratio by replenishing your resources on a daily basis.

The other reason you need to regularly get to sleep early enough is that Process C (your circadian rhythm) pushes REM sleep into the limelight. If Process S is dedicated to counting down the minutes until you get to sleep, Process C is counting the minutes until you wake up. Unlike Process S, which is completely determined by behavior (e.g., the time you woke up and how long you've been Doozering), Process C is driven by the internal circadian forces discussed in Chapter 2, which are, for the most part, out of your control. Remember that your circadian rhythm stimulates the morning rise in cortisol, and with it, REM sleep that evening. This matchmaking between a REV stress hormone and REM (a sleep state characterized by hyperactive brain activity similar to waking) is thought to help you wake up REVVING to go.

Here are the take-home messages:

1. The first part of your night is your ticket to restorative SWS.
2. The second part of your night is mainly dreamy REM sleep.
3. Both are important, so you need to get to sleep early to make sure you get a healthy portion of each one.
4. If you don't get to sleep early enough, REM sleep will take over and you'll have to wait until the next night to make up for your sleep loss; a false economy that will leave your Upstate/Downstate ratio unbalanced.
5. Upstate wear and tear is a daily problem that needs a nightly solution, so you can't actually make up for your sleep debt on the weekends. Getting to bed early brings you restorative SWS, while chronically late bedtimes can lead to Upstate REV, high blood pressure, buildup of brain toxins, and metabolic disorders.[19]

Why did nature set up your nightly rhythm with SWS coming before REM both in each individual ninety-minute sleep cycle and throughout the majestic architecture of a whole night? The truth is we don't know, but here is my theory:

Think about everything you've learned about the demands of the Upstate: it's chock-full of information, it's stressful, it's energy consuming; it's an emotional whirlwind; and for many, it's way too long. Doozering through a full day fills up your brain while simultaneously running down your battery, and that battery ain't gonna charge itself!

So, come beddy-bye time, the first order of business is to secure the information you want to keep by moving it from short-term to long-term storage, then to get rid of the crap you don't need by downscaling all your neural connections to baseline, and finally to replenish your resources so you are ready for the next Upstate. Given that REM sleep gets you as fired up as being awake, with brain activity high and REV arousal creeping up, REM is no time for protective or restorative processes. If REM came before SWS, there is a good chance you would overwrite all those precious new memories and they would get lost forever. You wouldn't condition your hair before shampooing, would you?

I hypothesize that REM comes after SWS because once you have secured your recent experiences into the library of your cortex, you still need to integrate those new juicy bits of info with the rest of your knowledge network. That's where the blasts of long-term potentiation and increased blood flow through the brain help you associate and make connections between old and new memories and ideas. Why do you think your dreams are so nonlinear, with your deceased grandmother playing basketball with that guy you just met who makes your guts feel all squiggly? You are putting together new experiences with older structures of knowledge. This is the reason REM slumber has earned a well-deserved reputation for birthing breakthrough insights, with famous artists and scientists crediting their eureka moments to end-of-sleep dreams. Paul McCartney dreamed the notes of "Yesterday" in 1963, heading straight from his bed to his piano to begin re-creating the melody; decades before that, Albert Einstein allegedly had a dream involving cows and electric fences that inspired his theory of relativity.[20] Whatever nature's secret reason for this SWS/REM cycle, it's as old as the trees, so best to honor it.

## The Slow Wave: The OG Downstate

Look long enough into the slow wave, and the Downstate will gaze back at you. During SWS, RESTORE is in its full majesty, with peak HRV throughout this sleep stage, while REV is taking a much-needed nap. This epic Downstate in both your brain and heart facilitates the refilling of energy stores; the laying down of long-term memories, and processing of the day's emotions. And though it may look like a simple blip on a sleep lab computer screen, the slow wave belies a tremendous fact, which is this: for half of every slow wave cycle, you are brain-dead.

I can explain.

A slow wave takes one second to complete, comprised of a half-second Upstate and a half-second Downstate. Yes, this is where the Downstate got its name! In SWS, when slow waves predominate, you are at the southernmost tip of the Downstate peninsula and your brain is literally turning itself off and forcing everything to just stop. Can you imagine it? The silence. The nothingness. Drink it in . . . that is you for a good portion of your night—the Custodian you, the Consolidator you, the Repairer you, the Replenisher you.

As the largest traveling wave of the cortex, the slow wave generally starts at the front of the head and moves to the back like a tsunami, lifting

## HELLO, FOUR P.M. CUP OF COFFEE...

It's four p.m. and every aspect of you is out of gas. And yet, you still have a metric ton of work and domestic duties looming over you before nigh-nigh.

Your buddies at work are headed hordelike to the coffee cart. The million-dollar question: do you join them? Of course, a shot of caffeine will give you the energy you need. Even just standing in line, smelling the java, will send *Get ready, it's wakey-wakey-eggs-and-bakey time!* messages to your brain. Do you consider the fact that caffeine can remain in your system for six hours or more? Or do you tell yourself you're invincible, nothing can threaten your ability to fall asleep?

Fast-forward to you, lying awake at two a.m., cursing that momentary weakness that's now preventing you from getting that hard-earned Downstate SWS. Maybe at some point you reach for that little orange bottle with the white cap and pop an Ambien. (Uppers by day, downers by night. You're such a rock star . . . ) This is your brain on caffeine.

Here's something to mull over as you stare at the ceiling: the molecules in your brain operate by making lock-and-key-like connections with little doorways in your neurons, called receptors. Nature designed the adenosine molecule (of ATP-to-ADP fame) to fit perfectly with the adenosine receptor, and when that door opens, your brain gets the sleepiness message. So, a long day of ATP-to-ADP Doozering creates a lot of adenosine molecules, which queue up for sleepytime. But caffeine molecules resemble adenosine closely enough that they can also make a connection with adenosine receptors, tricking them by sort of jamming the lock so the real adenosine can't get in. This is why drinking caffeine makes you feel wired; it monopolizes all of your adenosine receptors, so even if your brain is teeming with tiny yawns searching for a bed, your brain is getting the message that it's Upstate time.

If there is even a small voice inside your head wondering whether it's possible to get off the Keith Richards party bus, listen to it. As I have been preaching throughout this book, your natural rhythms are right there, inside you, waiting to get in sync with you. You can start by reducing the artificial go-tos for regulating alertness and sleepiness. If you drink caffeine or take any other stimulants, stop as early in the day as possible, noon at the latest. When you get sleepy in the afternoon, take a short nap. My first book, *Take a Nap! Change Your Life*, will help you do just that. YOU CAN DO IT!

everything up in its excitatory path, and then silencing all brain activity in one grand inhibitory sweep. Even though it's the slowest wave on the block, it has the honor of being the carrying wave for all faster frequencies, which are nested in its Upstate. You can think of the slow wave as a giant cargo ship transporting hundreds of smaller shipping containers at a steady pace across the ocean. During each Upstate of the slow wave, all of your different brain areas rush to send out messages in this sudden burst of communication. This narrow window ensures that all brain areas synchronize their firing, which increases the chance of successful information transfer because all the brain areas are riding the same Upstate wave. It's followed by the emptiness of interstellar space, during which every neuron in the brain takes a deep Downstate rest until the next Upstate opportunity. Scientists now understand this Upstate/Downstate rhythm as providing a temporal framework for all brain activity including the sweeping out of toxins, long-term memory formation, executive function reset, creative integration of ideas, and the building of all your knowledge networks.

Daily Downstate sleep, then, acts as a one-two punch, supporting two main functional categories: cognitive enhancement and brain cleaning.

## REPLAYING YOUR MEMORIES

As I explained earlier, sleep plays an important role in the integration of the day's experiences into our knowledge and memory networks. Whether you play piano, learn a new language, contemplate philosophy, or bird-watch, you need sleep in regular increments to not totally suck. To understand how the slow wave orchestrates this nightly consolidation, I'll explain a little about a groundbreaking series of studies showing how the exact neural activity pattern that supports thoughts and action during waking is replayed during slow waves.

Researchers stuck tiny electrodes that measure electrical firing into the hippocampus of rodents who were trained to run in a maze, and then continued recording the neural activity of those same hippocampal neurons when the rats fell asleep. What they discovered changed the course of sleep research: the neural pattern of firing during maze running was repeated during sleep, indicating that the rodent was likely dreaming of maze running.[21] Importantly, the replay only happened during the Upstate of the slow wave. Amazingly, during the Downstate of the slow wave the whole brain was silent. So, even rats go Downstating!

Remember, the hippocampus is only a short-term way station for new memories that need to be integrated into long-term cortical storage as soon as possible, lest they risk being overwritten by the next day's experiences. This process of transforming recent experiences into highly integrated, long-term memories occurs by replaying the memories through coordinated neural communication between key brain areas, including the hippocampus, thalamus, and cortex, during sleep. The neural trace of the memory in the hippocampus has to be sent, bucket brigade–like, toward the cortex by hitching a ride on sleep spindles traveling from the thalamus to the cortex. The thalamus, along with every other brain area, naturally coordinates its firing during the all-encompassing Upstate portion of the slow wave, making this supercarrier brain wave a rather nifty evolutionary mechanism for information transfer.

Think of the slow wave as a great passenger train that leaves the station at regular intervals. The spindle is the passenger and the hippocampal memory trace is the luggage. When the train pulls into the station, the Upstate is in full swing and all the passengers jump on the train with their luggage they are bringing to their final destination (long-term memory brain areas). After each train departs the station, the brain experiences the empty platform of the Downstate, which soon begins to fill up again with passengers (and their luggage) waiting for the next transport opportunity. In this metaphor, sleep is rush hour, when the important information you learned each day gets routed to long-term memory.

In my Sleep and Cognition Lab, we study how the hustle and bustle of the hippocampus-cortex train line during SWS leads to memory improvement, analyzing sleep EEG by counting the number of slow waves that have a spindle riding on its Upstate, as this is thought to reflect coordinated brain activity between three critical brain areas for memory: the thalamus, the hippocampus, and cortex. This coordination of widespread neural activity during the Upstate of the slow wave is believed to be the main mechanism by which long-term memories are formed.[22] In the lab, we find that the more these slow wave–spindle events occur, the stronger the memories upon waking.[23]

Slow waves, which originate and are largest in the front of the brain, are also beneficial for boosting cognitive functions that rely on Central Command, including executive functions. Your ability to focus your attention, hold items in your working memory, and have self-control is key to countless critical activities: remembering to take your medication every morning, following directions to a gas station, and holding up your end of a conversation.[24] Being awake drains power from Central Command, while SWS pumps it back up along with your executive functioning. Brain training apps that help keep your executive functioning sharp have the added benefit of boosting your slow waves in response to the training. The more you train, the bigger the slow waves, and the bigger the slow waves, the better the working memory. It's a good cycle to get into.

## Workin' Nine to Five (p.m. to a.m.) . . .

It's ten p.m. and there's a janitor bathed in fluorescent overhead lights pushing a broom down an otherwise dark hallway, whistling while he works. Is this the start of an '80s office comedy or is that your brain on SWS? For your sake, I hope it's the latter, because the second vital function of sleep is the starring role as your nightly custodian.

Sleep's role in brain cleaning was first reported in 2012 when a Danish neuroscientist, Maiken Nedergaard, PhD, and her team discovered that a group of large brain cells called *glia*, whose function up until that point was unknown, actually serve as the waste removal system in the brain, much like the lymphatic system in the body.[25] This system, which she termed *the glymphatic system*, is tightly coupled with Downstate slow waves. Prior to that point, scientists did not fully understand how the brain, which maintains its own closed ecosystem, removed waste. But these new findings revealed a plumbing system that switches on when the heart and brain are under Downstate control during sleep, pumping cerebral spinal fluid (CSF) through brain tissue to clean out toxins that accumulate from Upstate toiling. The glymphatic system itself also follows a circadian rhythm, only turning on during the deepest part of the Downstate night while you are asleep. This gives you another reason not to arrive fashionably late to the sleep party, lest you risk losing your chance at the best full-brain-cleanse in town.

One of the most critical custodial jobs of the glymphatic system is to prevent the accumulation of toxic proteins, such as beta amyloid and tau, which are the very material that form plaques in Alzheimer's disease. Disrupted sleep is, therefore, a major reason that people develop this devastating form of dementia. Without the deep nightly cleanse from robust slow waves sweeping waste from the hills and valleys of your brain, you get the equivalent of neural landfills that block these important tracts between the hippocampus and frontal lobe, polluting the natural pathways that keep your brain young and healthy. Indeed, age-related decreases in SWS put you at greater risk for dementia and Alzheimer's.[26] Even one night of sleep deprivation increases amyloid beta deposits in the brain; think of the damage incurred by chronic sleep loss. The reverse is also true: people with Alzheimer's typically experience chronic insomnia and excessive daytime sleepiness, both of which correlate with worsened symptoms.[27] The bottom line is that the more you lose touch with SWS, the more your glymphatic plumbing system clogs up, and the higher your chance of developing plaques and eventually Alzheimer's disease.

## Alcohol: A Pseudo-Downstate

I was chatting with another parent at school pickup about her career. She and her husband had just given up their secure jobs in finance to start a business together, which meant they were spending a lot more time in the same room. I asked her how she was dealing with this sudden togetherness, to which she offered one word: wine.

We live in an alcohol-soaked society. You almost can't escape its presence and temptation. It flows at workplace events, sporting games, and family picnics, and #daydrinking is a thing because, hey, it's five o'clock *somewhere*. Alcohol has even nosed in on gatherings that you wouldn't typically associate with getting tipsy, such as playdates and kids' birthday parties. It's our primary social lubricant and has become the critical test for US voters when casting their ballot for president: Do I want to have a beer with that candidate?

The question I'd like you to consider is "How is my drinking impacting my Downstate?"

Being married to a person who doesn't drink alcohol has given me an opportunity to interrogate my own relationship with drinking. Before Emily, I always drank a glass or two of wine or beer at the end of a long, tiring day—sometimes with friends at a pub, sometimes while making my kids dinner, sometimes after putting them to bed, with the rest of the night my own to privately slip away. I didn't think about why I drank, or whether it was necessary; I simply got into the habit of using alcohol to check out after being checked in all day. But, living with Emily, who, she says, quit drinking to save her life when she was twenty-four years old, forced me to question what I was doing. Why was I doing it? Did I *need* this drink right now or had I just let the rhythm of "It's five p.m. somewhere" take hold of my evenings? Was this drink replacing something missing in my life?

The first thing I noticed was that I was exhausted, and that when the end of the workday would finally arrive and the long night of parenting would then begin, I felt completely depleted and without the energy I needed to show up for my kids. It surprised me to realize that it was from this already wasted state that the desire to drink would arise. Opening the fridge to grab a can of beer, I was reaching for a numbing device that would take me from tired to not caring, from low battery to oblivion. I heard a voice inside my head say, "I am an adult and drinking is perfectly legal, especially in my own home. I work hard and this is my right. Mother knows best."

For many of us, alcohol has become a replacement for the Downstate. We work ourselves to the limit of our daily resources, until there is nothing left; yet we still have hours of service at home before we can fall into the void of sleep, and that void isn't even guaranteed. This doesn't work—we can't produce energy we don't have, and this makes us feel bad, inadequate, and overextended. So, we search for a buffer to put between us and our bad feelings, us and the noise, us and the demands; a way to cut ourselves off from the intimacy of the moment, the immediacy of human relations. Alcohol is one answer, taking the edge off the sharp stings of need. Though it may feel like a liquid Downstate, the problem with using it as a replacement for your natural restorative practices is the mission creep of this drug. As the F. Scott Fitzgerald quote goes, "First, you take a drink, then the drink takes a drink, then the drink takes you."[28] And, over time, numbing out requires more and more alcohol to do the trick, not to mention the hell it wreaks on your sleep.

Ask yourself one question: If your Upstates and Downstates were in the right ratio, would you need that drink? If you had had a full night's sleep, woke up in the morning to the sun in your face, made time for a workout or a lunchtime walk with a friend, ate healthy meals, and took a five- to ten-minute break during your day for some deep breathing, how would you feel at five p.m.? Would you need that beer or could you take a trip to the park to throw a ball around, spend some time in the garden, or practice a new hobby?

I spoke with artist Melora Kuhn about her relationship with alcohol. She stopped drinking eight months after her mother died because she felt numb and realized that she had been drinking nearly every night for the past twenty-five years. Along with dropping 10 pounds in the first month, she noticed many deeper, inward changes. She rediscovered her love of reading, starting with bell hooks' *All About Love: New Visions*, followed by every book hooks referenced therein. "Some days I would spend all day reading and skip painting in my studio altogether," she told me.[29] Without the nightly blurring of her mind with alcohol, her attention and endurance began to build, and she "started to feel like a scholar—reading, taking notes, digging deeper, writing, unpacking my own story by others' accounts, and really waking up." After about nine months of sobriety, she said she still felt "like a little pink nub of pure sensitivity, but the effects have been amazing. My skin is brighter, the bags under my eyes are less, and the fat under my chin is seriously reduced! My sleep is deeper, and generally uninterrupted, and I am more able to engage from a center I had a hard time contacting before. Not drinking has lifted a veil and been a practice in understanding why I drank and what it was encouraging me to avoid."

You don't have to give up alcohol entirely to become a Downstate Maven. You do, however, need to become conscious of your actions and discern those that are helping you maintain that vital Upstate/Downstate ratio, versus those that are hurting. It means mindfully choosing what is right for you in every moment.

## PUTTING IT INTO PRACTICE

Now that you know everything I know about sleep, it's time to put it into action. The following steps will allow you to optimize your nighttime behavior so you can reap as many benefits as possible out of your sleep, including improved cognition and emotional control; brain detoxification; and a recharging of your energy supplies on a nightly basis.

### Early to Bed

Let's begin at the beginning (of the night). The only way to get a full amount of purifying, restorative SWS and inspiring, integrative REM sleep is by getting to sleep early enough to afford time in the SWS dipping pool before you plunge into REM. This means going to bed by ten p.m. There is so much research that drives home the need for an early-to-bed attitude:

#### MEMORY

In terms of your hippocampus and memory functioning, size matters. Longer sleep duration is associated with larger hippocampal volume, and an early bedtime is the key. The earlier the bedtime, the bigger the hippocampus. And don't dupe yourself into thinking you can just sleep in to reverse the effects of a later bedtime. First of all, morning sleep is all REM, and second of all, the time you wake up is not associated with hippocampal volume.[30] It's the first part of sleep, the SWS sleep, that grows your hippocampus. If you want to extend your sleep duration, bedtime, not wake time, is the critical movable factor.

#### DEPRESSION

Attention, revenge bedtime procrastinators! (You know who you are, lollygagging on the phone, flipping through TV channels, and mindlessly refreshing social media instead of going to sleep.) Not only do you get less SWS, you're making yourself more vulnerable to depression by consistently putting off bedtime.[31] You also spend a whopping 451 percent more time on your smartphone in late evening compared with your nonprocrastinating counterparts.[32] On the other hand, people who get to bed earlier, and sleep longer, show fewer depressive symptoms.[33]

## FITNESS

Going to sleep later than ten p.m. increases daily caloric intake by about 250 calories, with the majority of those excess calories occurring at dinner and after eight p.m.[34] As you learned in Chapter 2, greater caloric consumption in the evening delays melatonin onset and bedtime, and also messes with your hunger and satiety hormones, increasing your risk for weight gain and obesity.

Getting to sleep early is as important for kids as it is for adults. Preschool-aged children with early weekday bedtimes are half as likely as those with late bedtimes to be obese as adolescents.[35] Critically, these effects were shown to be independent of total sleep duration.[36] Kids getting to bed later than eleven p.m. have higher BMIs and higher intake of energy-dense, nutrient-poor foods, such as cookies and chips, whereas those who hit the hay early consume more fruit and vegetables, plus the added benefit of less screentime and more physical activity.[37]

For dad-hopefuls looking to improve their sperm count, later bedtime negatively impacts semen quality. Research shows that aspiring fathers should consider adjusting their nightly routine by getting in bed before ten thirty p.m. and logging about eight hours of sleep.[38] Stay off of your screens, too; bedtime usage of smartphones and tablets has been negatively linked with semen quality.[39] Aspiring mothers, you're welcome.

## Stop Caffeine Early in the Day and All Liquids Three Hours Before Bed (yes, that includes alcohol)

In youth and young adulthood, RESTORE is under the control of your *forte* circadian rhythm, which inhibits nighttime urination, but as you grow older, those circadian signals weaken and you will find yourself needing to pee more and more overnight. Holding off on liquids three hours before your normal bedtime will reduce your need to get out of bed in the first place. Be especially wary of that afternoon coffee or energy drink, as caffeine will keep your mind and body awake far later than they want to be. Caffeine also revitalizes REV, which can cause increased heart rate and urine production exactly when you want the opposite effect.

Alcohol is one of the more common sleep aids used by adults, as it's a natural depressant and makes you feel sleepy; helps you fall asleep easier; and even may increase the amount of SWS in the first half of the night.[40] But drinking yourself to sleep, while surprisingly popular among those with insomnia, is the definition of counterproductive. First, the ability of a given amount of booze to knock you out will only last for about three to five days before you start to develop a tolerance and require even more alcohol to get to sleep.[41] This is a common path by which occasional drinkers rapidly find themselves slipping into alcoholism. The second reason alcohol makes for a lousy "sleep aid" is that even though it might be helpful in the passing out stage of sleep, it totally disrupts the second half of your night by reducing REM sleep.[42] This can lead to a chronic sleep problem called maintenance insomnia, meaning difficulty staying asleep or waking up and not being able to fall back asleep. My expert advice is this: don't vodka tonic yourself to sleep. And if you enjoy a single glass of wine or beer at night and it doesn't seem to massively disrupt your sleep, feel free to keep indulging, but consider shifting to a safer happy hour time zone between five and seven p.m. to give your body enough time to metabolize it.

## Try Melatonin

This wonder hormone is safe and available in practically every drug store in America. You can use melatonin to set your circadian rhythm and help your brain understand that it's time for sleep. The onset of melatonin release coincides with the setting sun and the vanishing of blue light from the horizon, so the secret to taking this supplement is timing, erring on the early side. Take it around one hour before your planned bedtime to give it enough time to build up potency.

Be sure to speak to your physician about whether melatonin is right for you. It's a good idea to start small (1 mg) and if that doesn't do the trick, gradually work your way up to an amount that's effective.[43] My avid quantified selfer friend Bill titrated his dose to 2.5 mg each night, which he says not only has improved his sleep, but it also boosted his daily HRV levels.

## TAKE BACK THE NAP!

If you read my first book, *Take a Nap! Change Your Life*, you might already be a nap aficionado, using your nap wheel to identify the best period of the day to nap yourself toward your goal, be it rote memorization, perceptual sharpening, or creative insight. For those of you without that prior knowledge, let's do a short primer to get your little nap toes wet.

Each sleep cycle lasts for ninety minutes, the first thirty minutes being mostly Stage 2, and the next sixty minutes being a ratio of SWS and REM. Your morning rise time will also affect the quality of your daytime nap, as it initiates your sleep pressure, which in turn determines how much SWS you'll nab. So, the timing of your nap will impact the ratio of your REM to SWS, with earlier naps having more REM sleep and later naps having more SWS. (Stage 2 is relatively uniform across the day.) The wise Prophet Mohammad, who was hip to the timing issue with naps, instructed that "Sleeping early in the day betrays ignorance, in the middle of the day is right, and at the end of the day is stupid."[44] All judgment aside, your nap length, the time you wake up and the time you nap will determine the type of sleep you get and the benefits you will see.

When deciding which nap is right for you, think about the goal of your nap: Is it a pick-me-up? In that case, a twenty-minute nap anytime during the day will do. Are you a student studying for an exam? You'll need an hour-long afternoon nap to snag more SWS. Are you an artist having a creative block? You'll need more REM sleep, so take an early nap around ten a.m. to stimulate

"If I take 5 mg, I toss and turn and have whacked out dreams and feel jet lagged the next morning, and my HRV is way toward the sympathetic side. Two and a half mg gives me a solid amount of SWS;[44] I wake up feeling great." His observation lines up with studies that show melatonin's cardioprotective role, mainly due to its antioxidative, anti-inflammatory, and antiapoptotic (prevents cell death) actions.[45] Since melatonin affects metabolism, it's also recommended to eat dinner early and wait at least two hours before taking it.[46,47,48] your dreamy free-associative networks. Are you planning an all-nighter either for work or play? Then, you'll need a thirty-minute disco nap in the early evening to decrease your sleep pressure and keep your brain and body stamina up as long as you need it. For a deeper dive into the napsphere, read my book and use the nap wheel available on my website to determine the perfect nap for you based on the time you wake up in the morning.

Of course, please nap *wisely*. Back to the Prophet Mohammad, who instructed Muslims to "Take a short nap, for Devils do not take naps."[47] I quite agree, but whereas a twenty-minute nap at any time of day will give you a perky Stage 2 boost, longer naps later in the day will plunge you into SWS and can let out too much sleep pressure, depleting the power of that first nighttime SWS wave and, with it, your ability to fall asleep. Also, some biological processes, including the glymphatic cleanse, are driven by circadian forces, so you want to be asleep at night in order to get the full treatment, and a late nap might sabotage that.

When it's nap time, do as Joseph Millar suggests in his poem "Venetian Siesta": "Making a hole in the afternoon" and drift slowly away. . . .[48]

> I know I'm getting away with a crime
> stretched out on the couch
> and listening to rain
> making a hole in the afternoon
> through which I can drift slowly away

## Control Your Light

Careful control of your light exposure across all 24 hours of the day will help your circadian rhythm cope with our modern world, which is busy doing everything possible to muck it up. On the early morning side, you need a solid dose of blue light to wake up the suprachiasmatic nucleus and entrain it to a new day. Modern America spends too much time in dim indoor light, which sends the wrong signal to your circadian rhythm and can mess with your alertness, metabolism, energy, and mood levels. If you

## THE GLOBETROTTER'S SECRET WEAPON: MELATONIN

Melatonin can also be a helpful sleep hack when travelling eastward across time zones, allowing you to advance your circadian rhythm to match the sunset at your destination. For example, let's say you're taking a direct flight from San Diego to JFK on Friday at noon. The flight takes about five hours, which will get you into New York at eight p.m. Eastern time (five p.m. Pacific time). That means that your melatonin onset will be delayed by three hours; when your NYC friends are getting sleepy, you are still raring to go. To minimize jet lag, you can start advancing your melatonin administration by thirty minutes five or six nights before your trip, taking your normal melatonin dose at eight thirty p.m. on Sunday, and eight p.m. on Monday, and so on, such that you have gradually shifted your circadian rhythm enough that it won't be too surprised when you head to bed three hours ahead of schedule on Friday night, followed by that monstrous seven a.m. Eastern time (four a.m. Pacific time) wake-up call. Early morning job interview? *Pas de problème.*

can't get outside first thing in the morning, research shows that anywhere from fifteen to thirty minutes in front of a light box at a consistent early morning hour can do wonders for daytime peppiness and cognitive sharpness and will improve sleep quality. Light therapy can decrease problems with falling asleep and staying asleep; reduce daytime sleepiness; and shift bedtimes and melatonin onset to earlier, more appropriate hours.[49] These effects have been seen across a wide range of populations. For example, sleep disturbances are commonly reported by cancer survivors, but using a light box for thirty minutes every morning for four weeks led to less time in bed staring at the ceiling, more total time asleep, and fewer middle-of-the-night awakenings.[50]

At the end of the day, the goal is to tell your big, beautiful suprachiasmatic nucleus that it's time to wind down. To do this, you have lots of light-based options. You could set up blue light blockers all around you, starting with computer filters, or blue light–blocking filters on your glasses or even contact lenses. Your phones and computers offer light filtering options, but their ability to affect your circadian rhythm have yet to be realized and they may just give you a false sense of security promoting more screen time.[51] If you use them, program them to turn on at 6pm and stay on until morning. While you are at it, set up the Do Not Disturb feature on your phone to eliminate the bells and whistles for the same period of time.

One study threw the whole circadian kitchen sink at a group of French Canadian night shift nurses by exposing them to forty minutes of bright light from a portable light box before their night shifts for one week, strategically timing their naps, and having them wear sunglasses to avoid bright light as soon as their shifts ended, typically at seven thirty a.m., removing them only before going to bed.[52] During the intervention period, nurses reported less fatigue, fewer work errors, better and longer sleep, and a more positive mood. Moreover, nurses with a preference for evenings (i.e., later chronotypes) reported the strongest benefits.

A few other fun ways to romance your suprachiasmatic nucleus include taking a stroll at dusk in an area where you will be exposed to late afternoon/early evening natural light; dining by fireside; lighting candles for your evening ablutions; and doing your best Corey Hart impersonation by wearing your sunglasses at night in any sort of fluorescent hellscape, from your local gas station/convenience store to the hotel lobby you just entered at ten p.m. after a long day of travel.

## Breathe Through Your Nose All Night Long

When James Nestor and his buddy spent ten grueling days mouth-breathing, they both experienced an onslaught of autonomic imbalance, including blood pressure spikes, constant headaches, general malaise, and a vicious onset of sleep apnea.[53] People with sleep apnea experience repeated closures of the upper airway, literally shutting off oxygen to the brain for minutes at a time. This triggers frequent awakenings, allows for virtually no deep SWS, and lets REV run you ragged all night. The lack of restorative sleep and prolonged hypoxia leads to excessive daytime sleepiness, poor fitness, and significant cognitive impairment of executive functions in both adults and children.[54] When Nestor finally removed the nose plugs and reclaimed his schnoz, all the negative symptoms, including the apnea, disappeared.

It's never too late to shut your mouth. The simplest and cheapest way to address this problem is to apply a postage stamp–size piece of tape to your lips before you fall asleep that will remind your lips to stay closed at night even if your jaw falls open. You can also buy strips made specifically for deterring mouth breathing during sleep, made with a gentle adhesive that stays put for long stretches but peels off without discomfort. Speak with your dentist or physician before starting, to make sure you don't have any medical conditions that would make this ill-advised. Better yet, speak with a nasal breath specialist, many of whom can be located online or in Nestor's book.

Practicing nasal breathing during the day will also train you to keep it up at night. Bring on the Downstate night . . .

## Have More Sex

I like to think of orgasms as blow darts, whisking you off on a nightly voyage to the Downstate. Whether you're with a partner or Lone Ranger style, think about sex as a great big Upstate romp in the hay, all brain areas fully activated as REV rides that pony all the way to the finish line. Every cell in your brain and body is running at max capacity, like a one-person orchestra performing *Ride of the Valkyries*. After the fireworks finale, RESTORE shuttles in the deep vagal comedown and it's lights out in the theater. The reason orgasms are such potent Downstate instigators is because your vagus nerve is directly connected to your genitals, bypassing most of the spinal cord. (In fact, many people with spinal cord injuries can still have orgasms for just this reason.) If you're wondering how scientists know so much about brain activity patterns during orgasms, it's because people volunteer in pairs or on their own to get down in a brain scanner while a bunch of scientists sit in a control room making small talk. Awkwaaaaard!

And the reverse relationship is also true; having robust Downstate sleep that thoroughly switches off REV is good for maintaining healthy plumbing in the sex department. About four or five times a night, proerectile RESTORE pathways predominate, producing nocturnal erections and labial, vaginal, and clitoral engorgement. Sex experts sound like Downstate aficionados when they refer to these events as a "battery-recharging" mechanism for the sex organs because they increase energy-rich, oxygenated blood flow to those areas. I know that shaking the sheets can sometimes be the furthest thing from your mind after a busy day that has sucked up your very last ounce of energy, but think about it as medicinal sex, like taking your vitamins, and have fun! You can even double your Downstate points by taking a little melatonin an hour before your estimated time of orgasm (ETO) to potentially enhance the duration of your ride into interstellar space.

## Be a Creature of Habit

Your body craves routine. Every cell in every organ has a clock that is looking for a consistent schedule to sync up to, whether it's your rise time or bedtime, your best concentrating hour, your prime workout hour, or your most efficient chow time. When you maintain a dependable pattern in your daily rituals, your brain and body perfectly prepare you for Upstate get-up-and-go actions and Downstate taking-it-down-a-notch calm.

Discovering your personal daily rhythm means coming into resonant frequency (a concept from Chapter 2) with the omnipresent, universal cadence of the Upstate/Downstate dance. By setting up these predictable daily markers, you are giving your personal orchestra of cells, neurons, and brain chemicals a downbeat to kick-start each movement or phrase of your day with as much energy and grace as possible. By honoring your nightly Downstate, your body has time to replenish resources, clear out toxins from your brain, and repair tissue, so the Upstate is as bold and beautiful as it can be. Similarly, when you stick to a pattern for eating and exercise, your body and mind can actually prepare themselves ahead of time for a big energy release or for receiving a bolus of fat and protein.

Your brain is looking for informative cues that will predict what is coming down the pike, so it can prepare your body. The danger of throwing it unexpected demands is grimly illustrated in many illicit drug overdoses. When a person takes a drug, such as heroin, in the same place and time with the same people using the same paraphernalia, the mind notes all these consistencies and gets the message that a specific amount of opioids, crack, meth, whatever, will soon invade the bloodstream, so it primes your organs to receive the assault. This consistent pattern develops drug tolerance such that the user in that same context (same companions, same time and place, same paraphernalia) needs a larger and larger dose to reach the same high. If the user takes this now high dose in a new context (different companions, time and place, or paraphernalia), none of the usual cues were sent to the brain to allow it time to prep the body for the impending physiological drug-induced tornado. This surprise blitz can overwhelm the organs of the body, sending them into shock and failure.

This same overwhelm happens on a smaller scale when you don't give your brain a predictable pattern for sleeping, eating, and exercise. When you treat your body to unexpected onslaughts of metabolic load (e.g., a midnight bowl of ice cream) or energic demand (e.g., hitting the hay at two a.m.), you catch it off-guard, forcing all Upstate subsystems to rouse their troops from a state of deep rest, which means that they will not be functioning optimally. This is why people who are able to stick to health habits, come hell or high water, live longer than people who are more prone to let their health habits exist at the mercy of their emotional swings.[55]

Although Hollywood has created the "crazy Jackson Pollock artist" trope of creatives who live in an upside-down, alcohol-soaked world of melodrama and mayhem, many famous artists and writers live the exact opposite life, rising at a consistent time each morning, forgoing fashion for a uniform, eating the same food at the same time every day, and rarely wavering from their long, daily constitutionals.[56] Rituals help automate life. Removing the busywork of thinking about trivial matters, such as what you will eat or wear, frees up more mental space for creating. These hardworking artists, and many successful people like them, understand that when you bring all your small daily habits into alignment with the overarching rhythm of life, you resonate with that rhythm, amplifying your energy, creativity, and effectiveness.

Yet another perk of habits: they drive us toward our goals in life. When we want to make a big change, the tendency is to declare some grand resolution—*I'm going to get in shape! I'm going to stop smoking! I'm going to be a better parent!*—and then attempt to will it into happening. But without detailed, recurring habits designed to help us reach that goal, we are destined to tread water, looking out at the horizon as our goals sink below the surface. The smartest habits are small, specific, and doable: walking for twenty minutes a day, four days a week, for instance, or eating an extra serving of fruits or vegetables with every meal. With repeated practice, they become built into our daily routine and eventually, we do them without thinking. In this way, eating less meat, taking the stairs over the elevator, or getting to sleep at a decent bedtime become as automatic as showering, brewing coffee or steeping tea in the morning, or checking email, and those new habits naturally lead to big-picture results.

Throughout the coming chapters, I'll offer a few *Golden Habits of Highly Effective Circadian Rhythms*. You know the old adage: Eating at the same time of day, exercising at the same time of day, and going to bed and waking up at the same time of day keeps the doctor away. Well, maybe that's not exactly how it goes, but it's the same idea, and mine works even better than apples.

## Golden Habit of Highly Effective Circadian Rhythms: Create a Sleep Habit

Your Downstate sleep rhythm thrives on consistency and ritual, so maintaining regular habits that occur at the same time each day will set your brain up to know when sleep is coming and set the groundwork for winding down. Choose a one-hour window for bedtime and wake time that you can stick to, on average, seven days a week. Start today by avoiding that afternoon caffeine injection so you can get in touch with your natural rhythm. Tonight, pay attention to when you first start to feel tired. That is your body's ideal bedtime. Most people push through it with screen time, alcohol, chores, or work. But, ignoring that first Downstate wave will make it harder to fall asleep when you want to as the next one might be hours from now, and you'll pay for it the next morning when you wake up feeling less than 100 percent. Make that first wave of drowsiness be the bedtime you shoot for, understanding that there will be missed days (date night, late night parties, work cramming sessions) but, on average, you'll want to strive to get to sleep somewhere within an hour of that time.

As for your one-hour wake time window, this may be harder to control, especially for parents of young kids, pet-owners, or people living in noisy, industrial areas. But do your best to choose a window that affords you a long enough sleep duration that you feel refreshed in the morning, usually around seven and a half to eight hours total (but this can vary widely). And try to wake up at a similar time on the weekends as on the weekdays, as dreadful as that might sound, otherwise you risk experiencing social jet lag, which you might recall occurs when you have a big discrepancy

**"FOR BETTER OR FOR WORSE, FOR RICHER OR FOR POORER, FOR EXTREME MORNING OR EXTREME EVENING CHRONOTYPE . . ."**

If you think it's tricky for a progressive Democrat to be partnered up with a right-wing Republican, you should see what life is like for a couple with different sleep rhythms, whether it's a morning person forced to share a bed with a night owl, or a napper shacking up with a nonnapper. Mismatched bedtime windows (*couples' sleep discordance* in sciencespeak) are seriously problematic, contributing to many Upstate ailments, including insomnia, increased sympathetic arousal and system-wide inflammation, and reduced opportunities for sex.[57] There are many factors that can contribute to why discordance can be so awful, including a Rooster (from Chapter 2) sacrificing his personal rhythms so as to spend more quality time with his Owl love, or that same Rooster retiring at the right time for him, but keeping one eye open until his Owl finally comes to bed, or just the busyness of the Owl beeping on the house alarm, walking up the stairs, showering, and then pulling the sheets off the already-in-bed Rooster. For a light sleeper, even small levels of arousal can ignite an Upstate flame, making it harder to fall back asleep.

This bedfellow problem is exceedingly common; when a mattress review company recently polled people about their sleep times, they found that more than half hit the sack at different times than their partner.[58] And the Better Sleep Council says that one in three Americans feels their partner negatively impacts their sleep.[59]

between your workday and nonworkday bedtimes and wake-up times. Social jet lag is a sign that your personal rhythm is out of sync with the demands of your work/family/public life, and has the same negative consequences on your health, cognition, and well-being as general sleep deprivation. Prioritizing your one-hour bedtime and wake time window is one of the best ways to treat this problem and get on good terms with Morpheus, the god of dreams.[57,58,59]

Before you head to sleep divorce court, try my go-to fix: ear plugs. They are simple, cheap, and act like blinkers for REV. If you go to bed earlier than your partner, they can work wonders at preventing unnecessary wake-ups. Look for sturdy ones that extend deep into the ear canal, or the fancy versions that are tailored to your own ear canal. If you are a single parent and concerned about not hearing your kids at night, I can relate. When I got divorced, I had a talk with my kids about my need for good sleep, and ear plugs. So, I asked them for a trial run to see whether I could wear the plugs and have them wake me up if they needed me. It's been four years, and I can say that I haven't slept through one night terror from my youngest and my oldest has woken me up each time she needs me.

I also encourage you to don eye masks to block out sudden changes in lighting that might normally rouse you. They also help if your partner likes to read in bed.

Here's another simple yet often overlooked idea: invest in separate bedding. Each of you gets your own duvet or comforter (this works best if you have a king-size bed and both buy a twin-size comforter). This way, you won't be disturbed by the sensation of the blanket being pulled as your partner slips into bed or tosses and turns. It also allows you to customize your temperature control; the hotter sleeper can use a lighter comforter. In addition, you can purchase a bed that provides each partner with a separate mattress so the insomniac partner's rolling and fidgeting don't become the other partner's problem.

# CHAPTER FIVE

# Exercise Your Right
# to Recovery

———————— • ————————

The last two chapters have focused on stimulating RESTORE in a very calm, relaxed way—deep breathing, yoga inversions, sleep scheduling, regulating blue light at night, and so on. Interjecting your Upstate daytime with these practices will develop the Downstate muscles you need to be at the top of your game and healthily manage stress (in traffic, in your doctor's office waiting room, in the throes of an argument with your spouse).

But exercise is a bit different. Instead of mindfully calming your brain and synchronizing your heart and breath, you can use your body to intentionally instigate the REV/RESTORE tango, and boost your heart rate variability (HRV).[1]

It's no coincidence that the physiologic changes that happen during a workout—a quickened heartbeat, blood flow to the extremities, laser-sharp focus on the task at hand—are the same as those that make up the fight-or-flight response; when you move your body in a way that gets your heart pumping, your sweat dripping, and depletes your energy (e.g., glycogen) stores, you are exciting REV and company.

Moving from low- to high-intensity workouts shifts control of the cardiac response even further into REV dominance, such that during full-throttle boot camp routines, the heart is under 100 percent REV control. In this activated state, the ultimate Upstate juice is glycogen, the main source of energy for skeletal muscles. Meanwhile, your heart is working hard to deliver oxygen- and nutrient-rich blood to thirsty muscles; the harder the workout, the faster the heart rate. In response to this sympathetic schvitz, postworkout your vagus nerve initiates an equal and opposite blast of Downstate activity (remember our Newtonian golden rule?), with the main objective being to return the cardiovascular and muscular systems to baseline. Ignited by the quick burst of REV provided by acute, intense exercise, RESTORE goes to work slowing your heart rate, cooling your body temperature, and relaxing your muscles.

Along with this short-term righting of the REV/RESTORE ratio that begins when you complete your reps or finish your run, there are longer-term HRV-enhancing results that transpire over a day or more that have wide-ranging advantages in terms of your athletic performance, as well as your cognition, sleep, and health. The heart is a muscle, so just like your quads or biceps, it makes sense that it would strengthen with repeated, intense use. And when your cardiovascular system grows stronger, that in and of itself unleashes a torrent of RESTORE gains. Exercise trains Central Command to have greater control of the heart via the vagus nerve such that it can dominate REV whenever necessary, leading to higher HRV in healthy adults as well as in people with weaker cardiovascular function. This exercise-induced vagal bump is cardio-protective, reducing your risk for future heart disease.[2] With strong vagal functioning and high HRV, your cardiovascular system can more flexibly adapt to the demands of each moment, quickly ramping up when you need oxygenated blood and down when you don't.

The exhaustion that comes from throwing around heavy tractor tires, taking a Spin class, or bench-pressing your upper limit of weight sends a signal to jump-start multiple other rejuvenating recovery processes, including the replenishment of exhausted cells with reparative, restorative nutrients; a tamping down of the stress hormone cortisol; and a boost in neuroprotective hormones, such as brain-derived neurotrophic factor (BDNF), which helps grow new brain cells.

The happy effects of the Downstate bloom that emerges from exercise can be seen across several categories. Join me for a jaunty tour through all the benefits of this great Downstate comedown, won't you? Go ahead and change into your workout gear now, because I'm pretty sure that halfway through this chapter, you'll be running out the door.[3]

---

**GYM RATS**

In my favorite study illustrating exercise's cognitive boost, researchers had one group of rats run on an exercise wheel and the other group remain sedentary.[3] Directly following an intense bout of exercise, the researchers transfused blood from the exercising rats to half of the couch potato rodents. Then, all the rats were given a memory test designed to activate Central Command. Amazingly, compared with the sedentary rats that didn't receive the blood transfusion, both the exercised and the sedentary rodents with the blood transfusion tested smarter, like little Einstein rats. Their brains also revealed evidence of more neurons and less inflammation. The scientists attributed these astonishing effects to exercise's ability to increase specific brain substances (such as lactate and glycogen) that enhance executive function, learning, and memory. All that just from getting a little sweaty. You'll find more evidence of exercise's link with cognition on page 137.

---

## Exercise Basics

Let's start by defining a few terms. You're probably familiar with the three levels of exercise:

- **Low intensity:** A casual walk, a stretch session, a beginner's yoga or tai chi class, bike riding, or using a cross trainer (a.k.a. an elliptical) at an easy pace.
- **Moderate intensity:** Brisk walking or walking uphill, a strenuous yoga session, weight training, jogging, cycling, or lap swimming.
- **High intensity:** Circuit training, vigorous forms of weight training, and moderate-intensity exercises kicked up a notch at heart-racing speeds, including sprints and laps in the pool.

Now, check out what these different levels of exercise can do for you.

### SLEEP

Exercisers sleep better, full stop. Anyone who's ever slept longer or harder than usual following a particularly active day, be it one spent running a race, touring a new city on foot, or chasing a child around an amusement park, will testify that extra physical exertion tuckers people out. But it goes deeper than that. A single bout of moderate-intensity exercise increases time in slow-wave sleep (SWS) and boosts the number of slow waves your brain produces across the night.[4] And as anyone just starting a fitness streak likes to tell whoever will listen, the immediate and short-term benefits you feel when you start lifting weights or taking regular walks spark a positive feedback loop that leads to more regular exercise and even greater improvements to sleep quality and quantity, and reductions in insomnia symptoms.[5]

Moderate-intensity exercise, such as walking briskly outside or on a treadmill or riding a stationary bike around thirty minutes, four days a week, is enough to help older adults with insomnia gain an impressive seventy-five extra minutes of sleep per night.[6] In one National Sleep Foundation poll, light-, moderate-, and high-intensity exercisers were all significantly more likely to declare they had a good night's sleep the majority of work nights of the past week compared with nonexercisers.[7] (High intensity was associated with the least amount of sleep problems and the highest sleep satisfaction.) In fact, comparing the magnitude of sleep improvement from sleeping pills versus exercise, researchers report that exercise produces the same and even greater benefits.[8] This is important because exercise is free, nonaddictive, and the benefits keep building, whereas sleep medications can be expensive, addictive, and typically stop working once your brain adapts to them. Committing to a regular exercise program can especially help sleep quality and insomnia symptoms in sedentary people who are at an unhealthy weight. On the other hand, avoiding exercise can exacerbate sleep disorders, including disordered breathing and insomnia.

But why does exercise act like an extended-release sleeping pill? It all goes back to the arc of the REV/RESTORE response. Vigorous exercise jumpstarts REV, and it takes a while for RESTORE to tamp down its twin subsystem. This is why trying to sleep immediately after a workout is ill-fated; your heart rate is high, your cortisol is jacked, and your autonomic nervous system hasn't transitioned out of Upstate mode. REV comes on quickly but takes longer to calm down. The goal is to time your exercise routine such that the postexercise RESTORE response synchronizes with the peak of your sleep pressure. (It's the Downstate version of the simultaneous orgasm.) Morning exercise is the most efficacious way to make that happen. When your postworkout RESTORE bloom overlaps with your SWS window HRV skyrockets, melatonin floods your brain, your core body temperature drops, and your heart finds a mellow groove, all of which set the stage for SWS-rich processes, including growth hormone release, protein synthesis, and restoration of cell structure and function.

Daytime exercise gives your autonomic nervous system enough time to override REV's excited blast, placing the Downstate wave right in time for beddy-bye. Compared with morning and afternoon exercise, intense aerobics too late in the evening elevates heart rate, blocking the aforementioned deep sleep climax.[9] In studies of both adults and children, exercising for thirty minutes at least four hours before bedtime at high and moderate intensity increases minutes in SWS and produces more powerful slow waves.[10] High-intensity exercise requires lots of energy (a.k.a. ATP, the smallest currency of energy in cells), which in turn builds up a bunch of the sleep-promoting molecule adenosine (shown in a rodent study) and boosts sleep quality in humans.[11] Just as with everything, it's all about rhythms . . . getting in tune with your exercise rhythm will have a direct benefit to your sleep rhythm. And don't forget the green exercise from Chapter 3; when you take your morning workout outside, Sol Invictus helps jumpstart your Upstate circadian rhythm, along with naturally extending your workout time as well.

Your muscles abide by their own circadian rhythm. Generally, people show increased strength and power in the afternoon and evening compared with early morning. This may explain why evening competitions have more world records broken, faster speed of first serves in tennis, higher swim stroke rate, and more.[12] These high-intensity or resistance exercises recruit more fast-twitch type II fibers, which are fatigable, exhaust glycogen stores faster, and are more susceptible to circadian rhythms.

Strength is highest in the afternoon and evening between five and eight p.m., and lowest in the morning between six and ten a.m., with differences ranging up to 18 percent for resistance moves and up to 11 percent for high-intensity exercise; quite a bit if we are talking competitive sports![13] These circadian differences in muscle strength don't appear to get weeded out with adaptation to a morning versus evening workout schedule, as a team of international researchers learned when they tried to adapt athletes to morning or evening strength-training over six months. At the end of the study, the evening training groups had still gained more muscle mass than the morning training groups, indicating that body building is truly an afternoon delight.[14] Mix in the circadian preference of the athlete (e.g., early, intermediate, or late), and you can see additional changes of over 25 percent in athletic performance depending on whether the athlete's personal circadian preference is aligned (morning Rooster competing in the early hours) or misaligned (Night Owl competing in the morning) with the time of the competition.[15]

On the other hand, endurance exercise like distance running and cycling at a steady pace involves keeping your breathing and heart rate elevated for prolonged periods and requires more slow-twitch fibers, which contract slowly but repeatedly over long periods of time and are less swayed by circadian influences. Studies of endurance, reaction time, and accuracy show little variation in performance between night and morning . . . but much more vulnerability to sleep loss.[16] For endurance sports, sleep is an independent predictor of winners and losers, even after accounting for the emotional toil of losing, with perceived exertion (how hard you think you are working) and time to exhaustion (when you decide to quit) as the driving forces for these decrements.[17] This suggests that sleeplessness impairs the athlete at the psychological and muscular level, speeding the road to exhaustion and early defeat.

The feeling of muscular fatigue during a workout is actually the depletion of glycogen stores in active muscles, and if your levels aren't brought back to baseline or higher—a process that happens during slow-wave sleep—you will tire more quickly the following day. So, if you have a bad night of sleep after a hard workout, you might find that you can't push yourself the next day due to early fatigue and shorter time to exhaustion, whereas extending sleep after a hard workout decreases perceived exhaustion the following day.[18] This means that a whole lotta losing can be chalked up to a lack of Downstate between trainings and competitions.

For all these reasons, sleep and circadian rhythms are a growing concern for athletes and their coaches. It's well known that athletes are a sleep-deprived bunch, thanks to demanding training schedules, travel, stress, family commitments, work and academic pressures (if they're students), and more, all of which costs them on the field, track, or court.[19] The home game advantage has even been directly linked to jet lag in the visiting team. (Eastward travel shows more impairment on sprint performance and fatigue than westward travel; rougher for the 49ers playing the Giants at MetLife Stadium.)[20] Many professional sport teams pay a sleep expert to advise them on bedtimes, light exposure, and exercise schedules. Luckily, you have me.[21,22]

## INFLAMMATION

Inflammation gets a bad rap. But the truth is that a little inflammation is a good thing, helping the body heal cuts and scrapes and sparking the acute immune response, crucial to fighting off cold viruses, flu bugs, and the like.

### USING EXERCISE TO RESET YOUR CLOCK

Night Owls suffer from daily misalignments between their internal clock and the clock of their kids, job, school, spouse, or the thunderously booming pre-sunrise garbage truck. If this is you, you might consider shifting to an earlier bedtime.

As someone married to an Owl, I know that this is a hard habit to break. Along with direct sun or light box therapy early in the morning to shift your circadian rhythm, you can also use exercise. Extreme Owls who engage in one hour of moderate-intensity morning exercise show earlier sleep and better mood and daytime functioning the following day.[21]

This clock reset works in the opposite direction too, whether you're planning to pull an all-nighter or taking a trip out west that would benefit from delaying your sleepiness and melatonin onset a bit. Studies show that moderate- or high-intensity nighttime exercise result in melatonin onset delays for both younger and older adults.[22] So, whether you're at home and want to get to sleep at the magic ten p.m. hour or gallivanting in some far-flung desert island, exercise timing matters. The former group needs to strategically schedule workouts early in the day so they don't inadvertently shift their melatonin sleepiness window to a later hour. The latter group can operationalize exercise to pump themselves full of Upstate juice into the wee hours, setting their internal clock to Kuala Lumpur.

The trouble starts when inflammation becomes a persistent state of affairs. And if you are constantly stressed, skimp on sleep, eat lots of sugar, smoke, have poor fitness, or are a couch root vegetable, you almost assuredly have chronic inflammation. That's because your immune system perceives those subpar conditions similarly to how it would a flesh wound or a virus that just snuck in through your nostrils; it sees a bad guy and tries to get rid of it by sending in proinflammatory white blood cells designed to disable and kill microorganisms.[23] That's good news if a paper cut on your hand opens up during cycling class and some gross germs on the handlebars sneak into your bloodstream. It's bad news, however, if you've adopted activities that your body inherently interprets as stressful (e.g., smoking, excessive sugar, late nights) and, as a result, triggers the release of search-and-destroy white blood cells that have been described in the medical literature as "grenades" that can blow up healthy tissue when sent to the wrong place at the wrong time.

The autonomic nervous system, and RESTORE specifically, is charged with keeping inflammation to a minimum by inhibiting proinflammatory cytokines. Unsurprisingly, lower levels of inflammation are associated with higher HRV, and HRV predicts levels of inflammation four years into the future.[24] However, chronic inflammation is associated with a slew of disorders of several body systems, including the circulatory (atherosclerosis, heart failure), endocrine (insulin resistance, metabolic syndrome), skeletal (arthritis, osteoporosis), pulmonary (chronic obstructive pulmonary disease), and neurological (dementia, depression) systems, along with many other adverse health conditions now considered chronic inflammatory disorders.[25] One inflammatory biomarker, C-reactive protein (CRP), has even been named an independent predictor of cardiovascular disease in middle-aged and older people, suggesting that having excessive amounts of CRP when you're younger increases the likelihood that you will develop heart disease when you grow older.[26] Here again, having lower CRP levels benefits your HRV, with specific improvements to the REV/RESTORE ratio.[27]

Why am I talking to you about paper cuts and microscopic hand grenades in the chapter on working out? Because consistent exercise dampens inflammation levels, and it does so in a dose-response fashion, meaning the more exercise you get (within reason—more on overtraining later), the greater the reduction in inflammation and improvement in HRV.[28] The reason this sudden burst of energy is so immune fortifying is that, with exercise, your body secretes anti-inflammatory cytokines in the muscle tissue that enhance the digestion and absorption of fats and increase glucose metabolism. A large population study called NHANESIII reported that those who engage in physical activity more than twenty times per month enjoyed a nearly 40 percent reduction in CRP levels compared to those who engaged in activity three or fewer times per month.[29] Several exercise intervention studies involving people with a range of diseases becoming more aerobically active for weeks at a time show consistent reductions in inflammatory biomarkers, independent of weight changes.[30] So, even though your body gets heated up with a hard workout, this eustress experience throws a bucket of ice water on any and all inflamed tissue.

## ENERGY PRODUCTION AND METABOLISM

Even though you might feel like slaying an entire cow coated in BBQ sauce after a mountain hike, research shows that exercise actually reduces appetite by suppressing ghrelin (the appetite hormone) and increasing leptin (the satiety hormone).[31] In addition, exercise increases glucose metabolism and insulin action, rendering your body better able to absorb nutrients from food and lowering your chances of type 2 diabetes. In one study, around thirty minutes of walking or body weight resistance exercises anytime between nine a.m. and three p.m. improved blood pressure and glucose concentrations in individuals with type 2 diabetes.[32] Interestingly, getting your steps in smaller bursts—a.k.a. "exercise snacking"—may be more effective at improving daily blood sugar levels, which can reduce metabolic syndrome risk. Exercise snacking involves breaking up a larger session into multiple shorter bouts, such as taking three ten-minute walks, one after each meal, instead of one thirty-minute walk. This produced greater glycemic gains in people with type 2 diabetes.[33] Just as getting good sleep decreases your craving for high fat and sugary foods, exercise has similar downstream effects, including improving the quality of your meals and reducing intake of carbohydrates and desserts.

## COGNITION AND EMOTIONS

Someone who embodies the full picture of exercise's benefits to the brain is my friend Wendy Suzuki, PhD, a professor of neuroscience and psychology at New York University. Wendy spent her life spelunking the inner workings of the hippocampus with all the Young Investigator Awards to prove it, and yet it took a whitewater river-rafting trip in Peru for her to realize that all that time staring into a microscope left her weak, out of shape, and kinda blue.[34] Upon returning to NYC, she hired a personal trainer, joined a gym, and though the hip-hop moves didn't immediately come naturally to her, something else did: a big, fat happy mood. This come-to-Jesus moment not only helped her turn her fitness life around, but her laboratory life too. She dumped her rodent lab and started focusing her research on the cognitive and mood-enhancing effects of exercise.

What struck this seasoned neuroscientist was the slew of perks that exercise serves up, including enlarging the volume of Central Command (prefrontal cortex) and enhancing every cognitive area that uses it (e.g., attention, working memory, problem solving, cognitive flexibility, verbal fluency, decision-making, inhibitory control, and emotion regulation as well as boosting the size of the hippocampus with improvements to long-term memory and motor and sensory skills to boot).[35] Think back, if you will, to the treadmill mice study I described on page 44, which revealed that there are specific brain substances that increase with exercise and have downstream effects on executive function, learning and memory.

Probably the most impressive among these substances is brain-derived neurotrophic factor (BDNF), which promotes the birth of new neurons in the brain, leading to smarter brains. In rodent studies, regular exercise appears to produce two to five times the number of new neurons compared with the brains of nonexercising rodents.[36] It's harder to study neurogenesis in human brains because it needs to be measured inside neural tissue. But circulating BDNF in the blood likely reflects levels in the brain, and by that metric, BDNF levels increase with exercise in an intensity-dependent manner. This means that the harder your workout, the more BDNF in your brain, the greater the neurogenesis and brain volume.[37] Importantly, these fresh sets of neurons are the ones responsible for the majority of memory improvements.[38,39,40,41,42,43,44,45,46,47,48,49,50]

## INEQUITY AND EXERCISE

Physical inactivity is rising across America, but it's especially insidious for some sectors of our society compared with others.[38] The reason for this unequal access to exercise is complex. One factor is economic status, with low income associated with decreased neighborhood safety and limited access to the necessary requirements of healthy, active living, such as community parks, sidewalks, and trails; as well as school programs that promote health education.

Another factor of systemic racial discrimination excludes certain groups from accessing healthy, enjoyable activities, some of which could even save their lives. Not so long ago, public beaches and pools were segregated for "Whites only." The legacy of that recent history exists today in the sparse number of public pools in Black communities, and of those that exist, many are overcrowded. The danger of this dynamic goes beyond limiting exercise opportunities: Black people drown at five times the rate of White people in the United States because fewer Black children learn how to swim compared to White children.[39]

As Mitchell S. Jackson points out in a Runner's World article, "jogging, by and large, remains a sport and pastime pitched to privileged whites."[40] The consequences of this segregation play out day after day in the experience of Black and brown individuals regularly and defensively modifying their behaviors so as to avoid being discriminated against, abused, and in some cases have their lives threatened or stolen while they are simply pursuing their basic right to exercise (or to bird-watch).[41]

Given the difficulty Black and brown people face when claiming their right to exercise, it comes as no surprise that underrepresented groups exercise less than their counterparts. These drastic reductions in exercise are found mostly in middle-aged Black and Latino people, the very people who, due to systemic inequities, have increased risk for chronic illnesses. More exercise could alleviate that risk.[42]

These bleak statistics along with his own personal experience led New York City mayor Eric Adams to turn his life around. The former police captain was in his midfifties when he woke up one day and couldn't see.[43] He rushed to his doctor's office where he learned that he had developed type 2 diabetes. His average blood sugar level was high enough that he should have been in a coma, with a hemoglobin AIC level—a lab test that shows the average level of blood glucose over the previous three months—at 17 percent, about three times the normal amount.[44] Although he was offered medication, he knew that the problem was lifestyle-related—he was at an unhealthy weight, used sugar as a pick-me-up, and honestly believed that ketchup counted as a vegetable.[45]

Rather than fill a prescription, he bet on himself and made some changes. He turned his office into a working gym equipped with a stationary bike, 15-pound weights, a multipurpose fitness tower and a TRX suspension trainer hanging on the door. He added a mini-stepper underneath his standing desk so he could stay active while working on his laptop. He dug deep into his spiritual practice of meditation and became a vegan, avoiding food "that has a face, mother or father."[46] He filled his office fridge with fresh fruits and veggies that he could juice or cook and enjoy right there at work. Within three months, his AIC level was down to a normal 5.7 percent.

At heart a community organizer, Adams took his personal breakthrough to his constituents.[47] He began publicly speaking out about the lifestyle changes he made and their lifesaving impact, removed sugary drinks and unhealthy snacks from the Brooklyn Borough Hall vending machines, helped bring Meatless Mondays to all New York City public schools, and wrote *Healthy at Last: A Plant-Based Approach to Preventing and Reversing Diabetes and Other Chronic Illnesses*.[48] He has also spoken out about the emotional toll incurred by systemic racism, connecting the dots between how factors as seemingly divergent as police brutality and lack of access to fresh produce all tie back to racial health disparities.[49]

"Having a serious ailment or serious disease, it hijacks your life," Adams has said.[50] "You're thinking about the next result, the next test . . . My goal is really to use my position as the borough president and any higher-profile position to empower people, to let us all know how we can control our health."

In terms of exercise intensity, cognitive performance increases no matter how low or high you go, but some studies show that moderate to high intensity makes the biggest impact on executive function, including attention, working memory, decision-making, and inhibitory control.[51] The perky effects of a single exercise bout can last up to a day, likely due to increases in lactate and glycogen, which both provide energy for the body but are also able to cross the blood-brain barrier and feed the brain, especially the Central Command and hippocampus, promoting cognitive improvement.[52]

In addition, due to its stimulating effects on REV, exercise promotes the release of cortisol, which can remain at elevated levels up to two hours postexercise.[53] Cortisol's effect on thinking is best illustrated as an upside-down U, also known as the Yerkes-Dodson law or the Goldilocks effect, with too little or too much being no good, while a moderate amount is *juuuuuuuust* right. With chronic stress, REV works overtime and cortisol levels run at a constant, irritating whine (keeping you Upstating way past bedtime and your Downstate restorative hormones at bay). Excessive amounts of cortisol are also corrosive for the brain and impair memory. But in moderate amounts, such as those produced during a game of tennis or a hot yoga class, it's beneficial for cognitive performance, with exercise-induced peaks in cortisol associated with higher blood flow to memory areas—good news for people worried about their forgetfulness.[54] In one study, a group of sedentary older adults recruited to participate in an eight-week yoga class showed better executive function and lower cortisol levels compared to their basic stretching counterparts.[55] Importantly, their change in cortisol levels as well as self-reported stress and anxiety levels predicted performance on the executive function tasks.[56] The same rewards have been seen in people with mild cognitive impairment, suggesting a potent nonpharmacologic intervention that improves executive control processes and may slow the way to dementia and Alzheimer's.[57]

Along with getting sharper, exercise also pumps you full of happy juice. Across all ages, it decreases tension, sadness, anger, and confusion, not just in healthy individuals, but in people with clinically diagnosed depression.[58] This mood boost is likely due to its strong enhancement of the feel-good neurotransmitter, serotonin. A few extra burpees or that final sprint lap in the pool blasts REV and bumps up your cortisol levels, making you more resilient to stress off the mat. In the lab, people have lower reactions to stress after they've exercised, suggesting that exercise may be a good buffer for the big and little dramas of life. In one all-ages study, completing thirty minutes of heart-pumping exercise increased feelings of being "energized" and "excited."

## With Exercise, All Boats Rise

You might think that you need to become a superstar triathlete to bring home the RecoveryPlus gold medal, but that is just wrong. Research shows that any amount of movement is better than no movement for all the earlier-discussed advantages. The critical thing is that you get off the couch, raise your heart rate, increase your circulation, boost your temperature, and flex and stretch those muscles. Whether your preferred workout involves a neighborhood brisk walk with friends, a solo early morning jog before the rest of the world wakes up, a sweaty group yoga class, or training for a triathlon, exercise is for everyone.

Too little information can leave a workout beginner without a clue as to how to get started, but too much can be overwhelming. All the gadgets and social pressure to keep up with the Joneses' steps can make you feel you're under a microscope and falling even the tiniest bit short of your daily goal can make you think you're a failure.[59] This causes many people to stop exercising altogether. My job is to give you just the right amount of information to get and keep you motivated, no matter where you fall on the exercise spectrum. Once you get a taste of the postworkout high, you'll find a little flame of motivation inside you to elevate your practice to the next level, fueling your upwardly mobile path to RecoveryPlus. Don't worry; it happens to everyone who doesn't give up.

For this reason, I'll introduce three different types of athletes: the Beginner, the Steady as She Goes, and the Lifer. Think about which best describes you and pay attention to specific information targeted to your athletic type. (If you're new to working out, avoid overwhelming yourself with details about measuring your $VO_2$ max. And if you're already a Lifer, you probably don't need prompts to pinpoint your fitness goals.) That said, there is the strong possibility that given the upward trajectory of Recovery-Plus you might change categories as you incorporate more and more aspects of the Downstate RecoveryPlus Plan. Beginners may graduate to Steady as

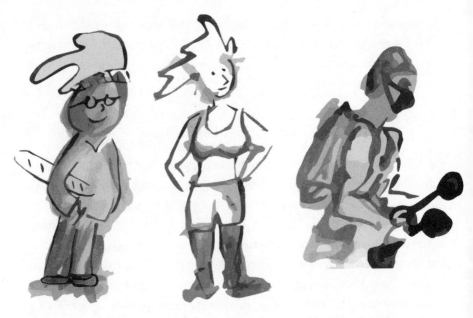

Exercise Types: the Beginner, the Steady as She Goes, the Lifer

She Goes, and Steady as She Goes types may find themselves signing up for half marathons and other Lifer favorites. You can always return to this chapter to take in more information as your fitness life evolves.

## THE BEGINNER

My friend Mikee is the baker in my little village on the Hudson. He's an expert fly fisher, a crackerjack knitter, and a maker of all things glutenous and delicious. A lifelong big guy, Mikee has enjoyed his fair share of chocolate brioches, and was a committed smoker of Lucky Strikes until his diagnosis of type 2 diabetes. After this frightening doctor's visit, Mikee turned to our friend Jon Nandor, a former Jiu Jitsu fighter-turned-gym owner and trainer of world-class mixed martial arts (MMA) fighters. Jon encouraged Mikee to start walking around the village ten minutes a day, which was about ten minutes more walking a day than he was used to. But guess what? He started seeing a difference in his energy levels and mood and became interested in pushing himself to the next level. Ten minutes led to fifteen, then he put down the cigarettes and picked up a little resistance training to reduce body fat and build muscle mass. In time, Mikee dropped the extra weight and brought himself back from the brink of diabetes.

I'm sharing Mikee's story as a way of saying you don't need to make a huge and sudden revolution in your life to see a change. Just ten minutes of walking around your neighborhood is enough to open a portal into a whole new world.

Our friend Jon helps people become and stay fit. After reading every book, trying every method, and working with every type of athlete, he has concluded that there are really only three important questions to ask yourself when embarking on a new workout routine:[60]

**1. What is your goal?** Mikee's goal was to turn his blood sugar around and lose weight. It wasn't to become a half marathoner, or to enter a body building contest; it was a straightforward, achievable goal to reverse his diabetes. Ask yourself, "What's my why?" It might be to lift your mood, to avoid the heart disease that's rooted deeply in your family tree, or to keep up with your grandkids. Stating your personal goal to yourself and to the universe will be your North Star when the turbulent storms of life try to throw your boat off course.

**2. What are you comfortable with?** Asking Mikee to join a swimming club or enter a jujitsu class would have sent him right back to his couch. But taking a ten-minute stroll around his beloved village was no problem; in fact, it quickly became even a welcome break from his day-to-day grind of watching dough rise. When figuring out what activities will jive well with your personality and lifestyle, think about what's doable and enjoyable. Maybe think back to what sports you played when you were younger; that might help you discover an activity you might naturally enjoy now. If you competed in gymnastics in high school, maybe try an Ashtanga yoga class as a way of gaining strength and flexibility while throwing in some scorpion tricks. Bottom line, it's got to come naturally or you won't do it.

**3. What can you stick to?** This is probably the most important question because exercise only works as long as you show up for it. If you own your own business *and* take night classes *and* have kids who barely give you enough time for your morning poopertunity; how are you going to squeeze in an hour-long walk? Overcommitting to an unrealistic goal will only serve up bad feelings about yourself when you inevitably can't cram it into your already packed schedule. Starting with an entirely doable, comfortable, and purposeful exercise strategy will ensure long-term stickiness and the growth trajectory you need.

## STEADY AS SHE GOES

This is me. I've been a runner my whole life, hitting the pavement in every city I've ever visited, from Prague to Pittsburgh. I never considered myself a particularly sporty person, never played on a team except the gay pool league in San Diego, and even then, my coordination sucked (coulda been the beer). At the same time, I've always loved hiking with my family and started running with my dog in high school. I ran a couple of half marathons in my early forties without seriously training for them and didn't die. Now in my late forties, if I don't get out for a run at least three times a week, I feel gross, stressed, and honestly kinda dumb. I also often supplement my runs with some resistance training, either with my favorite online workout or sneaking in some bicep curls underneath the camera while in a video faculty meeting at my standing desk.

If you're in this category with me, you might be feeling ready to challenge yourself to kick it up a notch. One way to do that is to start quantifying the length and girth of your workout by tracking your minutes and intensity. According to the American College of Sports Medicine, staying healthy (i.e., maintaining cardiorespiratory, musculoskeletal, and neuromotor fitness) requires a minimal amount of moderate- or high-intensity exercise: 150 minutes a week of moderate intensity, or 75 minutes a week of high intensity, or some combination of the two.[61] They also suggest a couple of sessions a week reserved for resistance training for the major muscle groups, as well as exercises that promote flexibility, balance, and coordination. For me, that translates to my runs lasting around an hour, with me putting the pedal to the metal for the last ten minutes every time, pushing my intensity from moderate to high. There are so many ways to fit these minutes into your own life. For instance, you could break the time up into twenty-five-minute chunks, reserving six chunks a week for moderate-intensity exercise or three chunks a week for high-intensity exercise, plus some yoga and weight training thrown in for good measure.

If six chunks of *anything* a week seems overwhelming, you may want to consider high-intensity interval training (HIIT). With this strategy, you stay in a high-intensity zone for a short burst of time, take a break to let your heart rate drop back down a little, then repeat. HIIT is more demanding than moderate intensity, but it's also more fun because you're constantly changing moves and recruiting different muscles. HIIT also enables you to push yourself harder because you know it will be over soon; a break is always just around the corner. HIIT is particularly effective for weight loss.[62] It's also a lot more time efficient—the mix of intense aerobic activity and strength-training pushes your heart rate toward its max capacity, strengthening it faster than a steady-state workout[63]—so you can trade in a thirty-minute moderate-intensity swim or jog for a seven-minute HIIT session. And you can sneak in a seven-minute workout just about anywhere, even between work meetings. As anyone with a job, a partner, a kid, a commute, a hobby, or an aging parent knows, time is money, so for people who are maxed out timewise, there's nothing sweeter to the ears than hearing that you can work out more efficiently.

Steady as She Goes types are primed to fully investigate the *what, when,* and *how* of their personal exercise regimen, which includes assessing individual fitness levels. As my long-legged friend Karen enjoyed pointing out when we used to run together, "This is your fast pace? I could walk that fast," which only goes to show that one athlete's sprint is another athlete's stroll in the park. There are several ways of measuring your personal fitness level and all of them have to do with gauging how efficiently your heart and lungs adapt to the present exercise demands. The simplest, gadgetless, mathless technique is called the Talk Test. While exercising, can you talk or sing without running out of breath? If so, you are in the low intensity zone. If you start "I Love Rock 'n' Roll" and can't get all the way through "so put another dime in the jukebox, baby" without gasping for air, you are in the moderate zone. And if all you can muster is a grunt for each downbeat, welcome to the bright lights and big city of High Intensity.

The next level of measuring your personal fitness requires a bit of math to figure out the heart rate range that you want to shoot for when getting your moderate- and high-intensity minutes in. Start by calculating your maximum heart rate (MHR; the maximum amount of times your heart should beat per minute when you exercise). First, subtract your age from 220.

### Maximum Heart Rate (MHR) = 220 – age

So, a badass forty-eight-year-old cognitive neuroscientist would have an MHR of about 172 beats per minute.

Next, let's figure out your desired target heart rate zone—the level at which your heart is being conditioned but not overworked. The American Heart Association generally recommends a target heart rate of 40 to 50 percent of your MHR for low-intensity, 50 to 70 percent of your MHR for moderate-intensity, and 70 to 85 percent of your MHR for high-intensity exercise.[64] When you are just starting out, begin at the lower end, and then as the call of your inner She-Ra or Rocky Balboa gets louder, start to push yourself to the higher RecoveryPlus range.

Here is how to determine your desired target heart rate zone. Let's say you are aiming for a target heart rate in the high-intensity range of 70 to 85 percent. First, calculate your resting heart rate (RHR) by counting how many times your heart beats in one minute when you are supermellow. Be sure to do this first thing in the morning while lying in bed. It's usually somewhere between 60 and 100 beats per minute for the average adult (an easy way to do this is to count for 15 seconds then multiply by 4).

Next, calculate your heart rate reserve (HRR) by subtracting your resting heart rate from your maximum heart rate.

### HRR = MHR – RHR

To find the lower boundary of you heart rate for high-intensity exercise, multiply your HRR by 0.7 (70 percent), then add your resting heart rate to this number. To find your upper boundary, multiply your HRR by 0.85 (85 percent) and add your resting heart rate to this number.

*Lower boundary of heart rate for high-intensity exercise =*
*(HRR × 0.7) + RHR*


*Upper boundary of heart rate for high-intensity exercise =*
*(HRR × 0.85) + RHR*


These two numbers represent your average target heart rate zone that you need to keep your heart rate within when you are doing high-intensity exercise.

So, that brilliant and sexy forty-eight-year-old with the MHR of 172 and a resting heart rate of 55 beats per minute would calculate her HRR by subtracting 55 from 172, which equals 117. Next, she would multiply 117 by 0.7 (70 percent) to get 82, then add her resting heart rate of 55 to get 137, to get the lower boundary of her target zone. Now, she multiplies 117 by 0.85 (85 percent) to get 99, then adds her resting heart rate of 55 to get 154. That's her upper boundary. So, her high intensity target zone is 137 to 154.

So, how can you gauge when you are working at a high (or low or moderate) intensity? The low-tech method is to stop in the middle of a workout and take your pulse by placing two fingers over your wrist or neck pulse points and counting the number of beats for 15 seconds, then multiplying that number by 4.

*Estimated heart rate = 15-second pulse × 4*


You usually need to stop exercising abruptly to accurately estimate your heart rate. When I try doing so, I usually lose count after a while and mix up my seconds with my heartbeats. This is where gadgets come in handy. A heart rate monitor hooked onto a chest strap is ideal, but a wrist-worn fitness band is also a great fitness accoutrement. Look for companies that explicitly have validated their measurements from the device against the gold standard of ECG; the more real science the better.

Getting back to our smokin', TCB forty-eight-year-old . . . During the last part of her sprint home, she counted 37 beats for 15 seconds and multiplied 37 by 4 to get 148. So, now she knows that her sprint speed was in the middle of her high-intensity range, meaning there's some room to grow. RecoveryPlus here we come!

### THE LIFER

There's no one who better encapsulates the Lifer ethos than my aforementioned friend Jon Nandor. Jon has dedicated his life to understanding how much he can stretch and push and squeeze from his body. On stormy days, Jon is out on his stand-up paddle board, battling the raging waves. On runs, he straps on extra weight and oxygen-restricting masks. He has tried every possible exercise method (except maybe Zumba, but that would be fun to watch) just to understand how it works and whether he could potentially incorporate it into his or his clients' training. Like Jon, any quintessential Lifer doesn't need to be told how to exercise, because he or she has already read every book on the topic. The Lifer has been measuring his or her max heart rate, max reps, max oxygen consumption, max everything in meticulous detail and experimented with every combination of training strategies with the singular goal of becoming better than s/he was yesterday.

The biggest gift I can give the Lifer is the gift of the Downstate, of reinstating the importance of recovery and training quality over quantity, and of underscoring the disaster that is overtraining. The promise is that the Lifer will emerge a more efficient athlete, one who can remain in the prime of his or her career long past the competition.

## The Exercise Pathway to RecoveryPlus

Whether you're a Lifer or Steady as She Goes type, the key to upping your game is optimizing exercise's built-in RecoveryPlus cycle. It involves three stages: *high-intensity training, compensation,* and *supercompensation,* in exercise physiology–speak. Honoring these three stages is critical for anyone whose goal is to get faster, run farther, lift heavier, swing harder, or live fitter.

The process begins with a hard workout, one in which you really push yourself. Just sticking with your same ole same ole workout routine is great

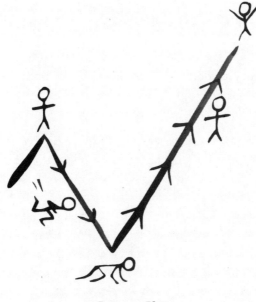

RecoveryPlus

for maintaining cardiovascular health and weight, but it will not get you to RecoveryPlus, whether your goal is to bump up to a higher lifting weight or nudge the numbers down the scale. Engaging in a single intensive training session that pushes the muscular and cardiovascular systems beyond their comfort zones is called *high-intensity training*, and it is chock-full of favorable Upstate activity. During this intense exertion, there's an initial breakdown of muscle fibers and a depletion of glycogen. In the hours following that workout (or days, depending on your fitness level), the body is busy rebuilding glycogen stores, repairing muscle fibers, and returning the cardiovascular system to its preworkout set-point. This Downstate period from peak fatigue back to baseline is known as the *compensation* period. But remember RecoveryPlus isn't just staying at your previous level of fitness, strength, speed, or dexterity; it's reaching beyond where you have been, pushing yourself to the next level of competence. For that above-baseline performance gain, you will need to enter the *supercompensation* period, where the extra Downstate gains happen.[65,66,67,68,69,70,71,72,73,74]

During supercompensation, your glycogen stores keep replenishing to greater than their former levels, filling up to a new set-point that you reached from that high-intensity training. The more intense your training,

## SHOW ME YOUR VO$_{2MAX}$ UGLY FACE

I've been called a man because I appeared outwardly strong. It has been said that that I use drugs . . . It has been said I don't belong in Women's sports—that I belong in Men's—because I look stronger than many other women do.[65]

These words belong to Serena Williams. Despite being one of the world's top athletes, Williams has spent her career on the receiving end of criticism for everything but her ability. She's won twenty-three Grand Slam Tennis Tournaments, (more than any tennis player, female or male),[66] seventy-two Women's Tennis Association titles, and four Olympic gold medals, so it's hard to disagree that she is the greatest tennis player of all time.[67] And yet people do.[68] This is nothing new. The shaming and critique of female athletes is practically a sport in and of itself. Vietnamese bodybuilder Amazin LêThi says, "We are seen as very nerdy, very geeky, very studious. So, we can't be good at sports. Our physique is different, we're smaller—so we're only good for the more traditionally 'feminine' sports—we can't be fast, we can't be strong."[69] Female tennis players, such as Belarusian Aryna Sabalenka, are ridiculed for grunting when returning 125 mph serves, and Women's National Basketball Association player Elena Delle Donne, a two-time MVP,[70] says that when she's covered in the media, comments like "Get back into the kitchen" and "[Make] me a sandwich" (along with "some really dirty, sexual ones that I'm disgusted by that I wouldn't even want to repeat") are the norm.[71]

We might as well be back in 1953, when the *New York Times* ran a story by sportswriter Arthur Daley in which he strongly supported the movement to eliminate women from the Olympics, declaring, "There's just nothing feminine or enchanting about a girl with beads of perspiration on her alabaster brow, the result of grotesque contortions in events totally unsuited to female architecture."[72] At most, women were encouraged to participate in swimming or fencing competitions, two sports that concealed the face of an ambitious, competitive athlete.

Our society tells women to be Nice. Feminine. Pretty. Thin. Quiet. We are allowed in the gym—actually, we're expected to be there, burning off calories—but explicitly and implicitly told to wear revealing, tight workout gear and stick to the cardio machines. In sports, female athletes can compete but need to look good doing it; no tense faces, noise-making, or overly chiseled biceps allowed.

The pressure is even more toxic for plus-size women. The track, weight room, or rowing studio haven't historically felt like safe spaces for this group, which in fact makes up more than half the US population.[73] Body positive activist Lindy West, author of *Shrill: Notes from a Loud Woman*, has described how defeating it can feel for a fat woman to see "many gyms have ads with people looking down at their fat rolls and frowning. Imagine entering a building where every person inside is working toward the goal of *not* looking like you."[74]

In my professional opinion, these outdated, sexist, misogynistic, racist norms can go screw themselves. It's time to reverse course and let our red-faced, messy-haired, sweat-stained sports-bra freak flags fly. No more makeup tutorials that show us how to apply concealer and mascara preworkout so we can look bright-eyed and bushy-tailed while we are showering our bike with sweat. No more alienating ads that always show plus-sized women as the Before model. No more shaming women because they're strong as hell.

Exercise pros rate an athlete's fitness level using a measure called $VO_{2max}$. It represents the maximum (max) volume (V) of oxygen ($O_2$) that your body can process and is assessed by placing the athlete on a treadmill or stationary bike while wearing what looks like a gas mask and gradually increasing the intensity until exhaustion is reached. The fitter you are, the greater your $VO_{2max}$. It's a grueling assessment, one that requires stamina and power. No one looks "cute" doing it. Women, the world needs to see your $VO_{2max}$ face—the face you make when you're pushing yourself to your limit, and all you care about is you doing you. It's okay to grimace. It's okay to be loud. You're a fucking beast, so look like one. Show us your $VO_{2max}$ Ugly Face.

the longer you need to rest so that your glycogen levels are even higher than they were yesterday, making sure your body is ready for the next vicious training session.[75] And glycogen isn't just filling up inside your body's muscles; the wrinkled gray muscle in your skull benefits, too, with specific increases in your hippocampus and cortex.[76] This is why exercise makes you smarter (remember those little Einstein rats?).

Intense workouts are the reasonable stressors I talked about in Chapter 1, fundamental to your growth as a sun's-out-guns-out Adonis. Reaching for your goal, be it finishing a 5K or cranking out a handstand push-up or dropping those extra pounds, requires a little bit of additional Upstate work on your part. Once again, I'm not knocking a low-intensity walk or a level three elliptical session. Those will help keep your heart in tip-top shape and all systems purring. But for blow-your-mind, Downstate-driven physical results—stronger muscles, faster times, upgraded endurance—you'll need to give up some blood, sweat, and, yes, even tears.

## When Less Is More

Widespread pressure to be faster, stronger, and more superhuman than the next person has driven gyms, trainers, coaches, and individuals away from following the natural rhythms of Upstate high-intensity training and Downstate compensation and supercompensation. This is reflected in the popularity of extreme boot camp, CrossFit gyms, and the oxymoronic *high-intensity power yoga*. These approaches share a common theme of encouraging maximum effort without much consideration of recovery processes. But the more these efforts push our bodies and minds to ignore best practices of safety and recovery, the worse the consequences. Studies show that intensive training without appropriate rest leads to something called *overreaching*, in which the accumulation of physical and psychological stress leads to compromised performance capacity.[77] Trying to cut short the Downstate process by working out too soon can put you on the fast track to injury, illness, and burnout.

Just like any chronic stress, continuation of training in an overreached state, as Lifers are prone to do, can lead to performance decrements and a condition termed *overtraining syndrome*.[78] Symptoms of overtraining can include increased vulnerability to injuries, impaired performance, irritability, disturbed sleep, depressed mood, general apathy, decreased self-esteem, emotional instability, restlessness, weight loss, loss of appetite, increased resting heart rate, and a poorly functioning immune system.[79] Recovering from this netherworld can take weeks to months.

The million-dollar trick to avoid overtraining and continue the ever upward trajectory of RecoveryPlus is planning your workout schedule around the compensation-supercompensation periods. Wait too long between workouts and your body will scoot back to baseline, losing the gains of the previous workout. On the other hand, tackling a high-intensity training too quickly, while the body is still attempting to reestablish healthy REV/RESTORE ratios and glycogen levels in muscle tissue, can further deplete the system. For example, even twenty minutes of moderate-intensity exercise during recovery can significantly decrease muscle glycogen by 30 to 58 percent.[80] Of course, an even higher exercise intensity would rob the body of glycogen concentrations to a greater extent. Instead, shifting into the low-impact lane during the compensation period can sometimes be the straightest road to success. One study showed that "easy" daily running doesn't further deplete muscle glycogen after a hard workout,[81] so choosing rest or an easy run allows your glycogen stores to fully replenish themselves.[82]

One of the best ways to assess your position on the compensation-supercompensation continuum is by monitoring your autonomic activity, either by heart rate or HRV, for clues that REV has successfully calmed down to preworkout levels. Elevated resting heart rate in the days following high-intensity exercise may suggest that the autonomic system is still laboring to bring itself back to a stable state and recovery is incomplete. On the other hand, a decrease in resting heart rate after aerobic training is a good indicator of improved cardiovascular health and generally greater physical fitness. Therefore, resting heart rate can be analyzed before and after training as an indicator of where you are on the compensation-supercompensation continuum and help you avoid overtraining syndrome.[83,84,85,86]

Similarly, HRV can be used to measure your position on the continuum. Studies of athletic performance that base their training programs on

**FROM OVERTRAINED AND NEARLY RETIRED TO WORLD CHAMPION: THE GLOVER TEIXEIRA STORY**

As an award-winning Jiu Jitsu fighter, Jon is now part of the training team for Glover Teixeira, the Ultimate Fighting Light Heavyweight Champion. At forty-two, Glover is the oldest first-time champion in UFC (Ultimate Fighting Championship) history and the embodiment of prioritizing the Downstate in the Lifer's training program.[84] As a young fighter, Glover hit it crushingly hard at every opportunity. To him, max effort meant max gain. But at thirty-five, a typical retirement age in his sport, he felt burned out and showed the telltale symptoms of overtraining syndrome: low appetite; sinking testosterone and increasing creatinine (waste products from muscles) levels; and, most troubling, his performance started to fall short of his younger competitors'. He recognized that he needed to make some changes or his lifetime dream of becoming a world champion would slip through his grip.

He underwent a full assessment of his training, recovery, nutrition, and sleep under the guidance of the UFC Performance Institute (PI), which targets elite mixed martial arts fighters. (Learn more about the PI's training approach in Chapter 9.) PI coaches explained that Glover was in chronic REV overexertion, and that he needed to focus more on his recovery. The workouts were so much less intense than his usual regime. "I felt guilty," Glover admits. "If they told me to take a day off, I thought, *Am I lazy? Am I slacking? I wanna be champion of the world and yesterday I didn't work so hard; how can I take another day off?*"

Hailing from a rural community in Brazil, his background was one of relentless Upstate Doozering. "My dad is a farmer; he wakes up every morning at four a.m. to milk cows. Our lives have been about hard work. It's a party hard culture, too, so your body gets no rest. You work, work, work. But you are not getting what you want."

Influenced by reading *The Power of Now*[85] and *The Seven Spiritual Laws of Success*,[86] which espoused the importance of doing less, finding flow, and the

RESTORE recovery using HRV have been shown to elevate performance better than the standard approach to training. In one study, moderately fit men were put on a four-week training program based on the following principles: If HRV was similar to or higher than the previous day's value, then each individual completed a high-intensity training session, but if HRV art of effortlessness, he developed a state he calls Rest Mode. "Rest Mode is being in nature, being calm, chill, paying attention to the universe. It means spending less time with friends and family. I miss a lot of birthday parties." It also means getting good sleep every night, which, historically, has been "the biggest problem in my career." He chalks up his sleep troubles to his balls-to-the-wall sparring matches (he can drop 7 pounds in one session), evening training schedule, and physical aches and pains.

To maximize his chances of getting eight hours of sleep, he spends twelve hours in bed every night (bedtime at nine p.m.) and ends his two-hour daily training sessions at one p.m. The week of the championship fight, he stayed in bed twenty hours a day to rest his body as much as possible. Rest Mode means "not doing much at all, not doing anything that will increase my heart rate. If I even go outside to feed the birds, my heart rate is going to stay ele-vated. I focus on my heart rate, my rest, my chill. I do breathing exercises and meditation." The benefits extend beyond the gym. "My wife can tell you that our marriage is better now that I shifted into Rest Mode. When you rest, you're happy."

He also dons wearable sensors that measure his heart rate, breath-ing, body temperature, sleep, and activity levels, which help him determine whether he is ready for a moderate- or high-intensity workout, or whether his system is still recovering and needs a low-intensity day. "When the device tells you that you're in the green zone and you perform better, or when it says you're in the red zone and you do worse, you start believing in the science," he says. The overall result is a wiser, more efficient, and sustainable approach that allows his body and mind to fully recover in preparation for the next Upstate onslaught. "Now, I win my fights because I combine all the technique work I've learned in the past with the right kind of training. I train less, but I'm happier, more chill, and stronger. Everything is better, and I got what I wanted." He certainly did.

was *lower* than the preceding day's value, each individual rested or com-pleted a low-intensity training session.[87] Another group of men followed a standard training program (HIIT training plus one day of rest per week), with no HRV data accounted for. Results showed that even though the standard training group ended up with more hours of training overall, the

HRV-guided training group showed two times higher running speed, along with higher HRV, underscoring the power of individualizing your training plan based on your autonomic recovery rate.[88] Given the mounting evidence for emphasizing recovery and utilizing body-heart training techniques that put quality over quantity, you would think that training smarter would be an easy thumbs-up for professional athletes. Think again.

## PUTTING IT INTO PRACTICE

We have covered so much ground in this chapter that I want to remind you of the main points and highlight the science supporting your Exercise Action Items. The first thing to remember is that exercise is a supershuttle to the Downstate because it powerfully sparks REV, which causes the vagus nerve to send in a RESTORE response. The trick is to time the workout such that the RESTORE recovery coincides with your nightly bolus of slow-wave sleep (SWS). Which leads to your first Action Item:

### Incorporate Intensive Morning Aerobic Exercise at Least Three Times a Week

Since exercise induces a stress response that first elevates REV followed by mollifying RESTORE activity, the time of day you get moving matters greatly. Late evening moderate- or high-intensity exercise prevents the nocturnal decline of core body temperature and heart rate, whereas morning exercise significantly increases HRV during SWS. It's during SWS that your most restorative sleep processes occur, including protein synthesis, clearance of toxins, downscaling of brain potentiation, and glycogen restocking—all the good stuff—so morning exercise-induced high HRV coinciding with SWS is the power band of restorative function and leads to greater Command Center functioning during waking, including greater executive functioning. If you are gunning to win the trifecta of the Downstate Derby, follow these steps: First, start your day with an intense morning training session. Second, make a date with yourself (and a partner, if available) to get down tonight. Third, take a small dose of melatonin an hour before your estimated time of orgasm (ETO). PAYOUT!

## Incorporate Resistance Exercise Three Times a Week, Ideally in the Afternoon

Muscle mass declines between 3 and 8 percent each decade after age thirty, and 5 to 10 percent each decade after age fifty.[89] This age-related reduction in muscle mass, known as sarcopenia, can weigh heavily on your metabolism. Lean muscle tissues use a lot more energy than fat, so are associated with higher body fat in adulthood, which in turn leads to higher risk for obesity and metabolic disorders, such as type 2 diabetes. Low muscle mass also means weaker bones (your muscles pull on your bones at various attachment points, stimulating them to grow stronger),[90] higher blood pressure, deteriorating cardiovascular function and lipid profiles.[91]

Resistance training is the best way to fight this slow decline. But, as with so many biological processes, timing matters. Since your muscles have peaks and troughs in functioning across the night and day, you can optimize your workout by banging out your resistance training in the afternoon, the best time of day for muscle mass building.

## Practice Nasal Breathing Throughout Your Entire Workout

I'm going to start with the good parts—and then let you in on the not-so-good parts—of practicing nasal-restricted breathing during exercise. The good parts: It increases oxygenation of blood through its action on nitric oxide (NO), a potent vasodilator, and carbon dioxide ($CO_2$), which helps bring more oxygen into muscle tissue. More oxygen means more energy, greater strength and speed and all that superhero stuff, but with less respiratory work, because nasal breathing slows your respiratory rate significantly. Breathing solely through your nose also allows for cleaner, warmer, more humidified air to enter your lungs, which, among other benefits, has been shown to reduce exercise-induced asthma. This is especially important for winter workouts. All in all, it's breathing the way nature intended.

Now for the not-so-good part: NASAL BREATHING WHILE WORKING OUT IS HARD. Inhaling and exhaling through your nose only during a light and easy walk feels great—you naturally take fewer yet deeper breaths and end up feeling calm and serene as a result. But difficulty begins to arise as you bump up your speed or start hitting hills. Suddenly you experience something called *air hunger*, which feels exactly like it sounds: the sense that you can't get enough air on the inhale, then can't exhale fast enough through your nose to catch your breath.

I won't lie; nasal breathing on a vigorous run is literally the most difficult thing I have done with my body since birthing a human. But I'm dedicated to it because I see the better athlete waiting for me on the other end. (I'm defining *athlete* as anyone who works out.) Nasal breathing for months at a time will make you a better athlete. In one study, nose-breathing Steady as She Goes–type athletes were given a graded exercise test designed to get them running on a treadmill at their max speed and oxygen uptake within six to ten minutes while breathing only nasally or orally.[92] Nose-breathers showed an economy of effort, meaning they took fewer breaths but had greater oxygen consumption. That translates into more energy left over for their muscles. They also consumed more carbon dioxide yet didn't perceive the run to be excessively challenging or experience air hunger. Carbon dioxide is actually really good for you—it increases oxygen uptake—but as I said before, most people aren't used to even small amounts of it because we're a society of mouth breathers. Increasing your carbon dioxide tolerance boosts fitness, allowing you to save your energy for the muscles involved in improving strength, speed, and accuracy of performance. Free divers, who can hold their breath in the water for up to ten minutes, eat carbon dioxide for lunch.

When I hit one of several hills on my run, I have found a way to keep my damn mouth shut—by groaning out my nasal exhale. The technique is not unlike that used to make yoga's ubiquitous nasal *ujjayi* breath. Yogic wisdom dictates that if you can hear it, you know you are breathing—the louder the better. Well, in my quest to improve my cardiovascular fitness, I have taken that message to heart. Everyone can hear me breathing; I sound like a grunting bull . . . a grunting Downstate bull. Oh, and also, all that forced air makes my nose constantly leak (especially during winter) and sometimes I blow snot into my shirt to keep my nose clear. It's full-on $VO_{2max}$ Ugly Face.

You can also consider incorporating the use of an external nasal dilator strip, which increases the flow of air through your nose and is prescribed for snorers and people with sleep apnea.[93] Studies in athletes using these strips show higher $VO_{2max}$ as well as longer time to exhaustion.[94] One caveat is that nasal breathing only works with practice and commitment;

you'll hear plenty of negative reviews from novice nasal breathers. Just keep calm, and nose-breathe on.

## Incorporate an Autonomic-Guided Exercise Training Plan

Instead of dogmatically sticking with a weekly set of hard, moderate, and easy days, base your daily program on your autonomic nervous system and the supercompensation framework. Studies have used this approach to guide daily decision making for when to push for a high-intensity training session.[95] With this individualized approach, you will measure your resting heart rate manually or use a wearable device, such as Polar or M-Wave, every morning before you get out of bed. These daily numbers will help you determine whether you should take it easy or go hard. Remember: high heart rate is an indicator of possible REV overdrive, whereas high HRV means that RESTORE is leading the charge, so regardless of which measurement you take, you will want to be clear that the goal is low heart rate (low REV) and high HRV (high RESTORE). The first reading will be your baseline; on that day it's a good idea to jump-start the system with a vigorous high-intensity workout. The next morning, take your measurements again. If your heart rate is higher than your baseline or if your HRV is lower, you are still in recovery mode and need an extra day of rest, which can consist of low-impact walking or an easy bike ride. On the other hand, if your heart rate is lower than or equal to your baseline or your HRV is higher than or equal to your baseline, then you are likely in your supercompensation mode and ready to push yourself to a whole new RecoveryPlus plateau. Before embarking on this new plan, it's a good idea to talk to a professional trainer or coach about how to incorporate autonomic training into your existing program to ensure you're getting the right readings and have a good idea of your options for low, moderate, and hard workouts.

## Exercise in Nature Whenever Possible, Ideally with a Friend, Family Member, or Pet, at Least Three Times a Week

When you move your body while out in nature, you light up RESTORE (your brain *loves* being outdoors), lowering stress levels and flooding your body with calming, euphoric hormones. Part of that has to do with the great outdoors' ability to draw you in with its diverse beauty and make you feel connected to the world at large. Outside, there is always something new to notice because the landscape changes in a natural cycle with the seasons, and you feel a sense of awe from the enormity of the big and small living things flourishing in the ecosystem.[96] As Susan Fox Rogers writes: "Perspective— that's what the natural world gives me."[97] These sorts of feelings may have a systemwide anti-inflammatory effect, which can protect against depression.

Exercising in nature also offers a multimodal, full sensory experience, as you're tasked with using all of your senses in a way that a treadmill workout doesn't. You need to watch out for twigs and rocks to avoid tripping; you smell the grass and flowers (and, without realizing it, inhale their valuable immune-enhancing plant compounds); you hear branches snapping underfoot and the wind rushing by your ears—a green workout stimulates every part of brain, sending vital nutrient- and oxygen-rich blood to all four corners, keeping your mind flexible and strong.

Exercising in green spaces (and blue! Bodies of water are just as impactful) tend to make the workout more like play than a chore. In one study, adults who hiked outdoors for forty-five minutes reported feeling more energized, happier, and calmer compared with those who walked for an equal amount of time on an indoor treadmill.[98]

And, of course, we bow down to the importance of natural light for sending our circadian rhythm the clearest message about whether we should feel alert or sleepy. Outdoor exercise is an easy, highly efficient way of letting that light into our brains.

To inject your outdoor adventure with even more Downstate goodness, do it with a friend, family member, or pet. Considering the effects of supportive relationships, love, and physical touch on your REV/RESTORE ratio, when you powerwalk, ride, Rollerblade, play ball, or do boot camp with a buddy, you reap those Downstate rewards as well. Exercising with a partner is also highly motivating and increases accountability. (It's easy to skip a solo morning workout because your bed feels so warm and cozy, but not so easy to ditch your friend who's waiting for you at the local park.) We all need human connection and exercise more than ever, so consider a weekly yoga class in the park, or a dog walk on the beach, or a meet-up to hike a local path.

# CHAPTER SIX

# You Are What and When You Eat

E ating and sharing a meal are two of the great pleasures of human existence. Cooking for loved ones, treating our friends to a special dinner
at a favorite restaurant, passing down food traditions from generation to
generation, and now the ever-evolving online recipes that allow for endless
updates and transformations . . . these are all part of the deep ownership of
and identification with what and how we eat. The foods of our families have
a global heritage that come in all sauces, all flavors, and all preparations,
and tell a rich story of our personal childhoods and our ancestors' histories
all at the same time. For me, the consumption of inherently Danish treats
like salty licorice, marzipan, and rye bread with liverwurst or herring, is
so inextricably linked with my upbringing and happy times with my loved
ones that I rank eating them as some of my most enjoyable life experiences
(while many non-Danes consider these delicacies something between dog
and cat food).

Just as teachers say, "There are no bad questions," there are also no "bad
foods," only spectrums of healthy to unhealthy preparations of food and
eating habits. This chapter is devoted to bringing to light what and how to
eat to best serve your own personal Downstate, as well as how to integrate
your eating habits with your daily Upstate/Downstate rhythm. Having the
best science-backed information on what and when to eat will help you set
up healthy nutrition habits that are eminently more sustainable than the
cycle of jumping on and falling off the fad diet wagon.

## The *Whats* of Downstate Eating

Contrary to the popular analogy that likens eating to fueling up a car with gas, there's far more to refueling than just pumping in whatever unleaded you can find. Much of our modern food supply has been processed to such a degree that it's lost any vitamins and nutrients that were present in the initial form (see: Cheetos, white bread, Frappuccinos); contains too many unpronounceable ingredients, most of which are preservatives; and is usually eaten in portions way beyond the actual physiological needs of the moment. Just like a bad germ, these not-found-in-nature ingredients or meal quantities beyond reason can stimulate an Upstate stress response, activating the sympathetic nervous system, inflammation, and oxidative stress (more on this later). Let's spend some time learning about how certain foods, many of which may be sitting in your pantry, desk, or gut as we speak, can trigger this Upstate uproar.

## Inflammation Starts with Eating

One of the first things to understand about food's effect on your Upstate/ Downstate functioning is that your brain considers anything you put in your mouth a foreign object, be it a bite of cake, a clutch of almonds, or a fistful of bacteria-infused sand. As a first responder, your immune system is in charge of monitoring all foreign objects that enter your temple, quickly determining whether they are friends or foes. Its first action is to mount a mild defensive response in case of bacteria or virus by releasing proteins called *proinflammatory cytokines* that cause a small blip of REV inflammation, and which also increase insulin, the substance necessary for shuttling glucose from food into the cells of your body so it can be used for energy.[1] This little stress blip is then followed by a protracted response from your RESTORE system, which reigns over the digestion process. The more food you eat, the more proinflammatory cytokines boost insulin release, and the more energy you have for your cells.

When you eat a reasonable and healthy portion of food, this closed system is mutually beneficial for both systems as energy is made for all cells including those of the immune system, which means that your ability to fight disease (immunity) and your ability to make energy (metabolism) are inherently linked, a concept called *immunometabolism*. And when you eat foods that are healthy and whole and ingested in reasonable quantities, the process of turning nutrients into usable glucose is a slow and steady process. Think of the factory conveyor belt in cartoons that either moves at its typical pace or, through some accidental or nefarious flip of the dial, gets turned up to high speed, pushing the machine past its comfort zone and sending the workers into a frenzy. That conveyor belt is your immunometabolic system, and when you eat whole grains, protein, or hearty vegetables, the system hums away at its optimal settings.

But, when you eat foods that are ultraprocessed, made from refined flour and filled with sugar, saturated fat, and preservatives, you send the factory into a dysfunctionally high-paced, stressed-out state with too much REV and precious little RESTORE. You see, those proinflammatory cytokines, while partly responsible for transforming food into energy, are actually the soldiers of your immune system, and sending preprocessed foods and lots of sugar down the conveyor belt puts your immune system on red alert and generates a sudden spike in glucose, leading to the release of too many proinflammatory cytokines. Those cytokines, in turn, signal the overproduction of insulin, and because the food keeps coming fast and loose, the insulin keeps flowing, desperately trying to keep up. Habitually consuming these foods creates a chronic state of Upstate inflammation and insulin resistance, where your cells start ignoring insulin and the sugar sits in the traffic jam of your bloodstream (i.e., hyperglycemia). Chronic inflammation and hyperglycemia are hallmark symptoms in people at an unhealthy weight or with type 2 diabetes. This situation can also trigger new chronic medical conditions, such as cancer, heart disease, arthritis, and more, or exacerbate existing ones.[2]

So, what's the difference between the small but crucial burst of inflammation that benefits insulin metabolic pathways and the chronic overdose that shuts it all down? Scientists believe that eating foods outside of Mother Nature's wheelhouse, or overeating, places too high a demand on your metabolic system, creating a constant Upstate with no breaks for restoration and replenishment of resources. This is the precursor for insulin resistance. In fact, the most cutting-edge treatments for type 2 diabetes are different variations on the theme of giving your insulin pathways a little Downstate vacation, a so-called "β-cell rest" (β-cells release insulin), which has been shown to reinitiate healthy insulin activity.[3] This is also why dietitians recommend eating three solid meals a day, which only stresses your immunometabolic system three times, instead of snacking around the clock, which overtaxes your metabolic conveyor. Just like every organ and system in your body needs regular Downstate breaks, your metabolism works optimally when it catches a break, too. More on the *When* of eating follows . . .

## Unchecked Free Radicals Can Lead to Oxidative Stress

Once insulin has moved glucose from food into your cells, the second step in metabolism is to turn that glucose into energy. Any process that turns fuel (e.g., wood, gas, or food) into energy using oxygen is called combustion. Just as you start a wood fire by blowing on embers, the fuel you eat requires oxygen to release the energy stored in the chemical bonds of the food's molecules. When your body converts glucose into ATP, the energy currency of the cell, oxygen helps break electron bonds and move them from one molecule to another. This process releases energy that is harnessed by your cells.

Under most conditions, oxygen plays nice, grabbing an electron from one molecule and giving it to another. Sometimes, however, this transfer doesn't work out perfectly, leaving some single electron oxygen molecules on the prowl for another electron with which to pair bond. Think of these single electron oxygen molecules as that guy or gal who, when single, is out at the bars drunkenly making passes at your girlfriends and boyfriends. You know the type. These scoundrel single electron oxygen molecules go by the rakish moniker *free radicals* and, just like every heartbreaker, they are highly unstable and go around stealing electrons and busting up molecules in the process.

For most things in life, moderation is key to well-being, hence the distinction between *eustress* and *distress*, where some amount of a substance, such as cortisol, or a process, such as a burst of REV, can be a sweet spot, while too little or too much can be toxic. So, too, with free radicals, which at eustress concentration levels do a lot of good for the body, including turning air and food into chemical energy, and are essential elements for proper immune function as they sail through the circulatory system attacking for-

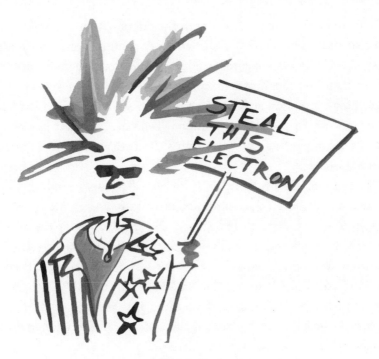

A Free Radical

eign invaders. They are also produced during exercise and contribute to the feeling of hurts-so-good muscle fatigue that brings on restorative healing.

However, left unchecked, they can start a chain reaction, whereby a growing army of rogue free radicals roam around, street ganglike, increasing inflammation and damaging tissue and vital biological processes, including injuring arteries and filling them with cholesterol plaques; interfering with cellular activity; breaking down collagen cell walls, which increases wrinkles; and even causing the death of healthy cells.

One of your main defenses against an overabundance of damaging free radicals is foods rich with antioxidant properties. Think of them as the yentas of the biological world, setting up free radicals with nice eligible electrons with whom to settle down. Antioxidation is one of many protective properties that come from *phytochemicals* (*phyto* is Greek for "plant"), chemicals that protect plants from the harshness of nature, shielding baby buds and sprouts from predators, nasty weather conditions, and pollution. They give plants their tastes, smell, and color, burning your tongue with capsaicin in habaneros, filling your house with the aroma of roasted garlic via allicin, tantalizing your eyes with the bright orange and yellow of the carotenoids in carrots and squash, and the dark purples of anthocyanins in blueberries. When we consume fruits, vegetables, nuts, legumes, and whole grains, their hearty antioxidant properties get passed on to us, including mimicking hormones, stimulating enzymes, interfering with DNA replication, destroying bacteria or binding to cell walls, and getting rid of free radicals, all of which protects us against heart disease, cancer, and many chronic diseases.[4]

Phytochemicals are found in a variety of plants, including broccoli, Brussels sprouts, carrots, collards and other leafy greens, mangoes, tomatoes, berries and cherries, red grapes, and more. Some spices also have phytochemical properties, including ginger, turmeric, grape seed extract, ginkgo, and rosemary, as does green tea.[5] Although commercials encourage us to cram supplements, the National Institutes of Health cautions against getting your phytochemicals through any means other than diet, as several studies of antioxidant supplements have demonstrated no benefit to health, and even some potential harm.[6]

As with everything, the right ratios of free radicals to antioxidants is key to health. When you overeat, eat foods high in sugar and unhealthy fats, or eat food made from ingredients that quickly turn into glucose, you end up with an overabundance of free radicals, a phenomenon called *oxidative stress*. A small amount of oxidative stress, termed oxidative eustress, can be helpful by stimulating your immune system, which in turn can regulate tissue growth and increase production of more antioxidant chemicals.[7] It may also protect the body from infection and disease via mild, short-lasting inflammation. However, long-term oxidative stress damages the body's cells, proteins, and DNA and instigates a cycle of chronic inflammation. And just like chronic inflammation, oxidative stress has been linked to several unwelcome diseases, including cancer, Parkinson's, Alzheimer's, type 2 diabetes, macular degeneration, and more.

Along with unhealthy portions and round-the-clock snacking, specific foods can be especially free radical-generating; these are the types of anti-Downstate foods your doctor always warns you about:

- Refined carbohydrates and sugars, which are quickly digested and absorbed, causing a rapid rise in blood sugar

- Preservatives in processed meats, such as sausage, bacon, salami, and cold cuts
- Animal products high in iron, such as red meat
- Overly heated cooking fats and oils

An occasional indulgence is fine—I'm not trying to be the donut police—but regular consumption of these foods can lead to an Upstate hellscape. (PS: The hot dog police already kind of exists . . . the American Institute for Cancer Research says the consumption of processed meats increases the risk of colorectal cancer and the World Health Organization has labeled red meat as "probably carcinogenic to humans."[8]) Alcohol, smoking, exposure to pesticides, and air pollutants also increase free radical production.

Inflammation and oxidative stress each have their own health risks, but they also have a combined effect of putting you in a perfect storm of Upstate stress. With a chronically poor diet, high stress, or a large infection, an ugly cycle of one-upmanship can occur, whereby oxidative stress triggers a large inflammatory response, which in turn produces more free radicals that can lead to further oxidative stress.

All this to say that what and how much we eat has a direct impact on our Upstate/Downstate balance and health. This is an exciting discovery, as it puts the power of the Downstate in your hands, with your diet offering one of the biggest opportunities for minimizing Upstate activation and maximizing Downstate recovery. Nutrition expert Wendy Bazilian, DrPH, RD, strongly urges her clients to balance out each meal with complementary foods that provide the right amount of protective phytochemical properties to match all the protein, fats, and carbs sitting on your plate. "It's a balancing act that you need to tackle on a meal-to-meal basis," she says. "You can't expect one healthy meal a week to make up for all the wear and tear building up during the week, creating potentially irreversible damage."[9] Just like sleep and exercise, nutrition is a daily Downstate practice.

## You Are What You Eat

Let's take a look at the two-way street that runs between the foods you eat and your mood, cognition, and sleep. Along the way, you will also be introduced to the downtown high-rise of microbes that live in your gut and can make your life heaven or hell depending on how well you treat them and also how well REV and RESTORE (the two sides of your autonomic nervous system) are getting along with each other. A full understanding of these relations will help you create a Downstate food vocabulary to live by.

## Foods That Make You Happy

Raise your hand if any of the following have ever happened to you:

You bake a quiche for a friend who lost a loved one.
You pop peanut butter cups like they're Tic Tacs when you're working under a tight deadline.
Your appetite goes on a walkabout when you're superstressed.
You crave homemade mac 'n' cheese when you've had a turd day.
You can't resist chocolate or a so-rare-it's-moving burger during certain times of the month.

You don't need to be a nutritional psychologist (yes, they exist) to know that food and emotions are as tightly paired as peanut butter and jelly. We eat differently when we're happy or sad, anxious or relaxed, tired or wired. This is why pandemic sourdough bread became, well, a pandemic. We self-medicate with carbs when we're sad or stressed in part because they trigger production of serotonin, acting a bit like edible antidepressants.[10] We can't resist grabbing the fifty-cent chocolate treat at the cash register because chocolate's trademark blend of sugar and fat signals the reward center of the brain to release dopamine, a euphoria-producing hormone that gives you a mild high, reminiscent of what you might experience on drugs or sex.[11] Feeling stressed and depressed also has the unfortunate outcomes of reducing intake of fresh, good-for-you foods and ramping up cravings for snacks, fast food, and sweets. Data from the Health Professionals Study showed that divorced or widowed men decrease their vegetable intake, which typically doesn't resume until after remarriage.[12] So, generally speaking, droopy moods not only wreak havoc on your Upstate stress response, they also make you crave inflammatory foods, throwing gas on the Upstate sympathetic fire.

And if crappy moods drive you to eat crappy foods, the vicious cycle can move in the opposite direction too, with certain foods wielding mighty influence over your moods, from sugar crashes to meat sweats, caffeine jitters to poutine hangovers. Much as stress and depression overstimulate REV and accelerate oxidative stress and inflammation, eating highly inflammatory, ultraprocessed foods—such as sugar, saturated and trans fats, vegetable oils, refined carbs and white flour products, fried foods, processed meats, and the like—has a similarly toxic influence on mood. In a study of postmenopausal women, higher sugar consumption was associated with increasing rates of depression, whereas higher consumption of dairy, fiber, fruits, and veggies was associated with sunnier dispositions. These inflammatory diets can also up your odds of developing anxiety.[13] Those who follow more Old World–type diets, heavy on produce and whole grains, light on ultraprocessed food, are 25 to 35 percent less likely to experience depression.[14]

Eating more fish boosts your omega-3 fatty acids, which is strongly associated with lower rates of depression.[15] In a study of medical students cramming for a big exam, three to four weeks of fish oil supplementation decreased REV and benefited circadian rhythms by lowering body temperature and cortisol levels. The more omega-3s present in the students' bloodstreams, the lower their inflammatory markers and depressive symptoms in response to the stress of the test.[16] Omega-3 fatty acids help us look on the bright side of life and have been used to treat bipolar depression, post-traumatic stress disorder, and major depression.[17]

You might also try taking up a green tea habit. Not only is the entire ethos and ceremony of tea drinking a daily Downstate habit worth fostering, but green tea is loaded with happiness-inducing polyphenols, feisty plant compounds that come in jewel-toned hues and give off a bitter taste. In a study of Japanese elders, daily green tea intake was associated with reductions in depression, and the more people drank each day, the happier they felt.[18] Consider making the switch from coffee, as green tea can also improve your sleep as it contains half the amount of caffeine. For those of you who are avoiding caffeine altogether, be aware that many decaffeination processes may remove a fraction of the polyphenols in tea and coffee—and some still remain, providing you with similar health benefits.[19,20,21,22,23,24]

## THE ALPHAS AND OMEGAS OF HEALTHY FAT

Your daily recommended portions of Downstate bliss require a good bit of healthy fat in the form of omegas-3, -6, and -9. Both omega-3 and omega-6 are *essential* fatty acids, meaning they can only be sourced from food, whereas omega-9s can be made by the body so don't need to be supplemented. The most important thing to remember about the essential fatty acids is that you want to have more 3s and fewer 6s. Omega-3s come from the ocean in the form of eicosapentaenoic acid (EPA) and docosahexaenoic acid (DHA) and are found in oily fish, such as salmon, mackerel, sardines, and anchovies, as well as walnuts, chia seeds, and flaxseeds, and some leafy green veggies, in the form of alpha-linolenic (ALA) acid. Omega-3s, DHA in particular, are responsible for the impressive feat of growing our brains to their modern size, thanks to early humans who lived by the Kenyan shores, feasting on catfish and inventing language, mathematics, and astronomy.[19] Omega-3s are critical for learning and memory by elevating BDNF in the hippocampus and promoting the formation and maintenance of neural cell walls.[20] They help you maintain a positive disposition by increasing the release of several mood-regulating neurotransmitters, and improve metabolism by using glucose more efficiently and decreasing oxidative stress and proinflammatory cytokines.[21] They're also important for maintaining healthy blood pressure and cholesterol.

Omega-6s predominate in vegetable and seed oils, such as soybean, corn, safflower, and mayonnaise. Eaten in small amounts, amid a backdrop of a diet heavy in omega-3s, these fatty acids can benefit cardiovascular function and blood clotting.[22] The danger here lies in the fact that the typical standard American diet (SAD) boasts far more omega-6s than necessary. Our ancestors—cave or otherwise—didn't eat French fries saturated in hydrogenated soybean oil, or sub sandwiches slathered in mayo. Up until the past couple of decades, the typical diet contained six to seven times more omega-3s, and five times less omega-6s, than we eat today, with the omega-6/3 ratio dangerously escalating from 3:1 in ye olde times to 25:1 in ye In-and-Out Burger times.[23]

Whereas 60 to 85 percent of omega-3s are used for making energy for the heart, brain, and muscles and for building proteins, with little stored as fat, omega-6s are mostly stored in fat with less used for active processing as for omega-3s.[24] Importantly, these two fatty acids compete for enzymes required to process them, which is why you want to keep the omega-3s high, or else they and all their good deeds will be usurped by the omega-6s. When omega-6 overcrowds the scene, the body turns into an inflammatory danger zone.

## Brain Food

The foods you put in your mouth have a profound impact on your memory, focus, executive functioning, and more, and whether you eat an apple a day or fries on every day that ends in -*y* can mean the difference between your brain aging robustly or ending up shrunken and forgetful.

To begin, join me on a quick spin through your memory's favorite parts of the supermarket, starting with the produce section. Dark leafy greens and cruciferous veggies, such as cauliflower and broccoli, feed the brain the phytochemical lutein, an inflammation-suppressing nutrient with serious antioxidant power.[25] Berries are also Downstate superstars, their red, purple, and blue tones evidence of *anthocyanins*, antioxidant-rich pigments with a unique ability to cross the blood-brain barrier. Anthocyanins enter the hippocampus and other memory and learning centers and scavenge for free radicals, those bully by-products of glucose combustion, causing neurons to age faster. Strawberries, raspberries, blackberries, blueberries . . . they taste delightfully different but act the same way in the brain, escorting free radicals out and preserving cognitive function in the process. Additionally, healthy sixty- to seventy-year-olds given polyphenol-rich extract from grapes and blueberries (600 mg/day) instead of a placebo for six months showed improved memory, especially in those people already showing some signs of cognitive decline.[26]

In the spice aisle, turmeric is the standout, turning your food into a psychedelic yellow feast via a potent anti-inflammatory substance called curcumin, a polyphenol that keeps you sharp while imbuing your curry with an earthy-sweet flavor. One study administered curcumin twice a day for eighteen months to people fifty-one to eighty-four years old who were experiencing mild memory complaints.[27] Their cognitive abilities were tested at the beginning and end of the study and their amyloid and tau signals (the proteins that develop into Alzheimer's plaques) were measured as well. The curcumin group showed improvement in memory, elevations in mood and attention, and brain scans showed less amyloid and tau accumulation.[28] Curcumin consumption, the study authors proposed, might be one of the reasons Alzheimer's rates are lower in India than in the US.[29,30,31,32]

## POLYPHENOLS: TOUGH AND PRETTY

Over eight thousand types of polyphenols have been identified in fruits, such as grapes, apples, pears, cherries, and berries, as well as red wine, tea or coffee, chocolates, and some herbs and spices, so I'll just highlight a few stars.[29] Flavonoids, the biggest group of polyphenols, are found in such foods as apples, onions, dark chocolate, and red cabbage and are especially Downstate-friendly, reducing blood pressure and LDL (bad) cholesterol.[30] Blueberries are particular stars in this polyphenol food category, with randomized control trials evincing cardiovascular disease prevention.[31] Adding supplements from tea extract to the diets of already healthy people has been shown to decrease the typical cardiovascular responses to a mental stress test, as well as lower cortisol, and increase relaxation; similar findings have been shown with intake of flavanol-rich chocolate and grape-wine extracts.[32] These studies suggest that polyphenols may help reduce Upstate overactivity and future onset of hypertension.[33]

Cacao provides epicatechin, a type of polyphenol shown to cross the blood-brain barrier, expand neural growth and neurogenesis, and increase memory in mice.[33] The same cognitive perks have also been seen in young, healthy humans, with daily cacao intake increasing executive function, memory, and attention.[34]

## Food That Helps You Sleep

Another late night, another early morning . . . your body and brain crave energy—a quick pick-me-up to get you through the next twelve hours. At the cafeteria, you could choose that salad bowl with some protein on top, light oil and vinegar, and a glass of water. It would be so easy . . . to . . . just . . . NOPE! Not today! Right now, you need energy, something solid, warm, and preferably very sweet or very salty to take the edge off the day; so, you reach for a candy bar or a plate of fries and a soda. We've all been there, so let me take that guilt off your plate when I tell you that it's not you, it's your bad sleep. Even a small amount of sleep curtailment completely messes with your entire relationship to food.

You've already learned that not getting enough zzz's dysregulates your eating hormones (ghrelin and leptin). It also shuts down the orbitofrontal cortex, a brain area responsible for helping you do the right thing even in cases where the wrong thing would feel sooooo goooood. A restless night leaves that brain area at half-mast, which makes sweet and soft food more compelling, while anything oaty, cruciferous, or complex seems downright disgusting.[35]

Beyond your brain telling you to eat high energy foods (sugary and fatty), the mere act of staying up late increases your potential eating hours, which can also contribute to weight gain. In the Nurses' Health Study, which followed middle-age American women for up to sixteen years, women who slept for five hours or less were 15 percent more likely to become obese compared with those who slept seven hours a night.[36]

Poor food choices can actually destroy your sleep. In a study of Japanese women, high amounts of confectionary and noodles were associated with poor sleep quality—the higher the carb intake, the worse the sleep—whereas higher consumption of fish and vegetables improved sleep. Not surprisingly, choosing energy drinks and sugar-sweetened beverages, skipping breakfast, and eating at irregular times were strongly associated with poor sleep quality.

Sleep stages also are affected by what you eat. Cramming a dinner of simple carbs (e.g., white bread, bagels, pastries, and pasta) into the last moments of your Upstate day will drive up your Upstate metabolic system just as it's trying to get some much-needed rest, resulting in more awakenings and significantly less slow-wave sleep (SWS).[37] On the other hand, a dinner featuring a small piece of high-quality protein is better for sleep by decreasing middle-of-the-night awakenings. Furthermore, when you follow a strict low-carb, high-protein diet for several days (à la Atkins, The Zone, or keto), SWS actually increases.[38,39,40,41]

## Inequity in Food Access and the Growth of Urban Farming

Knowing what you should eat is only the beginning of the fight for your health and your Downstate life. The next big challenges are access to that healthy food, and then the development of and adherence to healthy eating habits. One of the worst inequities in America today is the lack of access

Children's brains depend on healthy, nutritious diets to develop into functional adults. In 1969, my own brilliant dad, the late Sarnoff A. Mednick, PhD, set up the first longitudinal study to examine the impact of nutrition, exercise, and cognitive stimulation during early childhood on all the basic milestones of life.[40] The Mauritius Child Health Project set up nursery schools throughout this subtropical Indian Ocean island that provided children with a healthy breakfast, daily education, and time for physical exercise and play. Kids selected from all strata of society attended the nursery schools and were compared to a group of kids who grew up in the standard system of care on the island. His team has published hundreds of findings on these kids, who are now great-grandparents, looking at a wide range of topics, including the autonomic nervous system, mental illness, intelligence, omega-3 fatty acid intake, and more, with valuable data collection still going strong.

He was a pioneer in viewing the brain as a seed that grows into the sapling of adolescence and later the full-size tree of adulthood. A seed is vulnerable to environmental conditions that can harm its growth. So, too, the developing brain can be deeply disturbed in the womb by illness or stress befalling the mother, or in early childhood by malnutrition or other stressors. These "hits," as my dad called them, are conceptually the same as the Upstate overloads you have learned about in this book, and he showed that they predicted the emotional, mental, and physical makeup of who we become as adults. My dad and his colleagues were the first to show that early malnutrition resulted in lower cognitive abilities in adolescence, and predicted later aggression, and other externalizing behaviors, as well as mental illness.[41] They also probed the role of omega-3s in brain development and their potential use in preventing behavioral problems in later years. More recent studies have followed in my dad's footsteps, administering regular doses of omega-3 fatty acids to schoolchildren resulting in improvement in school performance, including higher scores on tests of verbal intelligence, learning, and memory after six and twelve months.[42] His groundbreaking work and others inspired healthy meal programs in preschool, such as Head Start, and the Black Panther Free Breakfast for School Children Program in elementary schools.

My dad understood how to prioritize the Downstate in his own life: he napped every day; loved hiking; traveled the world with my mom, Birgitte; was always ready for an excellent meal; and knew how to party just as well as he knew how to work. He is ever my inspiration for a life of perfect harmony between Upstates and Downstates.

to healthy food throughout communities of color and low-income areas across the country. For over twenty-three million Americans, it's not possible to buy the fresh fruit and vegetables that prevent chronic levels of Upstate oxidative stress and inflammation, because there simply are no grocery stores within 10 miles of their homes.[42] The local mom-and-pop shops that have always catered to the cultural culinary needs of their communities have recently and rapidly been run out of town by an invasion of convenience stores.

In low-income neighborhoods and communities of color, you'll find fast-food restaurants instead of fruit stands; instead of supermarkets, pharmacies peddle sweet and salty crap egregiously passed off as food. The worst bully of the convenience store model? The dollar store, legion in food desert communities, serving as the only food source for many struggling city neighborhoods and small towns by pricing out local groceries yet offering mostly cheap, plastic-packaged, ultraprocessed products loaded with preservatives, sodium, sugar, and fat.

Studies show that the closer you live to fast, ultraprocessed food, the less optimal your weight, whereas living nearer to grocery stores is associated with healthier weight levels.[43] The inequality in food access is popularly termed "food desert," but food justice expert Ashanté M. Reese, PhD, argues that the desert metaphor implies absence, a deficit-oriented approach that stigmatizes low-income communities of color, erases memories of now-shuttered local businesses, and ignores residents' existing efforts to resist exploitative policies.[44] Instead, food justice community activist Karen Washington prefers "food apartheid," which "brings us to the more important question: What are some of the social inequalities that you see, and what are you doing to erase some of the injustices?"[45]

Taking back your Downstate means taking back your right to fresh food, your right to local grocery stores and farmers' markets, your right to the earth and the fruits of farming the land. Over the last half-century, farming has become increasingly whitewashed, with Black farm ownership declining from 15 million acres in 1920 to 1 million acres in 2017.[46] About 15 percent of the US population is Black, yet just over 1 percent of farmers are. Instead of waiting for systemic change, the movement of young people of color establishing farms and urban agricultural communities is one of several grassroots solutions to food inequity being implemented.[47]

Jordan Thomas is one such man who ditched his job in supply chain management to become a farmer. Growing up in Columbus, Ohio, he remembers eating canned produce all week "and then on Sundays, after church, we would go to my grandparent's house and have fresh green beans, tomatoes, and cucumbers."[48] The striking difference in texture and flavor of the fresh-from-the-garden veggies and the soggy, tasteless canned food made an early impression.

Jordan's parents had rejected working the soil for complex reasons, including associations between agriculture and the trauma of slavery, and the push to become more "cultured," which Jordan interpreted to mean "more white." So, while his grandparents connected him to farming, his parents, aunts, and uncles eschewed it. At college, Jordan's strength and conditioning coach was the first person to ask him whether he knew where his food came from—did he know how it was raised, what ingredients he was putting in his mouth every day? Answering these questions led him to take a look at his community's disenfranchisement from food sources, the lost knowledge of farming and relation to the land that has always been deeply rooted in Black and Indigenous cultures. His brief postcollege stint living in the Bay Area exposed him to a revolution in urban agriculture, including rooftop gardens. Farming became his passion, with an ambitious goal of revolutionizing the food supply chain.

The COVID-19 pandemic revealed a broken system where millions of Americans sank into food scarcity while farmers, who didn't have a direct way of selling their produce to individuals, were dumping as many as 3.7 million gallons of milk each day, and a single chicken processor was smashing 750,000 unhatched eggs every week.[49] Jordan's solution: "I think we need to start moving closer to smaller garden spaces." In other words: think globally, grow locally. Instead of green lawns that are ubiquitous in most American suburbs, Jordan wants to see backyard gardens on every block that can provide fresh fruit and vegetables "for your street, your neighborhood, on a regular basis . . . What's the functionality of these large, green, useless yards, when we could be using that space to feed people, right?" Right.

Jordan now lives in Lexington, Kentucky, in a historically Black neighborhood that has been labeled a food desert. He is raising chickens and bees and turning his lawn into a kitchen garden, with future plans to buy land to farm. He is part of the growing movement of community gardeners and urban farmers who realize the Downstate value of growing and feeding locally, physically connecting to not just the earth but Earth, and eating whole, unprocessed foods that are in sync with the land and its seasons. Removal of food apartheids will also require policy changes, such as the Justice for Black Farmers Act, and funding for nutrition and gardening education in schools and community centers to help all children live and grow from equal access to the Downstate.

## The *Whens* of Downstate Eating

Along with what and how much you eat, recent research has discovered that *when* you eat is also critical because just like every system, your metabolism works better with nice long breaks. There are many different brands of this new nutrition movement. The two top players are *intermittent fasting*, in which you drastically cut down caloric intake on some days and eat normally on other days, and *time-restricted eating*, in which you make a daily habit of confining your eating period to a short window (usually eight, ten, or twelve hours), but don't change your calories. Both practices have anti-inflammatory properties, reduce oxidative stress, and benefit cardiovascular and metabolic health thanks to their potent Downstate stimulating properties.

These structured eating times bring us back to an old adage sung by the legendary Pete Seeger (who borrowed it from Ecclesiastes): "A time to every purpose under heaven."[50] Like everything else you do, your body's natural rhythm prefers a set period for Upstate intake and one for Downstate digestion. Daylight hours are meant to be devoted to energy-expensive activities such as hunting, gathering, and the consumption of food while the huntin' and gatherin's good. This is when your body *wants* to eat—it's already REVVED up, and 100 percent prepared to handle the barrage in oxidative stress and inflammation that comes with a turkey on rye. The rest of the time is meant for slowly building up these energy stores by digesting and extracting nutrients from food; making systemwide repairs, including decreasing inflammation and rebuilding cell walls; de-stressing via intimate and affectionate moments with cave-mates; and preparing ourselves for the next day's energy output. This is how the RESTORE system earned its "rest and digest" nickname.

Critically, specific aspects of repair and rejuvenation can *only* occur when you are not eating. This is when oxidative stress is corrected, protein synthesis is enhanced, new brain cells are formed, memories are solidified, and creative ideas are sprouted. This is key to understanding why expanding your Downstate period by severely restricting calories for an entire day or just restricting your mealtime window—to start eating at nine a.m., for example, and finish ten to twelve hours later—was invented by experts as a way of helping you reap more of the benefits of nature's activity/repose cycle. Your body will always prioritize consumption of nutrients over other processes, shunting the important restorative Downstate work to a time when feeding isn't available. This is the BIG WHY opening up a bag of potato chips at eleven p.m. is the equivalent of shaking REV awake after it's already turned in for the night.

Even though nobody likes to admit it, research shows that significantly cutting calories can slow aging by 50 percent, preserve white matter in the brain, and reduce the risk of multiple chronic diseases, including cardiovascular disease and cancer (in animal studies), as well as improve cholesterol levels, blood sugar levels, inflammation, and blood pressure in humans.[51] A landmark University of Wisconsin study put this on full display when researchers published photos of rhesus monkeys, some of whom had had their calories restricted by about 30 percent for twenty years, and some who had been allowed to eat whatever they pleased.[52] The free-for-all monkeys looked years older—wrinkled, hunched, and flabbier—than their calorie-restricted counterparts, and also had increased rates of age-related diseases, such as cardiovascular disease, diabetes, brain atrophy, and cancerous tumors. Hello, *Fast Food Nation*.

But for humans it's just not that easy to forgo all the social and sensual pleasures of a good meal. It's also clear that restricting calories by way of cutting out your favorite foods can leave you tired, hangry, and obsessively jonesing for pizza, cupcakes, or just a slice of toast. Enter intermittent fasting and time-restricted eating, the most successful methods of dieting because they focus on *when* you eat, instead of *what* you eat. Both hinge on manipulating caloric intake in a way that complements the human circadian rhythm as opposed to fighting it, but while the media tends to use them interchangeably, they are quite different.

## INTERMITTENT FASTING

If you've ever had an adorably fat squirrel cross your path at the beginning of winter, preparing for a long season of having its food buried in feet of snow, you've seen evidence of nature's built-in feast or famine framework. Fasting is a way of life for all species, including humans, who have developed cultural traditions around it, such as Ramadan, Yom Kippur, and Lent. As it turns out, abstaining from food for extended periods of time isn't just good for your soul, it's good for your health. In a study of Utah residents followed for about four and a half years, those who were "routine fasters," meaning they fasted one Sunday a month for most of their life in accordance with their Mormon religion, had a 46 percent lower mortality rate compared with nonfasters—even though both groups engaged in clean Mormon livin'.[53]

It turns out that eating like a mouse for an entire day puts a nice long pause on all Upstate shenanigans. Whether it's done once a week or once a month, the practice has been shown to dramatically reduce unhealthy accumulation of lipids in the blood; prevent chronic inflammation; calm immune system activation; and improve insulin sensitivity, lowering the risk of type 2 diabetes, along with expanding the life span, as we saw with our Mormon fasters.[54]

One reason intermittent fasting may work so well is that it provides RESTORE time off the task of eating, which reduces the creation of free radicals and oxidative stress. Fasting also "flips the metabolic switch" from sourcing glucose for fuel to using your fat and fatty acid–derived ketones, highly functional metabolites that increase when insulin levels lower.[55] As you know, eating carbs stimulates the production of insulin, which shuttles glucose into your cells to be used as energy or stored as fat to be used later. When you cut down on carbs, insulin doesn't get released and so your body starts using its own fat deposits for energy. Not only does this eliminate oxidative stress from eating, but high ketone levels also push the body into Downstate regeneration mode, enhancing all those processes that can only happen when your Upstate is hibernating.[56]

A University of Southern California study found that three months of a "fasting-mimicking diet"—five days of calorie restriction (approximately

1,100 calories on Day 1 and 700 calories on Days 2 through 5)—followed by no limits for the rest of the month successfully reduced various risk factors for age-related diseases.[57] The effects were strongest in subjects who had obesity and/or were unhealthy, with a study coauthor saying these folks might need to continue repeating the fasting pattern monthly to recover their full health, but for healthy, athletic individuals, twice yearly might be sufficient.[58]

So, with all these benefits, why don't we all spend more time starving ourselves for days at a time? One study illustrates the dilemma. An intermittent fasting challenge was given to a group of amateur weightlifters.[59] The outcomes were mostly great, with reductions in several Upstate sympathetic factors, including heart rate and blood pressure, as well as improved cognitive functioning in tests of prefrontal cortex executive abilities among the fasting athletes. Unsurprisingly, however, the starving weightlifters were also noted to increasingly be wearing their angry pants as the study dragged on, which puts the cost/benefit analysis in a slightly different light. Sure, you might be healthier and smarter, but you also may wanna punch people in the face at the slightest provocation, suggesting a lack of sustainability and sociability.

## TIME-RESTRICTED EATING

Cutting-edge circadian research shows that you can maintain your best fitness by keeping eating times strictly to Upstate daylight hours when your organs are more prepared for processing nutrients, fats, and sugars. Back in Chapter 2, you learned about the natural Upstate window early in the day when diet-induced thermogenesis (your body's natural calorie-burning mechanism), glucose metabolism, and insulin release are at their peak. By the afternoon, these systems are at half-mast, and headed downhill rapidly toward their much-anticipated Downstate. Hitting the pad thai late at night wakes the beast, but the beast is tired and not beasting so well. The glucose from your food stays in your blood longer, making it easier to be stored as fat, and you overstress your cardiovascular and metabolic systems. All of this leads to increased oxidative stress and inflammation. With a little planning, you could have feasted on that Thai food at seven p.m., successfully avoiding the REV onslaught when you are woefully unprepared for it.

Time-restricted eating was first introduced by circadian scientist Satchin Panda, PhD. In his book *The Circadian Code*, he explains that when his lab rodents were only given a short period of time to eat (six hours) every day, but were allowed to eat as much food as they wanted during feeding time, the animals remained fit and full of energy, whereas the animals who were allowed to eat around the clock consumed the same amount as the restricted groups but gained weight and began showing early signs of diabetes.[60] Rodents are nocturnal, meaning their systems are designed to Upstate with the moon and Downstate with the sun. For me, the craziest thing about Dr. Panda's research was that he could feed the time-restricted eating rodents the equivalent of Big Macs and French fries during their daytime to no ill effect, whereas the same meal in the round-the-clock eaters got them in serious metabolic trouble.

Next, Dr. Panda tested his phenomenal findings on humans, with similar results. His research team had patients with metabolic syndrome, a cluster of conditions including high blood pressure, blood sugar, and cholesterol, plus excess belly fat, restrict their eating times to a ten-hour window for twelve weeks.[61] Importantly, calories were not restricted. Usually the subjects would delay their breakfast by a couple of hours (waiting until around nine a.m. to eat, and yes, that includes morning coffee or tea) and shift their dinner an hour earlier (around seven p.m.), with a critical avoidance of late night snacking. At the end of the program, study subjects had lost weight and reduced their body mass index (BMI), and decreased their blood pressure and cholesterol levels. All by eating in accordance with their own circadian rhythms!

Thinking about when you need to eat to maintain your health offers promising new paths if you struggle with typical dieting scenarios that decrease calories without considering the whole person—your activity level, your genetics, your circadian tendencies—or give you a complicated algorithm of nutritional dos and don'ts that require a PhD to understand. Time-restricted eating and intermittent fasting work because they leverage the internal Upstate/Downstate rhythm that evolution set up trillions of nights ago in such a simple, straightforward way that even a caveman could follow it.

## Letting Your Microbiome Go to Your Head

Your guts and the microorganisms that live therein are central characters in forming who you are, from your bowel movements to your emotions. Since the day you were born, when you picked up your very first gut bacteria (called *probiotics*, meaning "for life") while passing through your mother's birth canal, taking your first sips of breast milk, or snuggling skin to skin, your gut microbiota have taken on a life of their own, developing a relatively independent ecosystem whose activity can be helpful, hurtful, or completely indifferent to its host (that's you!).

When they're helpful, boy, are they helpful. Your microbiome has its hands in nearly every aspect of your life. For example, your own cells can't break down certain nutrients, such as complex carbohydrates and starches found in grains, tubers, and legumes (e.g., chickpeas and beans), into usable chunks, so they get fermented in your intestines by microbes, turning them into smaller, more absorbable short-chain fatty acids to be used for energy. And if you hear the phrase "fermented in your intestines" and think "stink bomb," you'd be right. The gas released from this process is your main source for six-year-old dinner table glee and smelt-it-dealt-it jokes; in other words, that's where your farts come from. Truly, your microbiome is such an independent housemate that the next time someone accuses you of crop-dusting the room, you can honestly say, "It wasn't me; it was Gerald, my microbiome!"

Gut microbes also produce essential nutrients and support the immune system by forming a protective lining around the intestines that keeps pathogens out. Actually, they don't just support the immune system—they practically *are* the immune system, responsible for about 70 percent of your immune potential, and also benefit your mental well-being.[62] Microbiome-brain communication is primarily controlled by the superhighway vagus nerve, linking your gut health, good or bad, to the emotional and cognitive centers of the brain via RESTORE pathways. In fact, the microbiome is known as the second brain, with 90 percent of feelin'-groovy serotonin receptors residing therein.[63]

When your microbes are happy and they know it, your guts are in a state of *eubiosis*. The best way to make your gut bugs smile is through eating wholesome foods, especially those high in fiber or fermented (yogurt, kefir, miso, kimchi, kombucha, and sauerkraut); exercise; rest and relaxation.

But your guts can get out of whack, a.k.a. *dysbiosis*, from either a shortage of helpful microbes; an overgrowth of nasty ones, such as *Clostridium difficile*; or a lack of microbial diversity. Such circumstances can result from an ultra-processed, ultrafat SAD diet, excess stress, and unhygienic living conditions. And while a course of antibiotics can be helpful to kill the bacteria causing your strep throat or throbbing, infected wound, some bad bacteria don't give a rat's butt about your stinkin' drugs (e.g., antibiotic-resistant bacteria), plus you end up killing off good microbes in the process. Once you arrive in Dysbiosis-ville, expect a wide range of GI problems, a drop in immune functioning, and a breakdown of the intestinal lining (i.e., leaky gut). Thanks to the gut-brain connection, an inflamed gut means an inflamed brain. Studies of leaky gut patients show that pathogens can be transported from the gut to the brain via the vagus nerve, which is why dysbiosis has been linked with REV overactivity including high blood pressure and hypertension, along with a wide range of seemingly unrelated conditions, including obesity, allergies, autoimmune disorders, the family of angry bowel disorders, cancer, and such disorders as depression and autism.[64] (Thirty-five percent of people with depression have leaky gut syndrome.)[65]

Since your guts are inextricably linked with maintaining a healthy balance between REV and RESTORE, an important question is whether it's possible to treat the aforementioned disorders by altering the ratio of good to bad bacteria in the microbiome. Using our old friend the poop transplant, as I mentioned in Chapter 2, scientists have reported that healthy fecal suppositories decrease blood pressure in hypertensive animals.[66] But, before you start investing in a franchise of poop dispensaries, simply taking probiotic supplements can help too. Taken for several weeks, they can exert a positive shift in your overall gut homeostasis, with such Downstate effects as decreased blood pressure, improved immune function, and enhanced nutrient absorption. Probiotic supplementation has been shown to benefit people with clinical disorders, such as irritable bowel syndrome and depression, but they can also help *healthy* people stay healthy. Several studies have linked the *Lactobacillus casei* strain with increased clear-headedness, confidence, and elation—you know the old saying "Happy gut-wife, happy life."[67] Microbiome health is an evolving field, but the bottom line is that adding probiotics (or prebiotics, which are the foods that fuel the good microbes) to your daily Downstate health habit arsenal is an excellent way to boost RESTORE. The trick is getting the most effective strain or combination of strains in the proper dosage. Talk to your GI doctor, licensed naturopath, or registered dietitian to figure out the right combination for you.

**PUTTING IT INTO PRACTICE**

As you have read in this chapter, modern life has invented many ways for you to ignore and disrupt our Downstate recovery time, keeping your system REVVED up for longer than is healthy. Luckily, it doesn't take much to start honoring your rhythm by setting up eating and nutrition routines that support an Upstate full of energy and positivity, and a nice long Downstate to prepare you for tomorrow. Here are the highlights that will keep you as happy on the outside as you are on the inside:

## Eat Breakfast

Many of us, myself included, struggle with breakfast. I don't feel like eating right when I wake up, and a couple of cups of tea with milk and honey can take me all the way until noon lunch without a problem. But not all habits are good for you. And it turns out that breakfast is one of those things that you should get in the habit of eating. Skipping breakfast has been linked with type 2 diabetes, atherosclerosis (clogged arteries), poor cardiovascular health, higher BMI, more depression symptoms, and smoking, and as you have already learned, is associated with later melatonin onset and poor sleep quality.[68]

When you forgo the first meal of the day, you miss prime Upstate eating hours when your entire metabolic system is naturally geared up. It also inevitably means you'll be getting the majority of your calories when your system is already looking toward the sun setting on all Upstate functions.

Front-loading your calories during the peak circadian Upstate hours is key to maximizing your metabolic system when it's primed and ready to receive and process calories. You are like a factory whose most productive hours are from seven a.m. to three p.m., after which the early crew that started pumping out cortisol and heating up your core at five a.m. starts heading home to rest, leaving the system running at 50 percent until the skeleton crew arrives to turn everything down to a very low hum. By keeping your meals light at night, with majority protein, some healthy carbohydrates, and a bit of greens, your own personal factory will be whistling while it works. That is why I am eating a soft-boiled egg at eight a.m. while I write this section. After all, self-care starts with me!

## Eat Good-for-You Foods

Downstate nutrition can be enjoyed whether you are cooking Indian, Jamaican, Japanese, or anything in between, as long as you trade in the Upstate inflammatory foods for nutrient-dense, minimally processed, brain- and heart-healthy foods. The point isn't to force yourself to adopt a framework different from your cultural food heritage because that would be insulting and damn near impossible for many people to accomplish. It's to shift your key ingredients and basic guidelines to feature the following themes:

- Intake of fruit and vegetables at most meals
- Beans, nuts, and seeds on most days of the week
- More whole grains
- More fish, less red meat, plus a daily omega-3 supplement
- Less high-sugar, processed, and refined foods
- Healthy hydration with plenty of water and tea and limited fruit drinks, sodas, caffeinated beverages, and alcohol in moderation

The key to transforming your relationship to food, says Wendy Bazillian, is to prioritize the taste and enjoyment of the meals, such that you can stick with healthy eating for the long haul. For some cooks, adjusting their typical diet to include these ingredients and guidelines will be easy. But, for others it will be helpful to consider adopting entire meal plans that may be familiar or easy to prepare. As you've likely already heard, traditional, culturally specific diets such as the Mediterranean or Japanese diet promote longevity. These diets are the definition of Downstate, heavy on antioxidant and anti-inflammatory superfoods, including produce, seafood, nuts, seeds, and whole grains or rice, complemented by small amounts of lean meats and dairy and steering clear from sugars, refined carbs, and trans and saturated fats. Both make fine choices, and both should pave the way to favorable Downstate outcomes, such as sounder sleep and sharper cognition.[69]

If you want to up your game even more, check out the MIND diet, which combines the Mediterranean style with the DASH (Dietary Approaches to Stop Hypertension) diet. The MIND diet features fourteen standout dietary components, including leafy green veggies, nuts, beans, whole grains, olive oil, and wine, and specifically recommends limiting red meats (fewer than four servings a week), butter and stick margarine (less than 1 teaspoon a day), pastries and sweets (less than five servings a week), cheese (less than one serving a week), and fried or fast food (less than one serving a week).[70] It's light on fruit, although berries are recommended, and daily fish consumption is replaced with a prescription for at least one serving a week, which evidence suggests is equally neuroprotective.[71] In a study pitting the MIND diet against the stand-alone Mediterranean and DASH diets, all three seemed to confer cognitive protection when followed closely. (Steadfast MIND diet adherence, for instance, was associated with 53 percent reduced odds of developing Alzheimer's disease after four and a half years of follow-up, which is huge!)[72] But perhaps even more exciting is that individuals who followed the MIND diet to a moderate degree, meaning they sometimes ate a little more red meat than recommended, or indulged in some extra sugar a few times a week, still enjoyed a 35 percent reduction in dementia risk. This moderation effect was not observed with the other eating plans. So, if flexibility is important to you, the MIND diet may be a winner.[73]

## Try Intermittent Fasting

We've already run down the long list of reasons why fasting is so good for your physical, mental, and emotional health. And since you only do it occasionally, the great thing about fasting is that most of the time you won't even know that you are doing it, because you aren't! Anyone can make this eating regimen work, but I especially recommend intermittent fasting for people who have busy lives that include work dinners and late nights, travel, and variable schedules. For these people, spending the occasional day restricting calories will be a whole lot easier than trying to accommodate the daily shutdown that is required by time-restricted eating.

The shock and awe method is to just not eat anything once a week. There is something so simple about this: don't think, just get the hell out of the kitchen. But, for many this might be too distressing. Luckily, there are several more palatable versions of intermittent fasting, such as the 5:2 plan (you eat normally for five days a week and limit yourself to a single 500- to 600-calorie meal a day on two nonconsecutive days) or alternate-day fasting (you alternate normal eating days with days in which you consume 25 percent of your usual intake). These versions offer similar Downstate benefits, instigating the RESTORE effects of full-on fasting while preventing you from eating your own offspring.

Here are some tips for starting out. First, ease into the fasting practice by choosing a once-a-week fasting window that will not send you running for the hills, such as 16:8, which is sixteen hours of fasting (e.g., six p.m. to ten a.m.) and eight hours of eating (e.g., ten a.m. to six p.m.). Eating a meal is a social occasion so you will need to think about what fasting schedule allows you to still get the most out of your social life, be it family dinners, business lunches, or taco Tuesdays. On your fasting day, delay your breakfast slightly and drink lots of water, coffee, and black or green tea (hot drinks need to be straight up, no sugar or cream). During your eating hours, choose nutrient-rich, whole foods with lots of protein—foods that will give you energy over a long time and not spike your blood sugar. Also, keep busy, get your body moving outside with some moderate- or even high-intensity exercise, and gobble down water (with a slice of lemon if you are fancy) whenever you feel hungry. You know you are drinking enough water if your urine runs pale yellow to clear each time. From there you can gradually move into wider fasting windows, such as 18:6, 20:4, 22:2, all the way to the full-on OMAD (one meal a day) at 23:1. At first, you might feel a little tense about timing your meals and what you eat, but eventually your body will fall into a rhythm where you don't have to look at the clock to know when it's mangia-time or when it's time to leave the kitchen for the rest of the night.

For choosing your meals, it helps to get really clear on the minimal number of calories you need to consume. The website tdeecalculator.net is helpful for determining how many calories you need depending on your sex, age, weight, and amount of daily exercise (sedentary, low, moderate, or high). It also breaks down the ideal proportion of calories devoted to protein, fats, and carbs, depending on if you're shooting for a low-, medium-, or high-carb diet. For me, on days when I'm sitting all day working at my computer or in meetings, I would be in the sedentary category and need around 1,473 calories a day, whereas on exercise days I might need a few hundred more. If I was doing alternate day fasting, I would then alternate that number with about 1,100 calories every other day (1,100 is 25 percent less than 1,473.) Calorie tracking apps can help you figure out the type and quantity of foods that fit in your eating plan. (For instance, which are the most nutrient-rich foods that will keep you under 600 calories on your 5:2 plan?) Whatever you choose, your body and mind will thank you. As always, speak to your doctor to figure out whether a fasting approach is right for you.

## Time-Restricted Eating: Schedule Your Meals to Occur Within a 12-, 10-, or 8-Hour Window

Do this to give your metabolism a substantial Downstate on a daily basis. The best part about this scheduled eating regimen is that you can forget about counting calories and just focus on the time you start and stop eating each day. I recommend this practice for people who have steady schedules, who can control when and where they enjoy meals, and who don't do too much traveling that might throw off your circadian rhythm and require work dinners.

Although the goal is to get you down to a ten-hour eating window, a good way to ease in is by choosing a window that might not even feel like a window at all, say fourteen hours. So, if you wake up at seven a.m. and eat breakfast at seven thirty, eat all day, and stop at nine thirty p.m. For many of us, this will cut out that midnight snack that our inner Mr. Hyde likes to slip by us just before bed. Commit to this window and you will already be giving your Downstate a huge gift of repose. Stay on this schedule for a few days or even a week, then decrease the window by one hour, which can be done relatively painlessly by shifting breakfast thirty minutes later and dinner thirty minutes earlier. As you gradually expand your fasting window, you can either eat in the earlier part of the day and fast later or delay your first mealtime till the afternoon. I recommend eating first thing in the morning and then fasting in the afternoon/evening, as you will feel fewer hunger pangs, reduce your chances of getting hangry during the busiest hours of the day, have more energy and motivation for your workouts, and consume less alcohol. Remember to drink lots of water all day, tapering close to bedtime. You can gradually start moving yourself closer and closer to the 10-hour eating window that delivers fourteen hours of pure, unadulterated Downstate . . . the kind that can only happen when REV is tucked in bed and RESTORE has full reign of the kingdom.

## Golden Habits of Highly Effective Circadian Rhythms: Set Consistent Mealtimes

Just as your cat wakes you up to feed her at the same hour each morning, even on Sundays, your circadian clock is highly motivated by predicting when it's going to get some grub. Think about hunger pangs, which are really just the ghrelin hormone sending off signals to your brain that it's eat-o-clock. There is nothing inherent in the noon hour that requires nutrients; it's just the time you usually eat, so fifteen or so minutes before the lunch bell your metabolic system is setting itself up to receive a bolus of fat, carbs, and protein. If you moved across the country and started eating lunch in your new time zone, your circadian rhythm would take about a week to get the memo, but eventually your leptin alarm clock would reset itself to the new schedule. When you eat at random times across the day and night, your metabolic system can't prepare your body for caloric onslaught, which leads to inefficient metabolism, increased chances of weight gain, and even worsens your sleep.[74]

So, a golden habit for eating is to set consistent mealtimes and stick to them. Whether you're someone working with a fasting schedule or not, you can help your brain know that nutrition-is-coming-so-get-ready by always having breakfast, lunch, and dinner, as well as snacks at the same time every day. Another helpful way to work with your metabolic rhythm is to keep your meals consistent in quantity and quality. If you have your big meal in the middle of the day, stick with that pattern most days and only have a big feast at night on special occasions like date night or birthday parties. The added benefit of consistency is that you spend less time agonizing over what or where you'll eat and more time enjoying the meal and being productive in other ways.

# CHAPTER SEVEN

# Guess What?
# You Are Aging NOW!

———— • ————

As pesky young kids, we had it all: robust circadian rhythms that kept us alert all day, then helped us crash into a long, unbroken escape to Neverland each night, despite our cavalier use of such sleep blockers as caffeine and alcohol. Our Upstate action and Downstate repair systems were robust and required no attention; we worked hard and played hard, and our ability to bounce back was naturally the best it would ever be. Plus, we naturally tended to engage in activities that supported Downstate recovery by exercising and spending time outside in the bright sunshine. (Remember that feeling of invincibility against the forces of late night bar-hopping and two a.m. cheese fries at the diner?)

Aging, as I have gathered from a life researching this process, is about far more than counting the number of candles on your birthday cake; it's actually a process of erosion that can be determined by the actions you take or don't take to regulate your Upstate-Downstate ratios. In our thirties and forties, we hit the gas pedal on every aspect of life, reaching for new personal, family, and career goals that can have us scratching our heads in a "How did I get here?" Talking Heads kind of way . . . the beautiful house, beautiful wife, and all our accomplishments that we never would have thought possible in our youth. And though most of these reasonable stressors are wonderful and life-affirming and get us to reach beyond our comfort zone, the pressure to do it all and have it all can wear us down, and the telltale signs of an overextended life pile up: poor sleep, stress, never enough time for self-care.

Look around—we are all pulled in a million different directions, pushing ourselves to keep up professionally with our peers, alongside the endless well of need emanating from kids and parents (welcome to the Sandwich Generation). Financial obligations compound. We're besieged by spoon-fuls of crisis, terror, and danger on the news. Add to this the encroaching age-related changes to our sex hormones, sleep, metabolism, cognition, sex drive, and general health. No wonder anxiety and depression keep tapping on our shoulders urging us to lose the little hold on our sanity that we are maintaining. Each of these life experiences is a stressor that activates REV, requiring a mighty dose of RESTORE to balance us out. And though one stressor might be manageable, by the time we hit our thirties, we're usually juggling at least three or four at a time.

Given the crush of pressure, the first thing we tend to drop are the exact practices we so desperately need to replenish our daily resources, fill up our love-levels, and give ourselves the strength to leap tall buildings in a single bound. Like kids trading baseball cards, we swap Downstate favorites, such as daily walks, spending time with friends, and preparing healthy meals, for more common Upstate ones, such as sitting at a computer for hours on end, increasing nightcap pours, eating just-add-water foods, and hitting the pillow way past our bedtime. This slow creep into overindulgence in Upstate Parties and sedentary living only steepens past age fifty.

Ignoring our Downstate needs as we slide into our thirties and for-ties starts to bite back posthaste. Studies of cognitive abilities across the decades demonstrate significant loss to long-term and working memory, attention, logical reasoning, and processing speed manifesting in our thir-ties and steadily slipping downhill from there.[1] Starting at age forty, we begin to lose muscle mass, which translates to a weaker, less robust body that grows more vulnerable to falling and fractures.[2] In our fifties, under the pressure of runaway oxidative stress and inflammation, our once flex-ible and elastic arteries that were designed to squeeze and push blood to distant tissues and cells start to stiffen, leading to increased blood pressure and risk of cardiovascular disease.[3] One of the top complaints at this age is sleep disturbance, and a large longitudinal study has tied short sleep (six hours or less) in our forties and fifties to a thirty percent increase in risk for dementia thirty years later.[4]

Many of these symptoms of decay are all due to the gradual wearing away of Downstate functions and growing momentum of out-of-control

Upstate excess, including accelerations in oxidative stress, chronic inflammation, and mounting autonomic imbalance. As we age, three Upstate markers—suppressed RESTORE, inability to dial down REV, and reduced heart rate variability (HRV)—worsen.[5] The slippery slope starts when we let go of our Downstate self-care practices in our thirties and forties and become a midlife or older person who dedicates almost no time to Downstate-regulating activities.

Yes, there are the rare folks in their seventies and eighties, such as my Aunt Nancy, who zips from activity to activity, throwing on sneakers for her morning constitutional around her tree-lined neighborhood before meeting up with friends for lunch at her favorite vegetarian café, followed by a lecture at the local museum. But they are the exception, not the norm. And to avoid this rapid swerve into pathological aging that has taken over our modern society, we have to build in Downstate time as early in our lives as possible . . . and continue to nurture it in perpetuity.

All this to say that if you're in your thirties and think you can skip this chapter, you might want to reconsider.

Let's take a look at the main anti-Downstate culprits accelerating the downhill go-cart across the decades. But, worry not, because it is never too late to start getting your Downstate on and this chapter is chock-full of evidence that doing so will keep your engine running smoother and longer.

## Autonomic Imbalance

Autonomic imbalance is at the heart of the aging process. In young, healthy people, the two branches of the autonomic nervous system are in equilibrium. But, this exquisite and much-needed balance starts to get out of whack as we age. The overall result is that REV dominates because RESTORE can't muster its natural defenses the way it used to, resulting in worsened cardiovascular control, decreased HRV, and a state of autonomic imbalance that can lead to greater risk for heart disease, depression, diabetes, and dementia.[6] One of the main reasons the bottom drops out of RESTORE is that you lose the protective shelter of nightly slow-wave sleep (SWS) with every increasing decade starting in your twenties.[7] Instead of an overnight train whisking you away for a "cardiovascular holiday," sleep becomes more like the local train, making disruptive stops that jerk you awake all night, and your daily make-things-right dose of restorative sleep simply doesn't happen. Contributing to the autonomic imbalance is an increasingly overactive immune system in older adults, which promotes inflammation. As mentioned in Chapter 1, this *inflammaging* is caused by a breakdown across several pillars of health, including metabolism, regenerative processes, immune response, gut microbiome, and adaptation to stress, which strongly predicts risk for chronic disease and mortality.[8]

Getting older also means spending more time alone as partners and friends die, family moves away, and mobility decreases, all of which can spell loneliness. Being alone and frail can feel stressful and unsafe if you can't rely on your youthful brawniness and mental faculties as you used to and there are no cave mates around to make you feel protected. Loneliness speeds up age-related physical deterioration, with more rapid decline in your ability to get around.[9] Loneliness can inflame stress, such that everyday challenges—for instance, getting to the grocery store or figuring out bus schedules—can instigate adverse inflammatory and REV responses, worsen immune function, and lower HRV. Among healthy adults aged forty to eighty-five, lonelier people with lower HRV have shorter telomeres, caps at the ends of chromosomes which, like your palm's life line, can be used to predict longevity.[10] Shortened telomeres are associated with pathological cellular aging and more severe response to immune challenges.[11]

One of the best antidotes to the heightened REV and cardiovascular strain seen in lonely aging people is boosting RESTORE activity.[12] Retrieving your Downstate autonomic wingmen from the abyss is relatively simple and yields excellent results. Remember the Action Items from Chapter 3—your tickets to Vagus, baby? When practiced throughout life, these pro-RESTORE habits have the power to slow the aging process. Mindfulness practice in older populations, for example, increases HRV.[13] Slow, deep breathing in older adults can reduce blood pressure, especially in individuals with hypertension; it also increases endurance, muscle strength, and lung capacity.[14] An intervention study that had older adults practice HRV biofeedback for three weeks (just six 30-minute sessions), reported improvements in depression, anxiety, and attentional skills, with several participants reporting better stress management and sleep quality.[15]

## Sleep

You have already learned how healthy sleep goes hand in hand with successful memory and executive functioning. Well, as you grow older, these two processes stay in lockstep with each other, which means that you could be in the lucky minority of people who sleep like a stone and remember like an elephant . . . or you could be in with the rest of us, whose sleep and cognitive processes start to decay into a drunk stumble as the years go by.

Beginning in their midthirties, many adults find themselves counting too many sheep when they lay down to sleep, then feel inexplicably wide awake for a couple of hours starting at 2:43 a.m., give or take. The sleep you *do* get can feel less restorative because of those middle-of-the-night awakenings and less time spent in deep SWS, leading to what sleep researchers call *fragmented sleep*. One study estimated that age-associated disruptions in sleep contributed to a loss of about thirty minutes of sleep per night each decade, beginning in our forties.[16] Worst of all, a significant decline in slow waves begins in middle age, with those all-important frontal cortex slow waves ebbing most dramatically, taking with them the critical foundation for Central Command executive function, long-term memory, and self-regulation. Studies have shown that the decline in slow waves across the years is directly related to neural degeneration, including atrophy of the prefrontal cortex and reduced communication between the hippocampus and cortex.

This is bad. Just like any muscle that dwindles without constant training, when you don't use your memory and executive function networks, they stiffen, shrink, and can't do their job. You really don't want these brain areas shutting down chit-chat with each other because it leads directly to memory and executive function failure. And without powerful slow waves washing away the unforgiving cobwebs made up of proteins, amyloid-β, and tau night after night, these substances become the plaques and tangles associated with Alzheimer's disease. This is not just a problem for patients who currently have mild cognitive impairment (MCI, a milder form of dementia) and Alzheimer's disease; cognitively normal older adults with poor sleep show signs of Aβ and tau plaques and tangles, especially if they lack robust slow waves and sleep spindles.[17]

The longer this spiral continues, the harder it is to engage these cognitive networks when you need them, such as when remembering which pills

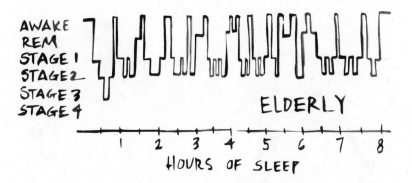

A Typical Progression of Sleep Stages Across the Night in Elderly Adults

you already took today, how to get across town, or what you went upstairs to look for. As the communication between your brain's memory areas (hippocampus–frontal cortex) worsens, memory problems mount, and like the proverbial dog, you're less able to learn new tricks. Instead, you start relying on old habits and rote procedures that have been long drilled into your memory, thus requiring much less brain power to carry out: going to the same shops, buying the same foods, taking the same route home, watching the same shows. This is exactly why cognitive neuroscientists recommend that you never stop pushing yourself to stay intellectually engaged and curious.[18] Learn Italian after you retire; join Road Scholar to stay socially active; attend lectures on topics that have always interested you; use different routes to get home without relying on your GPS; play games that challenge you; try to remember that actor's name without Googling it. These actions will be the motivational wind you need to steer your boat toward new and exciting destinations after middle age, while at the same time flexing and flushing out your hippocampal–frontal cortex networks well into your later years.

All of these problems start and worsen because the sleep and circadian Downstate mechanisms put in place to keep you functioning optimally are foundering. And if you have the job or the family duty to care for pathologically aging people, their sleep problems substantially increase your own caregiver burden.[19]

Significant hits to your circadian systems become apparent after fifty, likely due to a combination of factors. First, your brain activity decreases. Neuron-to-neuron communication slows; blood doesn't flow from the

**The Vitality of Slow Waves Affects Brain Function and Cognition.**

body to the brain with the same youthful joie de vivre as it used to; and you have that shrinkage and rigidity I mentioned in regions of the brain responsible for learning, memory, and executive function.[20] The suprachiasmatic nucleus, the main driver of timing signals to the brain and body, starts to peter out after age fifty, making it harder to stay awake or asleep when you want to.[21] Age-related changes have also been identified in the visual system that impair the processing of blue light, which is exactly the type of light your circadian rhythm needs to shake you awake and keep you peppy all day.[22] Older people also tend to lead a more sedentary, indoor lifestyle, resulting in a deficiency of bright light during the day. In fact, research demonstrates that middle-aged adults only receive approximately fifty-eight minutes of bright light per day, whereas older adults in assisted-living facilities fare even worse at thirty-five minutes per day.[23] All of these small changes add up to reduced and delayed melatonin and core body temperature changes, the two most important circadian "It's Downstate time" signals. If you can't see well, or you're shut indoors all day, you miss the crucial cues sent by the bluish rising morning sun and the rosy-red setting sun at night. This is one reason that older individuals tend to awaken earlier, feel tired throughout the day, hit the sack earlier, then experience fragmented, unrestful sleep throughout the night. Together with autonomic imbalance and decreased deep sleep, that brings too much REV and not enough RESTORE, and you find yourself in an Upstate wasteland.

The effects of these changes are thrown into stark relief in my lab, where we have hooked young people and seniors up to electrodes to measure their brain activity and HRV as they fall asleep. In healthy young adults, we typically see a steady shift from light to deep sleep with a long luxurious soak in SWS that is matched with skyrocketing HRV. But in the sixties-and-up set, many have almost no slow waves and no change at all in their HRV from wake to sleep. These are otherwise healthy individuals, with no major chronic health conditions, but they fail to provide evidence of any meaningful slow wave activity and RESTORE regeneration as they sleep.

This doesn't have to be you. We know it's possible to slow the age decline by getting your sleep ducks in order. Sixty percent of MCI patients have a history of sleep problems, but treating sleep disturbance during mid-life delays the onset of the disease.[24] So, even if you are nowhere close to showing signs of impairment, the earlier you set up a Downstate-oriented approach to your sleep, the better your chances of never receiving that MCI diagnosis in the first place. Getting to bed early will put you in the right time frame for soaking up as many SWS hours as possible, and adding a little melatonin to your evening ritual can also improve your sleep quality.[25] Meditation that includes deep breathing increases SWS and HRV.[26] Exercising also boosts SWS, and the brains of exercising older adults show greater communication between memory brain areas (hippocampus and frontal cortex) than their nonexercising peers, which is also reflected in more flexible thinking.[27]

Another major reason that we lose deep SWS and the precious slow waves therein is that the circadian control of our bladder, which is trained to keep things flowing during the day and zipped up all night long, starts to fail, making us feel the need to pee multiple times a night, increasing fragmented sleep and eliminating slow waves. Reducing your liquid intake three hours before bedtime will help here.

Also, remember that you are the boss of your circadian rhythm and can make it sit, stay, and roll over with consistent habits and light cues.

One study found tailored lighting for nursing home and assisted living residents decreased sleep problems, increased their sleep amounts, and reduced depression.[28] Another study showed that just four weeks of an in-home tailored lighting intervention, including morning light boxes and reduced evening blue light, boosted sleep efficiency and reduced depression in older adults.[29] Let's make sleep and circadian rhythms your dog.

## Exercise

Thirty-one million adults aged fifty or older are inactive.[30] To put that in perspective, the sixty-five-plus population currently numbers close to fifty million in the US alone. That's a lot of sedentary seniors. This inactivity is downright dangerous, as it can lead to muscle and bone loss, unhealthy weight, hardening arteries, increased risk for Alzheimer's disease and early death.[31]

On average, you will lose 1 to 2 percent of lean muscle mass *every year* after age forty.[32] Sarcopenia has been linked with physical limitations and disability, dementia, and brain atrophy.[33] In fact, in a study of those aged forty years and up, people with low muscle mass and strength were six times more likely to have cognitive impairment.[34] These results are saying that it's not just the loss in overall muscle mass, but it's the loss of muscle *strength* that leads to cognitive decline, even more of a reason to drive up RecoveryPlus with a strength training class or video once a week. Indeed, physical deterioration appears to precede and lead to cognitive impairment and risk for Alzheimer's disease, as both kinds of poor functioning share common underlying states of low-level chronic inflammation, oxidative stress, and depression.[35]

If you're one of those people who have kept up their fitness levels since they were young, you've been doing yourself a huge favor, cognitively speaking, as people with relatively high levels of endurance, whatever their age, tend to perform better on tests of thinking and memory than people who were less active.[36] In a longitudinal study of older adults, those who exercised three or more times per week were more likely to be dementia-free at a six-year follow-up.[37]

But it's never too late to turn your fitness life around and still see benefits. Researchers tracked fitness levels and memory clinic enrollments of a group of people in Norway for twenty years, they found that people who spent a lifetime dedicated to exercise were 50 percent less likely to develop dementia, but even the subjects who started the study out of shape and gained fitness after middle age showed the same substantial reduction in their subsequent risk for dementia.[38]

Scientists even recommend a specific amount and type of exercise for maintaining your physical and cognitive fitness through the decades. There's the inescapable ten thousand steps recommendation, but recent longitudinal studies of middle-aged adults show that the benefits begin at seven thousand daily steps reducing your chances of dying early by 50 percent compared to those with fewer steps, with the longevity reaching 70 percent less chance of early death in the nine thousand–steppers.[39] And if you are minutes guy or gal, a similar study from Denmark showed that 2.5 to 4.5 hours a week of exercise increase longevity by 40 percent compared with less active people.[40] If you are this type, try interval walking, which involves repeated cycles of cranking up your heart rate to about 90 percent of your maximum for four minutes by increasing the incline of your treadmill or speeding up your gait, followed by three minutes of easy walking. One study had sedentary men and women aged seventy and up engage in either interval walking or gentle stretching. Memory performance and physical endurance improved only in the interval walkers. This fits exactly with what you learned in Chapter 5 about jumpstarting REV with a hard enough kick-in-the-pants workout to generate a robust RESTORE response, and all the goodies flow from there. These positive outcomes from exercise also apply to Older You, including boosting your HRV, regulating your circadian rhythm's release of melatonin, and increasing your SWS.[41] For people with physical immobility, well-controlled studies of chair-based exercises have shown similar improvements to strength, cognition, and depression.[42]

Exercise also brings people together outside, hitting three Downstate targets in one go. My sister Amy visits with many of her friends on vigorous walks around her neighborhood when the weather is warm and jumps on cross-country skis with her husband, Joel, when it snows. After her divorce, my friend Emmy joined the Sierra Club and turned into a monster backpacker who is either hiking or planning her next expedition with a whole new group of comrades.[43,44]

## TAKE A LOVE BOAT CRUISE TO THE DOWNSTATE

As I have said, sex is exercise too! But with age, it's common for both men and women to experience loss of interest or an inability to get and stay aroused. For some people, it's a welcome change. Nature and adventure writer Susan Fox Rogers said that the loss of sex drive after menopause was the best thing that happened to her, as it freed up her mind from hunting around for who, when, and where 24/7, which she replaced with an insatiable birding habit, authoring a couple of books to show for it.[43] But for those who feel frisky at age sixty and beyond, having a rich and plentiful sex life well into your eighth and ninth decades has secondary benefits for Central Command, as studies have shown that executive function is higher in people who are more sexually active.[44] And if you need a little help heating up the lower chakras, get ready because when you increase HRV, as will no doubt happen while following your Downstate RecoveryPlus Plan, your ability to get turned on both physically and psychologically warms up too. Check Chapter 3, where I describe autogenic training, which has specifically been used to help return warm feelings to your erogenous zones, and Chapter 8, where I will guide you through the autogenic meditation.

## Nutrition

A diet filled with McFood isn't a sound idea for anyone, but at least when you're young you have a RESTORE insurance plan in the form of an inherently active lifestyle, plenty of SWS, and time outdoors bathing in circadian-regulating sun. If you aren't careful, those natural protections can get stripped away with each passing decade, and what was bad for you at age twenty-five becomes potentially ruinous at age forty-five. Your tools for combatting oxidative stress and inflammation are simply not as *fuerte* as they used to be.

Aging is often accompanied by a reduction in the amount and variety of fiber-containing foods. Fiber is food for Gerald, your microbiome, which, in return, produces health-promoting short-chain fatty acids, low levels of which may also be linked with stereotypically age-related conditions, such as reduced appetite, vitamin D deficiency, and more.[45] Lower fiber intake also leads to decreased microbial diversity (and a corresponding overabundance of some of the unhelpful bacteria strains, such as *C. difficile*), which is detrimental not only to gut health itself, but has been associated with worsening frailty (a geriatric syndrome characterized by weakness, weight loss, and low activity that renders rollerblading down the boardwalk fully out of the question).[46] Fortunately, eating fiber every day can slow and even reverse common age-related changes, such as muscle loss and obesity. When Australian researchers followed people aged forty-nine and older for a decade, they found that those who ate the most fiber were nearly twice as likely to age successfully—defined by the research team as "being free of disability and chronic disease (coronary artery disease, stroke, diabetes, and cancer); having good mental health and functional independence; and having good physical, respiratory, and cognitive function"—than the low-fiber group.[47] Mortality was lower in the high-fiber group too.

With each passing decade, an anti-inflammatory diet becomes more important. I've already sung the praises of a diet that's heavy on the produce, nuts, beans, whole grains, and olive oil while reining in sweets, butter, cheese, red meat, and fried food. This plant-forward approach has proven Downstate benefits in terms of reducing oxidative stress, preserving cognition, and enhancing sleep, along with being environmentally friendly.

What I'm telling you, then, is that eating as you would while on a Greek Isles vacation, including veggies doused in olive oil, broiled salmon with a side of couscous, and a glass of red wine will help you stay lean, strong, and sharp. Kind of a no-brainer.

The traditional Japanese dietary pattern, which includes lots of soybean products, fish, seaweed, vegetables, and green tea, can check off plenty of boxes on your Downstate Bingo card too. The fatty acids in the fish and isoflavones (beneficial plant compounds) in the tofu, edamame, miso soup, and other soy products are known to positively impact cognitive function and show promise in reducing dementia odds. Higher soy intake can help you sleep longer and harder, which may have to do with the fact that isoflavones behave similarly to estrogen in the body, and estrogen, as any woman in the throes of menopausal insomnia will tell you, is vital for good sleep.[48] Eating the Japanese way is also linked with less physical disability and is one reason so many Okinawans are able to achieve centenarian status.[49]

And to help keep your microbiome teeming with a diverse array of good bacteria, make sure to include fermented foods whenever possible; grab a tub of yogurt at your local grocery store; or, as the hippies at my college did, make your own bacterial petting zoo in a mason jar full of kombucha starter or kefir grains.

## I Am Woman, Hear Me ROAR!

Although the Downstate is 100 percent relevant to both sides of the sex spectrum, I'm going to spend some time talking to the half of the population who has been dealt an all-aces hand when it comes to rhythms. The crazy thing is some of us don't even know what a gift it is! This is because for most of written history, women have been told by doctors, scientists, university presidents, magazines, and even other women that the very fact that we were born with these natural rhythms is a problem; that girls' brains are deficient in some critical thinking area; that menstruating makes us unqualified for positions of leadership; that menopause is a disease; and that wrinkles aren't sexy. These perspectives have dominated the public and academic discourse, encouraged toxic standards of femininity, and promoted overflowing shelves of books that tell us that all we have to look forward to after age forty-five is sickness, loneliness, and dying. Like my tween daughter's T-shirt says: *First of all, NO! Second of all, NO!*

Being a woman is an awesome experience for so many reasons. One of the most profound is that during our reproductive years, we are in sync with a natural rhythm that imbues every day with an extra layer of color. I like to think of our monthly hormone rhythm as a microcosm of the rhythm of an entire year: the fertile spring starts just after menses with a great big burst of the sex hormone estrogen; the verdant summer is a lush phase of both estrogen and progesterone; then just like the leaves on the trees, during the fall, all sex hormones plunge, preparing us for the how-low-can-you-go hormone dance during the dormant winter menstruation. Each of these phases takes approximately seven days, rendering the cycle more or less the same as a lunar cycle (though whether the moon phases influence the reproductive cycle is still up for debate).[50]

Yes, hormones can make some women more vulnerable to swings in emotion, sleep, body image, cravings, and cognitive ability, particularly as estrogen and progesterone drop during the "fall" of our monthly cycle, or during menopause. But they are also what make us as strong, smart, and powerful as we are, and they protect our minds and bodies during the reproductive years.

But when they eventually ebb, women become especially vulnerable to a wide range of problems, all of which point to an inability to maintain a strong Downstate. Understanding the ways in which the Upstate/Downstate cycles are particularly programmed in women and how they change across the life span is the best way to ensure you're ready for these changes as they occur.

## HORMONES DROPPIN' LIKE THEY'RE HOT

Both females and males have plenty of the two main sex hormones, however, testosterone is usually considered the "male sex hormone" because when present in larger amounts, more masculine sexual behaviors are displayed, whereas estrogen is usually considered the "female hormone." Estrogen is found in large amounts in the prefrontal cortex and hippocampus, which explains why women tend to have superior short-term and long-term memory, verbal skills, and perceptual speed and accuracy compared with men.[51] In fact, studies from my lab have shown that while we are riding high on estrogen and progesterone during the spring and summer menstrual phases, we also have the most powerful slow waves and sleep spindles and the highest level of memory consolidation to boot, compared with our winter phase (menstruation) when these sleep processes and their cognitive benefits weaken.[52]

When hormones take *la plungée* (e.g., during major transitions such as the days before menses, postpartum, and perimenopause), women are more prone to mood disturbances and depression, cognitive impairment, sleep troubles, and physical ailments.[53] A primary reason for these negative outcomes is that along with our hormones, our Downstate recovery systems also take a nosedive. Women are 1.5 times more likely to report sleep disturbances than men, particularly the week before menses when sex hormones are in free fall, as well as other premenstrual symptoms, including breast tenderness, swelling, headache, sudden mood changes, irritability, depressive mood, and changes in eating habits.[54] Any number

## BEING A WOMAN AND . . . HOW INTERSECTIONALITY CAN CHIP AWAY AT YOUR DOWNSTATE

Social inequality starts when we are young and has a major influence on our Upstate/Downstate balance throughout our life spans. Exercise is one of our lifelong tickets to the Downstate, but from birth, boys are encouraged to be more physically active and stronger than girls, whereas verbal skills and emotional intelligence are fostered in girls.[55] As a consequence, girls often become more sedentary than boys as early as age six, and the majority of girls partake in almost no physical activity outside of school gym classes throughout adolescence.[56] In general, women are less likely to meet federal physical activity guidelines (aerobic and muscle-strengthening activities) across every age group compared with men of the same age groups.[57] The impact of exercise inequality is far reaching, with higher rates of exercise in men associated with higher education and household income.[58]

Along with sex-based barriers, racial barriers can impact your health, a phenomenon termed *intersectionality*, whereby multiple types of discrimination build upon one another.[59] In general, exercise is promoted in well-educated and wealthy White men above all other categories, with women of color having the least access to exercise likely due to low socioeconomic status and a lack of availability of leisure time, autonomy, or flexibility in the workplace, as well as poor access to childcare.[60] These differences start early, with Black American girls engaging in the lowest amounts of physical activity, a gap that widens during adulthood.[61]

Women typically experience higher levels of stress than men due to many factors, including greater responsibilities at home, microaggressions at work,

of these symptoms combined seriously curtails Downstate deep sleep and increases risk of insomnia, unrefreshing sleep, tiredness, nighttime awakenings, and unpleasant dreams.[55,56,57,58,59,60,61,62]

The last week of a woman's cycle can be autonomic misery as well. The transition between fall and winter (i.e., the three days before your period starts) brings on deficits in RESTORE activity and increases in REV arousal, leading to autonomic imbalance. In addition, problematic relations with eating may also occur at this time, such as eating for emotional reasons and with less control. More snacking and unhealthy foods translate to glass ceilings, as well as the income gap, and stress eats away at their most precious Downstate commodity: sleep. Importantly, when women are in the same pay bracket as men, the sex differences in sleep are cut half, which is a strong argument for equal pay (as if we needed any). In addition, many women are single parents, working for lower wages, and have a lower income-to-needs ratio. This is especially true for women of color, as Black women have lower sleep quality than White women do, and this relation worsens as social economic status declines.

In the face of social inequality and the lived experience of one thousand little cuts delivered from the slights, threats, and advancement denials that impact women of color on a daily basis, Audre Lorde, Angela Davis, and others have urged a commitment to *radical self-care*. After her cancer diagnosis, Lorde wrote about how living as a Black lesbian in our world had robbed her immune system of the resources it needs to protect her from disease. "I had to examine, in my dreams as well as in my immune-function tests, the devastating effects of overextension. Overextending myself is not stretching myself. I had to accept how difficult it is to monitor the difference. Necessary for me as cutting down on sugar. Crucial. Physically. Psychically. Caring for myself is not self-indulgence, it is self-preservation, and that is an act of political warfare."[62] Note the difference she draws between stretching and overextending, self-preservation and self-indulgence. At its heart, radical self-care honors and uplifts all Downstate practices such that they are at eye-level with forces of the Upstate: not dominated, rather in the right ratio.

greater oxidative stress, inflammatory responses, and weight gain. In sum, the hormone transitions are some pretty clear and predictable beacons in a woman's life that can have a significant influence on long-term health and happiness.

Now here's the rub: these fluctuations happen monthly. Us girls know that once a month from the time we are twelve-ish, one week before bleeding, many of us lose our proverbial shit. Not all of us, but some of us definitely. What *Our Bodies, Ourselves* didn't tell us is that this is in large part due to a slump of our Downstate RecoveryPlus system: a lack of deep sleep, lower RESTORE activity, decreased exercise, and poor eating habits. We also know that these deficiencies are entirely predictable and preventable with only mild adjustments to daily life. Yet, it always amazes me that my female friends and I seem so caught off-guard when that time of the month comes around! We get into fights with our partners, eat crappy foods, decide to forgo exercise for the scintillating option of moping in our sweats, and we NEVER think that the emotional sinkhole we find ourselves in might be due to a drop in hormones. REALLY? Not until there is actual blood in our pants and the telltale cramps and aches does the light-bulb go on.

With a little forethought and planning, we can do better. By tracking where we are in our menstrual cycle, and how we feel in the days leading up to each bleed, like the seven-day weather forecast, we can predict when we will need to pay extra attention to our healing recuperative Downstate processes.

## POSTPARTUM BLUES

Another female-only factor that sends us on a hormone roller coaster is pregnancy, during which estrogen concentrations increase by a hundred-fold, then plunge rapidly after delivery.[63] Again, it's the sudden ramping up and down of hormones that affects us the most. The massive phys-iological and hormonal changes from pre- to postpartum can throw women out of balance in body and mind. During pregnancy, sleep distur-bances rear up during the first and third trimesters, including increased rates of insomnia, disordered breathing, increased nocturia (peeing), and physical discomfort. Once Baby is home, a full night of sleep will be all but a distant memory until she or he can sleep through the night, and even then, many of us sleep with one eye open, just in case . . . (Interest-ingly, studies have shown that mothers can make a split-second switch from deep rest mode to TEN-HUT mode at the sound of their baby's cry, whereas fathers seem immune to this "gift," the outcome being that moms typically lose more sleep than dads).[64] Unsurprisingly, the risk for postpartum depression skyrockets, thanks to intense hormonal fluctua-tions and subpar sleep.

## MENOPAUSE

As we reach the end of our reproductive years in our late forties and early fifties, our hormones start to lose their cyclic regularity, granting us all a golden ticket to Ms. Toad's Wild Ride Through Menopause. The 'Pause has the power to change every aspect of our lives, including access to the Downstate. As with menstruation, the great transition of menopause can affect some women like a feather dropping, whereas others feel as if a grand piano fell from the sky and landed right on their head. Hot flashes are caused in part by a sudden, uncomfortable burst of REV that wrenches one from deep Downstate sleep and impairs memory function.[65] One friend described the sensation as a sudden feeling of having a burning flame inside her. But, even without hot flashes, RESTORE can significantly decrease and HRV alongside it.[66] Memory complaints occur during menopause, and without the protection of sex hormones, this population of women becomes more vulnerable to age-related cognitive diseases, such as dementia.[67] Age and sex are two of the three major risk factors for Alzheimer's disease (genetics is the third), with women having a twofold greater risk after age seventy-five.[68] And whereas cardiovascular risks are reduced premenopause, postmenopausal women have equal if not greater risk for hypertension and cardiovascular disease compared with men, and similar findings have been shown regarding climbing rates of obesity.[69]

The important news here is that these changes that can negatively affect women across their life span are manageable and even somewhat avoidable. I'm not saying you can stop PMS with yoga or deep breathe away your hot flashes, but with a little planning, you can modify your risk factors in ways that enhance better sleep, boost RESTORE functions, and well-being at every age. Studies show that freshly menopausal women receiving noninvasive acupressure or practicing rejuvenating techniques, such as yoga, qigong, and meditation, all show improved sleep, lower REV, and greater RESTORE.[70] Some women benefit from adding hormonal support to soften the changes associated with aging. I know several women who swear by the stash of hormones they keep in their medicine cabinet that they take "when necessary," which they say is usually when they have had a bad night of sleep.

Wherever you are along the life span, taking a women-centric approach to understanding your Upstates and Downstates will help you gain insight into how to best support your whole system naturally.

## Yes, Men Age Too

Although men don't fall off the hormonal cliff like their XX peers, there's enough evidence to say that men experience their own personal abyss as their strength, virility, and motivation begin to wane in their forties and fifties. A study examining functional limitations in midlife men aged forty-five to fifty-nine reported that 40 percent of the group faced some level of difficulty with basic activities, including lifting, bending, squatting, walking, climbing stairs, rising from a chair and bed, and other self-care activities.[71] In the aged fifty-five and older group, that number rose to around 70 percent. Some of you may also have heard of the term *andropause*, or male menopause, to describe an unhappy grab bag of symptoms that happens to many men in their forties and fifties—among them, loss of sex drive and erectile dysfunction; difficulty sleeping and increased daytime tiredness; mood swings, depression, and irritability; loss of muscle mass and reduced ability to exercise; fat redistribution (such as developing a large belly or gynaecomastia, which is enlargement of breast tissue); as well as cognitive impairments, such as poor concentration and short-term memory loss; and a general lack of enthusiasm or energy. And although testosterone does decrease two percent each year starting in the thirties, it rarely gets low enough to account for all of these negative trends, suggesting there are other causes to blame.[72]

If it ain't hormones giving men trouble, what might be the source of these little valleys? Science has only recently begun to explore this question because for a long time it wasn't okay for men to acknowledge that age took a toll on them at all, as many of these changes conflict with society's standard notion of masculinity. In fact, the more a man subscribes to the 1950s definition of manhood as a self-reliant, dominant, emotionally and physically tough, risk-taking Superman, the lower the chances that he will ask for help when he needs it and, as a result, the greater his health risk.[73] American men die nearly five and a half years earlier than women, and they die at higher rates than women from twelve of the fifteen leading

causes of death.[74] Experts in men's health suggest that one of the promi-
nent reasons for men's shorter life spans is that society's gender roles pressure men to put their health at risk, including smoking, excessive drinking,
and dangerous sexual and driving decisions; putting work before self-care;
and avoiding help from medical and mental health professionals.[75] With all
of these Upstate excesses, it isn't surprising that the majority of individuals under age sixty-five who die from heart attacks are men.[76]

But it doesn't have to be this way.

You probably won't be surprised to learn that you can chalk up a lot of
men's age-related deterioration to an overabundance of Upstate stressors
without the proper amount of Downstate restorative processes. Considering sleep, my own lab has shown age-related loss of SWS and more frequent waking throughout the night, both of which are greater in men.[77]
Looking deeper into this loss, sleep science has found a specific decline in
slow waves that happens to affect men much worse than it affects wom-
en.[78] In particular, beginning in their midforties, men show more loss of
the frontal lobe slow waves, the ones from Chapter 4 that are important
for Central Command executive functioning and memory, which can make
them specifically vulnerable to age-related memory loss.[79]

Generally speaking, men swing more toward REV than RESTORE,
with lower HRV and a greater tendency toward autonomic imbalance, and
higher blood pressure between the ages of twenty and sixty. (Women's
blood pressure surpasses men's postmenopause.)[80] Cardiovascular disease
is also higher in men.[81]

Altogether, though, there is a lot to be positive about when it comes to
improving men's health because so many of this group's inherent risk factors can be turned around via simple Downstate lifestyle changes. It's time
to stop listening to those tired and harmful masculine standards that look
down on maintaining a healthy diet, and that say meditation, yoga, or mod-
erating your drinking isn't manly. The fact is that excessive alcohol consumption leads to sexual and erectile dysfunction, not to mention weight
gain and poor sleep, whereas keeping fit and trim helps men maintain their
let's-get-it-on juju.[82] Men also need to take more time for relaxing Downstate activities. A Finnish study of middle-aged men showed that rates of
Alzheimer's disease went down as trips to the rejuvenating sauna went up,
a benefit attributed to regular self-care more so than just the circulatory

### INTERVIEW WITH A BLEARY-EYED, FORTY-SOMETHING VAMPIRE

For years, I've gotten together with a few other families for Friday night BBQ. Our kids play and the adults talk. One of them, Carlos, let me in on a personal battle he was having with insomnia, giving me a firsthand view of its toll.

Carlos is a top executive at a company who was orchestrating the sale of the entire South American wing of this massive beast of a business. Work-related stress was at an all-time high, plus he was flying once or twice a month to South America, along with raising two amazing kids with his wife, Paula. On travel weeks, he would often depart on a Sunday for a day of travel, arrive at his hotel at dawn, shower, and head straight into turbulent and tense executive meetings for four days. He would take the red-eye back to San Diego Thursday night and head straight to the office for a full day of work on Friday. This may sound like a nightmarish schedule and indeed it was, but when he was just a little bit younger it wasn't a problem. When he hit forty-five, however . . . Something. Just. Broke.

When Carlos would return home from work each night, the only thing he wanted to do was sleep, but he also didn't want to abandon his post as father or bail on his only quality time with Paula after the kids went to bed, so he'd struggle to stay awake until ten p.m. Although he had no trouble falling asleep, exhausted as he was, at two or three a.m. his eyes would open, usually because his son had cried out, and that, as they say, would be that, sleepwise. Even if he tried going to bed at eight p.m., his internal clock would wait for five hours and then wake up at midnight, so no help there. In retrospect, Carlos believes the stress of waking up in the middle of the night to catch his weekly flight thrust him into a cycle that habitually roused him at that time *every* night, and once awake, the wheels of obsessive thinking about not being able to fall back asleep would take over, preventing rest of any kind. He spent two years in this ever-worsening situation. "It became the biggest problem in my life," he says. He never stopped functioning or doing what needed to be done, but every day would be the same: tired by day, sleepless by night.

Carlos tried different strategies, such as sleeping pills, which would work at first but lose effectiveness after a couple of weeks. He tried melatonin, CBD, and THC, none of which made a significant dent in the problem. I put him in touch with the UC San Diego sleep clinic and he spent a night hooked up to electrodes—a night he remembers fondly because it turned out to be the best sleep he had gotten in years, which is actually pretty typical for people visiting a sleep lab. Think about it: no kids, no psychological reminders of that tortured three a.m. arousal. Away from his home environment, he was also away from the prison that had become his circadian rhythm.

To treat his maintenance insomnia (middle of the night waking) the sleep doc put Carlos on a sleep restriction schedule that limited time in bed to five hours (e.g., eleven p.m. to four a.m.) every night in an attempt to force his brain to associate time in bed with sleep, not with being awake. "It was difficult, and I never really did it the way I should have," Carlos admits. "I always cheated by not getting out of bed at four a.m. exactly. So, I gave up on that." His sleep crisis became all-consuming, repeating cycles of nightly hope for rest met with daily confirmation of failure. His tiredness made him unhappy, irritable, and short-tempered with his kids, and left no time for his relationship with Paula.

Then, COVID-19 hit and everything changed, but maybe not the way you might think. Carlos's company moved his job to Mexico City, so the family left San Diego for a new life. Permitted to work remotely, released from international travel responsibilities, and with newfound time to devote to exercise, and manage his own schedule, his sleep problems dissolved. He believes getting regular daily exercise was one of the most critical changes he made. At first, he started slowly, going for a light walk or bike ride a few times a week, and eventually got into taking an early morning swim for thirty to forty-five minutes, seven days a week.

"The pandemic forced me to completely change the dynamic that had been creating my sleep problems, and there was this drastic change that happened seemingly overnight that really got me over the hump." he said. Carlos's example illustrates an important point, which is that getting unstuck from a broken record habit sometimes requires a massive disruption to bump you out of the well-worn groove established in your circadian rhythm. Before taking on his Downstate practice of incremental shifts in habits, he needed to make a big shift that would disrupt the very firmament of the Insomnia life he wanted to change. If you have been walking down the same street and falling into the same gaping pothole over and over, it could be due to circadian dysregulation, a drug or alcohol addiction, an abusive relationship, or a habitual psychological trigger, you might do better choosing to walk down a different street all together. Chapter 8's section entitled "What's Your Why?" (page 216) will guide you through a list of helpful questions as you embark on your transformational way.

benefits of heat.[83] Exercise is a great way to naturally increase testosterone levels, with resistance training slightly edging out aerobic training.[84]

Finding a way back to feelings, broadening awareness of how emotions manifest in the body, and learning skills to manage unwanted feelings, are especially important for men on their RecoveryPlus path.[85] Any therapy or mindfulness training that focuses on emotion regulation, including dialectical behavioral therapy skills training, emotion-focused therapy, acceptance- and mindfulness-based therapy, and emotion-regulation therapy, will do the trick.[86] Taking these steps will turn self-care into a Downstate Maven strategy that will help you be a better person, friend, son, brother, father, or partner.[87]

## The Straight Story:
## To Age Well, You've Got to Respect the Downstate

Aging doesn't have to come as a package deal with chronic disease, fractured sleep, weakened muscles, and dozing mid-conversation. You can turn these ramifications of aging into the tired clichés they deserve to be by aging fearlessly—not in a Suzanne Somers, take-fifty-supplements-a-day-and-slather-your-body-in-yam-cream kind of way, but in a way that acknowledges the natural systems in place that support both sides of the activity and repose scale.

Think of the classic image of a street scene in modern day Havana, Cuba, filled with mint-condition Chevrolets and Fords from the 1950s. How do you think these cars have survived so long and remained solid enough to serve as a main source of transportation for many Cubans? Their owners don't run them into the ground and then throw their hands up and leave them by the side of the road. Quite the contrary; everyday Cubans have become expert automotive mechanics who know every subengine and how to keep each one purring through careful daily conditioning. I'm going to ask you to think of yourself as a 1958 Chevy Impala: You need to take care of your subengines! And the best way to do that, the best way to stave off many of the undesirable symptoms often associated with aging, and perhaps avoid some of them altogether, is by committing to the Downstate RecoveryPlus Plan. In the next chapter, I will show you how to do just that.

PART THREE

# Hitting the Reset Button

Now that you're ready for action, Part 3 will give you what you came here for. Chapter 8 introduces my four-week Downstate Recovery-Plus Plan, an evidence-based, multidisciplinary program I have developed that encompasses the most up-to-date scientific findings available.

Each week will be devoted to one of the four Domains of Action, the systems and activities that directly support Downstate function: the autonomic nervous system, sleep, exercise, and nutrition. Next, you'll be ready for Chapter 9, "Everything You Always Wanted to Know About the Future of the Downstate (but Were Afraid to Ask)," which will answer any and all questions you might have about the most cutting-edge, highly experimental Downstate-restoring methods of the future. Part 3 will end with me driving home the messages woven throughout the book—the importance of choosing the Downstate, valuing it, overcoming resistance (both personal and societal), and making peace with your resistances, fears, and insecurities (your inner NO!) instead of avoiding them or going with the Default options of life.

Is it far easier to come home from work, crack open a beer or can of rosé, order takeout, and watch TV until midnight than it is to prepare a real meal that's finished by seven p.m., watch just one episode of your favorite Japanese gangster series, do your deep breathing exercises, and tuck yourself in bed by ten p.m.? Hell, yes. But you will start small, adding only one Downstate action at a time, so your life will not feel as if it requires a full makeover. You will celebrate each "little w" (little win) on your way to the "BIG W." As Janelle Monáe eloquently sings, "To be victorious, you must find glory in the little things."[1] In time, these little Downstate activities will take firm root in your life, which will help you grow stronger branches with each daily Downstate practice. Before you know it, tending to your Downstate tree will be part of the widespread health boundaries you habitually set for yourself.

# CHAPTER EIGHT

# The Downstate
# RecoveryPlus Plan

———————— • ————————

Congratulations! You made it through the science jungle and now you're ready for action! The next steps will operationalize all you have learned and create your own uniquely tailored Downstate RecoveryPlus Plan to bring yourself back in sync with your natural rhythms. The Plan is divided into four areas of functioning that each promise to take you to your own private Downstate Wonderland. I call them the Domains of Action: Autonomic, Sleep, Exercise, and Nutrition. Think of them as the four legs supporting the stability and strength of the Downstate, with a list of Action Items under each domain, each item steeped in the science you've learned about in previous chapters.

The Plan is progressive, meaning in Week 1, you begin by setting in motion one Action Item from the first Domain, *Vagus, Baby*, and spend the week making it operational. In Week 2, you continue your progress on the item from Week 1 and add an Action Item from the next Domain, *Join the Rest-o-lution*. In Week 3, you keep up practicing the first two health habits while adding something from *Exercise Your Right to Recovery*. After adding an Action Item from *You Are What and When You Eat* in Week 4, you will be officially running a complete Downstate RecoveryPlus plan on all four cylinders.

Keep in mind that each Action Item promotes Downstate recovery, so you can't go wrong, no matter which one you choose. Here's an example of what your month might look like:

**Week 1:** Slow, deep breathing for five minutes every morning or evening

**Week 2:** Setting a bedtime and wake time window that you stick to seven days a week + slow, deep breathing every morning or evening

**Week 3** Exercising at least three times a week at consistent times each day + setting a consistent bedtime and wake time window + slow, deep breathing every morning or evening

**Week 4** Scheduling your meals to occur within a twelve-, ten-, or eight-hour window + exercise at least three times a week at consistent times each day + setting a consistent bedtime and wake time window + slow, deep breathing every morning or evening

On their own, each Action Item might seem small, but they are mighty. And combined, these small fixes to your everyday habits have the power to make life more supported, productive, organized, and fulfilling. When you stick with your Plan, you'll resonate with a universal rhythm that has guided all living things since the beginning of life on the planet. You'll feel greater well-being and connectedness to your body and emotions, greater patience and love for people around you, and that spark of energy that comes from getting in touch with nature and your own wild, natural self. Last but not least, replenishing the Downstate will lead to widespread improvements in health, including boosting heart rate variability (HRV), deepening your slow waves, improving fitness, and reducing risk of everything from heart disease and unhealthy weight to diabetes, cancer, and early death.

## What's Your Why?

Embarking on a life change, big or small, can feel exhilarating, frightening, and altogether too difficult. One of the primary reasons why we put up so much resistance to change is that adding a new activity, or putting the kibosh on an old, unwanted behavior, requires overriding the deep trenches our daily habits have worn into our psyche. Remember that starting a new health habit takes a massive top-down wave of Central Command energy to turn our intentions into actions.

Study after study has shown that the key to success lies in finding the motivation within—what I call figuring out your *why*—then determining and clearly stating your personal long-term goals to yourself, your community, and the universe. That's because once your intentions become explicit to you and everyone around you, the steps to your goal become clearer, and if you subscribe to any woo-woo philosophy, there's something to be said for putting your intentions out into the universe and seeing what comes back. I have been making a good-luck, black-eyed pea soup every New Year's Day for many years. Part of this ritual involves speaking my intentions for the year out loud, along with my highest hopes for those I love, as I chop the veggies and ham and stir them into the cauldron (it's very witchy). Identifying your *why* makes it easier to stick with the daily habits that are aligned with those goals, and to avoid behaviors that hurt them. You will also find that by sharing your goals with the people around you, they respect your personal health boundaries more and may even set up their own goals, the magic and beauty of social networks.[1] And by getting in touch with your highest aspirations, existing habits in conflict with those aspirations are thrown into stark relief—"My main goal is to get more sleep. Why am I watching Netflix every night until 11:59 p.m.?"—and that helps get you where you want to go.

So, to set yourself up for success with your Plan, I'd like you to do a bit of guided self-inquiry. Get a journal, a white board, or even a canvas, and something to write with—your favorite pen, markers, whatever feels good in your hand. You can even speak into a recording device. The point is to interview yourself in the privacy of your own soul and take note of your answers to these questions in whatever way inspires you and allows you to return to them again and again. Personally, I like to talk to myself out loud. If you want to try it, take a walk in the park, wherever you can be free to let this conversation with yourself really happen. In stating out loud or writing down these answers, you'll start to understand your own aspirations, and will have a living document or a mental reference to look to as you embark on your Plan, as well as a motivational force for when you find yourself slipping off-Plan.

Ask yourself these dig-deep questions:

- What do I value most in my life?
- What are my priorities?
- If I think about the future, what do I want for myself?

- If I was successful with the Plan, what would that look like?
- What does it look like when I'm not living out my values as fully as I would like?
- How are my current behaviors supporting my values and future goals?

The answers to these questions can help you figure out what motivates you.

Next, I'd like you to think about your internal resources and strengths (e.g., perseverance, patience, optimism) that will help you build a sense of empowerment, something you will rely on when the going gets hard. So please also answer these questions:

- Think about a time you made a big change in your life. How did you do it?
- What personal strengths do you have that help you succeed?
- What encourages and inspires you?
- Who are the people in your life who can support you through change?

One of the biggest challenges might be making yourself a priority: making room for yourself at the table, giving your needs and your desires equal weight to everyone else's, and believing that your worth is measured in more than what you do for others, and beyond external rewards. You may spend the majority of your life pretzeling into ridiculous contortions to make everything right for other people. You may be so used to running on empty because the concept of securing your mask to your own mouth and nose (à la the Oxygen Mask Rule of flying) before assisting others has never crossed your mind. You may look at your very full life and think that there isn't a single moment that can be sacrificed for your Downstate Plan. You may think that you have too many people depending on you to take time away from Doozering to be able to meet your own Downstate needs. Whatever story you have in your head that gives you an excuse to let life wear away at your health, cognition, and happiness, and eat away at your potential for RecoveryPlus in the Upstate, stop listening to it. Start listening to your body, start caring for your brain. Let the rhythms of nature be your coach. This is your life. Find your own rhythm and breathe into it.

## The Structure of the Plan

Although the Plan is organized into four weeks based on the four Domains of Action, there is nothing magical about this time frame. It sometimes takes more than one week to make a habit stick; and it's far more important for each practice to become embedded into your life in a way that is dependable and symbiotic than it is to keep up the pace of the Plan. The Downstate RecoveryPlus Plan works best when you optimize it to the timeline that suits your individual pace. Maybe the best approach is for you to take on one Domain a month, or even spend a whole season working a single Action Item into your life. Indeed, research on the time it takes to form a health habit shows a wide range, between 18 and 254 days with an average of 66 days.[2] That's because we are each equipped with a specific constellation of strengths and challenges. As such, each personal path takes the time it takes. Don't waste energy thinking about that perfect you that would have done things "better." She or he doesn't exist except between your ears.

How do you choose an Action Item? I suggest you select one that speaks to you or that you are curious about, or simply whichever one feels most convenient for your busy schedule. Try picking an easier Action Item in the beginning and working your way up to items that are more challenging for you. Sometimes it might seem that one Action Item is at odds with another in the same Domain. For example, eating breakfast might seem to conflict with time-restricted eating or intermittent fasting. But there are always ways of making these Action Items work together; you just need to be flexible. If you commit to eating breakfast and fasting one day a week, just skip breakfast on your fasting day. If your time-restricting eating means your meals occur within a ten-hour period, make breakfast the first meal and start fasting earlier in the day.

Once you've chosen your first Action Item, take at least a week to integrate it into your life before moving on to the next one. Of course, after reading Parts 1 and 2 of this book, you might be keen to jump into the deep end and adopt more than one Action Item right from the start. That's understandable and I love the enthusiasm. But at the same time, research shows that one of the reasons people have a hard time sticking with new habits is they set expectations too high for themselves and then, if they can't meet their demanding goals, they become disappointed and give up. Think of learning to juggle. A beginner would not be able to maintain more than one or two balls in the air, so she starts with throwing and catching just one and then introducing a second when ready. So, too, with the Plan—adding too many Action Items at once before settling into a comfortable rhythm with each one on its own can defeat the whole thing. So, setting yourself up for the big W's includes giving yourself the opportunity for a lot of little w's along the way.

Now, let's meet your Domains of Action . . .

## DOMAIN 1: Vagus, Baby

### ACTION ITEM #1

**Practice slow, deep nasal breathing.** The simplest way to instantly boost HRV and RESTORE is by slowing down your breath such that your inhale syncs up with the rhythm of your heart rate. Breathing through your nose for both the inhale and exhale ensures that your respiration is at its most efficient, giving enough time for your body to soak up oxygen from your inflated lungs and extending your tolerance of carbon dioxide. Nasal breathing also sends warm, moist, filtered air into your body, reducing dryness in your throat and pollution in your lungs. (Goodbye, runner's asthma!) The practice involves five counts on the inhale, five counts on the exhale. At a minimum, practice it for ten minutes every day—five minutes as part of your wake-up ritual and five minutes during your bedtime decompression ritual. Slow, deep breathing is Central Command's secret weapon, bringing inhibitory calm and control over REV, so you can remain cool under pressure.

### ACTION ITEM #2[3]

**Practice HRV biofeedback.** For this Action Item, you will need a device that can measure your heart rate and breathing rate, providing feedback to help you match your physiology with the information on the device. There are many systems to choose from and the market is constantly

**FOREST BATHING**

No forest? No problem. You can practice *shinrin-yoku*, or *forest bathing*, in the park. Just follow this short guide, adapted from Dr. Qing Li's book *Forest Bathing: How Trees Can Help You Find Health and Happiness*:

**Step 1**—Ditch your phone or other distractions, so you can be fully present.

**Step 2**—Leave behind any goals and expectations. Your only goal is to wander, allowing your body to walk wherever it wants.

**Step 3**—Take occasional pauses, investigating blades of grass or leaves, or noticing the sensation of the ground beneath your feet.

**Step 4**—Find a comfy spot to sit and listen to the sounds around you. Take in the sights and smells. As Dr. Li writes, "Let nature enter through your ears, eyes, nose, mouth, hands and feet. Listen to the birds singing and the breeze rustling in the leaves of the trees. Look at the different greens of the trees and the sunlight filtering through the branches. Smell the fragrance of the forest and breathe in the natural aromatherapy of phytoncides. Taste the freshness of the air as you take deep breaths. Place your hands on the trunk of a tree. . . . You have crossed the bridge to happiness."[3]

As a reminder: If you're practicing forest bathing with others, avoid talking until the end of the walk.

expanding, so do your research and figure out which one is right for you. My lab and many others use the HeartMath HRV biofeedback system for conducting HRV research. Their findings are published in peer-reviewed journals, reporting benefits to sleep, self-regulation, cognition, and stress management, with favorable results in professional sports and workplace environments.[4]

ACTION ITEM #3

**Connect with nature once or twice a week.** One of the best ways to decrease stress is to take your concerns to Mother Nature. She is big enough and strong enough to handle all of your tribulations. While you become absorbed in the massiveness of the trees or the grand emptiness of the desert and find a new perspective on your place in the universe, you'll breathe cleaner air and awaken all your senses. Visit a park, take a walk in the woods, stroll along a river or beach—the goal is to get yourself somewhere with an absence of buildings around you and no cement under your feet.

### ACTION ITEM #4

**Practice meditation three times a week.** Meditation engages your mind and heart through a wide range of approaches. There are very specific practices that coordinate body movements with breathing, such as qigong, tai chi, and yoga, whereas others guide your mental meandering, such as mindfulness, Vipassana, or Shoonya, which teaches conscious nondoing. Although meditation practices often get lumped together, there are significant differences between them, so I encourage you to explore various practices to help you decide which one suits you. You can study alone, in a group, with a teacher, at a workplace offering, or with a guided meditation app.

### ACTION ITEM #5

**Do twenty minutes of inversion poses three times a week.** When you get into a position where your head is below your heart, gravity does the work of draining the blood and lymph from your feet, legs, hips, sex organs, and GI system, filling up your chest, throat, arms, fingers, and, of course, brain. This position is less taxing to your heart and pushes oxygen and nutrients to that big old brain of yours. Options include basic yoga moves, such as Legs Up the Wall Pose (*viparita karani*), Supported Bridge Pose (*setu bandha sarvangasana*) done on bolsters, Downward Dog (*adho mukha svanasana*), shoulder stand (*salamba sarvangasana*), and headstand (*sirsasana*). Start with short sessions of seven minutes three days a week, morning or night, and gradually build up to twenty minutes. You can also start by lying on a bed with your lower half propped up with pillows. Remember, if you have high blood pressure, check with your doctor before attempting inversion poses.

ACTION ITEM #6

**Engage in consensual physical connection as much as possible.** You need to feel connected to people at a very basic level to function well. The most immediate way to send this message to REV is through human touch, which says, "Hey, look: I have friends that are so close to me that we're touching!" But when you are lonely and isolated, REV gets on edge, like a dog that thinks it needs to constantly secure the perimeter and attack any and all who approach its house. Consensual human touch tells that barking, growling, teeth-baring dog that it's okay, you are in charge and that you have friends who would come to your aid if you needed help. There are so many ways to fulfill this basic need: holding hands, sharing a hug, or walking arm-in-arm with friends and family; sitting close while watching a show or gazing at beautiful scenery; having sex with a partner with whom you feel safe; even joining a cuddle party where consensual adults engage in platonic sensual touch. A loving pet can also provide that grounding presence of another being who needs your comfort.

ACTION ITEM #7

**Practice autogenic training daily.** This mind-body practice is a useful tool for enabling Central Command to gently nudge RESTORE into a more dominant role. The key points of the practice are to bring heaviness to the muscles to increase relaxation and warmth to the abdomen and extremities to increase blood flow throughout the body, to steady the heart and breath, and to shift your energy away from your busy mind.

There are many versions of autogenic training, from short and sweet to longer and more detailed. I have chosen to offer the short and sweet version here, as it has been shown to be equally effective at increasing HRV along with other Downstate benefits.[5] If you're interested in exploring this training more deeply, I encourage you to read the *Relaxation and Stress Reduction Workbook* by Martha Davis, Elizabeth Robbins Eshelman, and Matthew McKay.[6]

Autogenic training's primary goal is to transform yourself into your own calming force, your own protective guardian, your own facilitator of physical relaxation. You will want to learn the key points by heart and then

## AUTOGENIC TRAINING SCRIPT

Take a few slow, deep, abdominal breaths before you begin mentally reciting the phrases. Imagine the sensations in each phrase happening in the body as completely as possible. Passively note what's happening in your mind and body. If you notice your mind drifting, that's fine; just gently return your focus to the practice. With repetition, you will drop into your body with more and more ease.

Repeat the following phrases to yourself six times, inserting a long pause between each one:

My left arm is heavy and warm, my left arm is heavy and warm, my left arm is heavy and warm, my left arm is heavy and warm, my left arm is heavy and warm, my left arm is heavy and warm.

I am calm and relaxed.

My right arm is heavy and warm, my right arm is heavy and warm, my right arm is heavy and warm, my right arm is heavy and warm, my right arm is heavy and warm, my right arm is heavy and warm.

I am calm and relaxed.

My left leg is heavy and warm, my left leg is heavy and warm, my left leg is heavy and warm, my left leg is heavy and warm, my left leg is heavy and warm, my left leg is heavy and warm.

My right leg is heavy and warm, my right leg is heavy and warm, my right leg is heavy and warm, my right leg is heavy and warm, my right leg is heavy and warm, my right leg is heavy and warm.

I am calm and relaxed.

My heartbeat is calm and strong, my heartbeat is calm and strong, my heartbeat is calm and strong, my heartbeat is calm and strong, my heartbeat is calm and strong, my heartbeat is calm and strong.

I am calm and relaxed.

My abdomen radiates warmth, my abdomen radiates warmth, my abdomen radiates warmth, my abdomen radiates warmth, my abdomen radiates warmth, my abdomen radiates warmth.

I am calm and relaxed.

My forehead is cool and relaxed, my forehead is cool and relaxed, my forehead is cool and relaxed, my forehead is cool and relaxed, my forehead is cool and relaxed, my forehead is cool and relaxed.

I am calm and relaxed.

My breath is deep and even, my breath is deep and even, my breath is deep and even, my breath is deep and even, my breath is deep and even, my breath is deep and even.

I am calm and relaxed.

My body balances itself perfectly, my body balances itself perfectly, my body balances itself perfectly, my body balances itself perfectly, my body balances itself perfectly, my body balances itself perfectly.

I am calm and relaxed.

Remain in this deeply relaxed state for a few more moments. This is a magical time when you are highly suggestible and able to plant seeds of your intentions, so think of a succinct phrase that captures one of your goals, maybe about one of the Action Items you are working on. For example: *I cultivate my Downstate by going to sleep at ten p.m. every night.* Bring yourself back to the present moment by deepening your breath and slowly moving your limbs, rotating the wrists and ankles and taking a gentle stretch. Say to yourself, "When I open my eyes, I will feel refreshed and alert." Then, make the transition to your daily activities.

---

Adapted from Martha Davis, Elizabeth Robbins Eshelman, and Matthew McKay, *The Relaxation and Stress Reduction Workbook*, 6th ed. (Oakland, CA: New Harbinger Publications, 2008).

use them to bring relaxation to any part of your body that needs it. You can start by writing down the main phrases or recording yourself speaking them with the goal of eventually committing them to memory. When starting, give yourself ten to fifteen minutes twice a day to build the skills that will allow you to activate it quickly, whenever you want. After the first few weeks, you can reduce your frequency, but make sure you're sticking with the practice at least three days a week. Once you've mastered it, you can make the practice your own by focusing on specific areas that need warmth and increased blood flow, such as an injured shoulder or your erogenous zones, or go in the opposite direction to cool down your revved-up mind by increasing circulation to a distant body part, such as your feet. You can also truncate the phrases to those that most efficiently deliver you into deep relaxation.

I suggest practicing somewhere quiet and safe so you won't be disturbed. You can sit upright or lie down—whatever allows you to feel most comfortable, preferably where your limbs don't touch any other parts of the body.

## DOMAIN 2: Join the Rest-o-lution, Deepen Your Sleep

### ACTION ITEM #1

**Early to bed, every night.** Slow-wave sleep (SWS) is perfectly positioned at the end of your busy Upstate day to sweep you off your feet, wash all the cobwebs out of your brain, deepen the neuronal bonds that hold your memories, repair and grow your muscles, restore levels of glycogen in the body and brain, promote widespread protein synthesis, and let RESTORE reign supreme, unhindered by REV's uppity blustering. Why would you want to miss that show? By going to sleep late, you do. The solution here is to get to bed by ten p.m., just in time for the Downstate opening credits to roll.

### ACTION ITEM #2

**Take naps three times a week between one p.m. and three p.m.** We are not made to function at maximum velocity and top performance across the whole day; instead, we deteriorate significantly when we keep working, and only a nap can restore our functioning . . . and even improve it to the same extent as a full night of sleep. Taking a twenty- to thirty-minute nap presses the reset button on your alertness and wipes the desktop clean of information build-up. A sixty-minute nap includes the rejuvenating powers of SWS, which is as important for your body as it is for your memory and executive functioning. A ninety-minute nap includes REM sleep, increasing your creativity and sensory abilities and building on the SWS benefits by integrating your new memories with the rest of your prior knowledge.

### ACTION ITEM #3

**Stop caffeine early in the day and all liquids three hours before bed. (Yes, that includes alcohol.)** We've talked about the reasons for limiting caffeine and alcohol; you'll also want to limit *all* liquid three hours before bedtime to avoid putting any undue pressure on your bladder during the night. Getting out of bed to use the toilet is one of the biggest sleep disruptors for older people.

### ACTION ITEM #4

**Take a nightly dose of melatonin.** Taking melatonin is not like taking a sleeping pill; you aren't knocking yourself in the head with a knobby caveman club and falling into oblivion. It's been shown to be safe for children and older adults alike, but always talk to your doctor before starting to take any supplements. The effects might be subtle enough that you may not be sure it's working because it doesn't immediately send you into an amnestic coma or cause you to wake up in a hotel with no memory of getting there. Try at least a week of a consistent dose and then ask yourself whether you're sleeping better than before you began taking it, or compared to the weekly averages in your RecoveryPlus Daily Journal (see pages 238 and 273).

### ACTION ITEM #5

**Control your light exposure.** Your circadian rhythms' primary language is light. The goal is to communicate with it in terms that it understands.

Large amounts of blue light bring on a rousing chorus of "Wakey Wakey, Eggs and Bakey!" and low amounts of blue light bring on a whispering "Rock-a-Bye-Baby." The sun is the OG circadian messenger, so simply spending fifteen minutes outside in the early morning is adequate. Sitting in front of a window in full sun may not give you the same circadian jolt. New windows are made to block the sun's rays, limiting the appropriate signals to your brain. If you are stuck indoors or you live in a winter wonderland that doesn't get enough bright sunlight, you can invest a little money in a full spectrum light box that you can turn on each morning while you eat breakfast, read, or partake in your favorite sitting-still activity. This is surprisingly powerful stuff, so no more than fifteen or twenty minutes is necessary.

Once you've set your circadian clock with the morning light signals, turn your attention to your evening lighting situation, which is also completely under your control. By six p.m., the lights of the universe naturally move into the orange and red spectrum. You need to mimic this shift in your home by turning off all fluorescents and LEDs with blue hues. Invest in warm lightbulbs or candles for your evening bedtime/bathroom rituals and orange-tinted nightlights for any middle-of-the-night bathroom trips. Minimize or ban blue light by using filters on your screens and blue light–blocking glasses. If you can't control the light around you, such as if you are arriving at night to a hotel with wakey wakey lights, wear dark sunglasses, like a mobster.

**ACTION ITEM #6**

**Keep a consistent bedtime and wake time schedule.** Consistency is a golden sleep habit of highly successful circadian rhythms. For this Action Item, you will commit to a one-hour window for bedtime and wake time (e.g., a bedtime of ten to eleven p.m. and a wake time of seven to eight a.m.), Monday through Sunday. Of course, there will be times when you stay out later or enjoy a lazy morning in bed, but as long as you get back to your rhythm the next day, you won't do any lasting damage to your circadian rhythm's internal clock.[7,8,9]

## SET UP A SLEEP DEN

The phrase "sleep hygiene" refers to the collective health boundaries you keep to enhance and deepen your sleep, and a good Sleep Den is the backbone. All the restorative Downstate Action Items in the world aren't worth a hill of beans without creating the physical space for them to get their proper start.

Here are my top eight tips for designing your Sleep Den:

1. Keep it cool. A too-warm bedroom can leave you sweaty and restless, and a higher core body temperature is a sign of REV arousal and can suppress restorative SWS.[7] Anywhere between 60° and 69°F is optimal for restful sleep.[8] To artificially create a big difference in temperature between your extremities and your core, try the following: lower your thermostat, strategically arrange your bed covers and body position (e.g., letting your feet and arms peek out of the covers), or even take a warm shower or bath right before bed (as your body temperature drops back to normal afterward, you'll feel sleepy). See what combination works for you.

2. Wear earplugs. Whether your neighbor plays loud music, your partner snores, or your kid talks in her sleep, nighttime noise keeps REV sentineled all night long. Earplugs are cheap, easy, and effective at helping you sleep because the calm stillness they provide gives your highly gullible sympathetic nervous system the "all's well" message. Look for ones labeled with a noise reduction rate (NRR) of at least 30 decibels.[9]

3. Make the bed a sacred space. It's hard to think of your bedroom as a sleep sanctuary if you also associate it with financial spreadsheets, difficult talks with your employees, social media metrics, or gruesome ax-murderers. The bed is for sleep, relaxation, and sex. That's it. Resist the urge to bring your laptop into bed. All tech should stay out of the bedroom, period.

You are not a lab rat pressing a lever for pellets, so stop treating yourself like one by letting your phone be the first thing you reach for every morning. Waking up to your phone jacks up REV the moment your eyes flutter open, robbing yourself of one of the most sacred Downstate moments in your day: the liminal space between dreamtime and waking. Keep the phone in another room and wake up with an old-school alarm clock (with no lights or one with red or orange numbers), giving yourself the gift of choosing how and when the day begins, and keep it turned away from your face so the light

*(continues)*

**SET UP A SLEEP DEN** (*continued*)

doesn't interrupt your sleep, and so you only look at the time when you are finally ready to greet the day. Speaking of light . . .

4. Block out light. Any light that seeps into your room overnight, whether from a streetlamp, passing car, or the earliest peek of sun, has the ability to shine through your closed eyelids and arouse your suprachiasmatic nucleus. Invest in blackout curtains and/or wear a comfortable eye mask. If you tend to get up in the middle of the night to use the bathroom or tend to a baby, purchase a warm-tinted nightlight to avoid having to turn on any bright lights.

5. Clear your mind before bed. They call it "doomscrolling" for a reason: when you start reading scary or upsetting news right before bed or scouring social media for the latest schadenfreude-inducing gossip, you get sucked into a vortex of negativity that spells doom for that night's sleep. After a long day, your Central Command is exhausted from evaluating every incoming stimulus and regulating and inhibiting every one of your knee-jerk reactions. So, like any smart person, it's gone to bed, and left you *Home Alone* in the hands of your amygdala. Hmmm . . . is this a good time to write a letter to your boss whom you feel disrespected you or to start that big relationship talk with your significant other? JUST SAY NO! Reserve late night for reading an enjoyable book or magazine or having a quiet conversation with your partner or a friend. Keep a journal for writing down what you did that day and what you have on your plate the next; doing so will reduce the open loops in your mind. Write down ten things

# DOMAIN 3: Exercise Your Right to Recovery

### ACTION ITEM #1

**Exercise for thirty minutes at least three times a week.** This Action Item is intentionally vague because exercise needs depend on what type of athlete you are (from Chapter 5). The Beginners will spend their thirty minutes three times a week in an easy walk around the 'hood, graduating to interval walking, whereby they push themselves to walk in sequences you are grateful for that happened that very day. When you fill your heart and mind with grateful thoughts, you banish the kvetch.

6. Declutter your nightstand. If your goal is to fall asleep with an uncluttered mind, it makes sense that the last thing you lay your eyes on before turning out the lights be as uncluttered as possible. Set up your bedroom with the least amount of furniture and mess possible so that it is a clean canvas on which to paint your Downstate dreams.

7. If you aren't sleeping, get out of bed. Your bed is for sleeping, relaxing, and shakin' the sheets. Don't spend hours tossing and turning because, like Pavlov's dog, doing so will condition you to associate lying in your bed with, "Oh good, it's time for worry." If you find yourself awake for twenty or thirty minutes, get up, grab your journal, and by the dim light of a candle or a nightlight start writing everything on your mind. Write until you feel done and/or tired—only then should you return to bed. Do this as many times as you need to until you fall asleep.

8. Read a dense book. I'm not talking about a Stephen King thriller or anything that is going to pique your curiosity, your worries, your envy, or your emotions generally. This should be a book that you find mildly interesting, but maybe it's a little too philosophical, or too historical, or too hardcore astrophysics. Turn down the room lights with only a small reading lamp that can be easily switched off, get cozy in bed, start reading. When you first start to feel the heavy lids and the loss of focus, don't fight it. Turn off the lights and ride the slow wave home to sleep.

switching from high to regular pace throughout their session. For Steady as She Goes types, workouts can follow the CDC guidelines of 150 minutes a week of moderate-intensity exercise (brisk walking, doubles tennis, bike riding on flat terrain) or 75 minutes a week of high-intensity exercise (jogging, singles tennis, basketball, bike riding with hills), or some combination of the two.[10] This group might also throw in a couple of sessions a week of resistance training, plus exercises that promote flexibility, balance, and coordination. Lifers will see this Action Item and skip to the next.

ACTION ITEM #2

**Exercise in the morning for regulating your weight and in the late afternoon for muscle building.** Your metabolic and muscular systems have different circadian rhythms, so it makes sense that they work most efficiently at different times of day. Studies show that morning aerobic exercise naturally promotes weight loss, as your metabolic system is at its peak and ready to burn calories. Additionally, morning exercise lowers daytime hunger pangs more than afternoon exercise.[11] On the other hand, your muscles tend to get stronger and build faster when you save the dead-lifts and hammer curls for the early evening. This is a good Action Item for Steady as She Goes types and Lifers who want to add circadian science to their Downstate workout plan so as to get the most out of their hours in the gym.

ACTION ITEM #3

**Use your autonomic system to inform your workout schedule.** Studies have shown that using your own body's data, in the form of resting heart rate, can be more informative than preset traditional workout schedules, because it tells you whether you have sufficiently recovered from your prior workout to go hard again today, or whether you need an extra day of recovery. All you need for this Action Item is your resting heart rate (explained in Chapter 5). At the beginning of the week, measure your baseline resting heat rate in the morning and write it down, then kick things off with a hard workout to jump-start REV. Each morning thereafter, measure your pre-workout resting heart rate in the exact same way as the baseline condition. If your heart rate is the same or lower than baseline, you can push yourself with another moderate or hard workout. If, however, it's higher than your baseline on any one morning, you need a little more time to recover from your last hard workout to build up your glycogen stores and reduce REV. On rest days, you don't need to go total sloth on the couch; low-impact walking is a great alternative.

ACTION ITEM #4

**Practice nasal breathing throughout your entire workout.** Nasal breathing is the secret weapon of athletes who want an edge over the competition, or just want to be the most efficient athlete they can be. I have made nasal breathing its own Action Item because it's that important, but also because it's going to take you a while to get used to. The early stages of nasal breathing are not easy and there aren't any shortcuts. Just shut your mouth and grunt like a Downstate bull, focusing on the exhale. It takes time to transform your physiology, but that time will be well worth the gains as you tranquilly run past the wheezing mouth-breather spewing germ clouds with every gasping breath.

ACTION ITEM #5

**Exercise in nature whenever possible, ideally with a friend, family member, or pet, at least three times a week.** You've learned about the independent benefits of being in nature and of exercise. Well, together they are greater than the sum of their parts. And it's a lot easier to get a friend to join you if you're going for a walk in the park or at the beach rather than walking on abutting treadmills. Research shows that exercising in nature makes it feel more enjoyable and less of a slog, so you're more likely to stick with it and commit to longer sessions without even realizing it.[12]

ACTION ITEM #6

**Exercise at a consistent time each day.** Just as with eating and sleeping, throwing on running shoes or diving into the pool at the same time each day lets your body know when it needs to gird its loins and prepare sufficient usable energy for you to expend energy. A consistent workout schedule isn't just great for your metabolism; studies have shown that people who exercise at consistent times each week engage in longer and more frequent workouts at the gym or pool, and therefore have a greater chance of meeting the recommended 150 minutes of moderate exercise a week.[13] So, block off time in your calendar for workouts and don't let anything but an emergency knock you off your schedule. This is called Respecting the Downstate.

## DOMAIN 4: You Are What and When You Eat

### ACTION ITEM #1

**Eat breakfast every day.** Your metabolism, insulin, body temperature, and REV are all riding high as the sun comes up, optimized to extract the greatest amount of nutrition and energy from the food you eat. In fact, people who eat half of their calories earlier in the day are healthier, smarter, happier, and more well rested than people who eat at night.[14] So, if you are someone who tends to skip breakfast, this is the Action Item for you. You can make breakfast a big deal by sitting down to a plated meal, or just have a bowl of boiled eggs in the fridge that you peel and eat with a dash of sea salt on your way out the door. Whatever works, just start putting breakfast into your schedule. The long-term goal is to make breakfast and lunch your main meals, with dinner the lightest meal of the day. This will give you more sustained energy levels across the day, decrease hunger pangs, maintain your weight, reduce REV at night, and help your sleep quality.

### ACTION ITEM #2

**Eat good-for-you foods throughout the day, every day.** Your body is your temple, the only one you get in this life, so this Action Item will prompt you to carefully consider each and every morsel that you put into this precious vessel. You have two choices:

A. You can stick with the traditional diet of your cultural heritage, while simply focusing on these ingredients and guidelines:

- Daily intake of fruit and vegetables
- Beans, nuts, and seeds on most days of the week
- More whole grains
- More fish, less red meat, plus a daily omega-3 supplement
- Minimal sugar, ultraprocessed, and refined foods

- Healthy hydration with plenty of water and tea and limited fruit drinks, sodas, caffeinated beverages, and alcohol in moderation

B. You can adopt a specific meal plan that promotes all the best features of nutrition while limiting the ones that increase oxidative stress and inflammation. These include the Mediterranean, Japanese, or MIND diet. Do your research and choose the one that feels easiest to stick with.

## ACTION ITEM #3

**Practice intermittent fasting.** There are many different versions of intermittent fasting—alternate day, 5:2—all providing similar long-term benefits, so choose the one that works best for you and your lifestyle. After a few weeks, your body will adapt to this schedule of eating, and the changes you see and feel will be the hard evidence you need to keep going, all of which will transform any rough patches you experience into renewed dedication to preserving your personal health boundaries.

## ACTION ITEM #4

**Schedule your meals to occur within a twelve-, ten-, or eight-hour window.** The priority here is to eat in the daytime when your Upstate system is naturally active and to stop eating in the evening when Upstate systems are waning, giving RESTORE uninterrupted time to do its thing. Studies have shown excellent health results from all different restricted eating windows, but the shorter you can make it, the better. And remember, this Action Item is not about *what* you eat, but *when*, so you have a lot of freedom in your food choices. Once you get the whens of eating working for you, you can then add Action Items that guide the whats of eating.

## ACTION ITEM #5

**Set consistent mealtimes.** Putting any edible item in your mouth will do three things: increase REV, trigger inflammation, and boost oxidative stress. The key to healthy nutrition is to keep these three reactions to food under an optimized level of control, and one of the best ways of doing this is by taking your meals at the same time every day. Your body does a lot of pregame prep for the big meals, priming you for getting the most nutrition and energy from your foods. Help it by providing food at predictable times. Skipping meals or snacking at random times throws your system into a state of unexpected stress that, over the long term, leads to weight gain and extreme swings in energy levels. Make each mealtime a stable, predictable daily event and a strong Downstate will follow.

ACTION ITEM #6

**Buy your food at farmers' markets once a week, join a CSA (community-supported agriculture), or plant your own vegetable garden.** This Action Item is good for your and the planet's Downstate. Unlike the packaged goods sold by the food industry, you won't find nutrition labels or lists of health claims on food sold at farmers' markets. Farm food is what your great-great-grandparents ate, and it don't need no stinkin' labels. Preparing meals with in-season produce gets you in touch with the Upstate/Downstate cycles of nature; increases the freshness, taste, and quality of the food; and seasonal eating benefits metabolic health most likely because ripening on the vine, rather than a refrigerated warehouse, allows all those rugged phytochemicals to become fully expressed the way nature intended.[15] Growing your own also gets your hands in the dirt and your body moving, and inspires the awe of eating something you planted. Priceless.

## Better Living Through Self-Experimentation

There is no better argument to keep you doing good things for yourself than cold, hard data, and now you have the opportunity to turn yourself into a lab rat and a scientist all at the same time. Remember those lab reports in middle school? Well, they are really not that different from the lab journals that real scientists use during an experiment to record their results and see the expected and unexpected changes from baseline or placebo. In this spirit, here is your Downstate RecoveryPlus Daily Journal that allows you to measure your baseline and then see how adding each Action Item has affected your day-to-day performance goals.

**First, measure your baseline.** Get yourself a lab notebook. I prefer basic composition books with lined paper, but you can get as fancy or techy as you please. The RecoveryPlus Daily Journal (see pages 238 and 287) is set up for a week of data collection, so you can use this page as a template and draw your own versions into the pages of your journal, make many copies of this page and paste it into your journal, or build your own app. Start with the second page, and always put the daily journal on the right-hand page, leaving the left-hand page open for any comments about your day. Start off with collecting one week of preassessment data to take the pulse of each area of your life that you want to elevate.

**Record your experimental data.** After a week of baseline assessment, start your Domains of Action items. Remember to write the date of the first day of the week and then describe the specific Action Item(s) that you are working on that week (e.g., baseline, intermittent fasting, etc.). Before bedtime, you will assess how your day went on a 1 to 7 scale (1 = worst ever and 7 = best ever; be sure to use the whole range of the scale so the experimental effects really pop out) for each outcome variable, except sleep. When you wake up in the morning, answer the questions about your sleep and how well you stuck to your Plan over the past 24-hour period (Plan Adherence). Then, get on with your day. That's it!

**Evaluate your results.** At the end of the week, look over the trajectory of your data. Do you see the numbers going up compared with your preassessment week? The variables that show increases are the aspects of your life that are reflecting RecoveryPlus, whereas the numbers that stayed the same or went down aren't. These fluctuations might depend on how much you stuck to your Plan (Plan Adherence), so pay attention to those numbers too. Check out which specific areas of your life modulated the most with which Action Items. Did your sleep improve? Or how well you regulated your emotions? How did the variables interact and affect one another? For example, when you tightened up your eating routine, did you see benefits to your emotional stability, sleep, or cognitive sharpness? Create averages for each week, so you can compare across weeks and examine how each Action Item altered your outcomes. How did adding two or more action items together compare to when you just focused on one?

# RECOVERYPLUS DAILY JOURNAL

DATE: _____

ACTION ITEM(S): _____

RESPONSES:

| 1 | 2 | 3 | 4 | 5 | 6 | 7 |
|---|---|---|---|---|---|---|
| WORST EVER | BAD | SLIGHT BAD | NO CHANGE | SLIGHT GOOD | GOOD | BEST EVER |

| OUTCOME VARIABLE | DAY 1 | DAY 2 | DAY 3 | DAY 4 | DAY 5 | DAY 6 | DAY 7 | AVERAGE |
|---|---|---|---|---|---|---|---|---|
| MENTAL SHARPNESS | | | | | | | | |
| PRODUCTIVITY | | | | | | | | |
| BEHAVIOR REGULATION | | | | | | | | |
| ENERGY | | | | | | | | |
| EMOTIONAL STABILITY | | | | | | | | |
| PHYSICAL HEALTH | | | | | | | | |
| SLEEP QUALITY | | | | | | | | |
| PLAN ADHERENCE | | | | | | | | |

Make this RecoveryPlus Daily Journal your own by adding variables that you are interested in tracking, such as your HRV; steps; how well you got along with others; what sleep aids, alcohol, or other drugs you used. Add specific notes to yourself about your day on the left side of the journal. Did something happen that made one day particularly great or extra difficult? Did you have any insights that you want to jot down? Did you have any memorable dreams? This is your space to record your Downstate Maven journey, to fine tune your progress, and to chart your future course.

## Help! I've Fallen Off the Downstate Wagon and I Can't Get Up! (how to deal with off days)

Your Plan will not shatter into a million tiny pieces or collapse in a puddle of regret if you stay out all night or get the occasional extra buttered popcorn at the movies. If you're traveling—one of the biggest challenges for maintaining health boundaries and getting enough Downstate time—it's okay if you end up skipping a workout or extending your ten-hour eating window to shovel in deep dish in Chicago or gelato in Milan. To deal with these ups and downs, you need to factor a few off days here and there as you adjust to the #DownstateLife.

The two most important things to hold sacred are the habits you have worked hard to develop and the long-term goals you've set up for yourself. This means that when you find yourself in a disrupted state, do whatever token gesture you can to acknowledge the Downstate habits you've committed to following. If you're traveling and don't have time for a full forty-five-minute workout at the gym, do a seven-minute HIIT workout in the hotel room at the usual time just to keep the rhythm, sympathetic schvitz, and health boundary intact. By keeping this consistent schedule come hell or high water, your brain and body will know you mean business and be ready to climb back on the Downstate wagon as soon as you get back home. The same goes for the eating, sleep, and autonomic domains. The point is to keep the ritual consistent so that you can jump back into your Plan as soon as you are ready, rather than send your brain and body the message that you are losing control, falling off the Downstate wagon, and getting judgmental with yourself. As my wise friend Alex John used to tell me:

## DEEP DIVE INTO OUTCOME VARIABLES

The Daily Journal contains outcome variables related to areas of functioning that we typically assess in the lab, with one additional empty space meant to encourage you to add your own variable(s), plus an overall daily rating of Plan Adherence. These variables are formulated to capture your subjective sense of the primary areas that the Downstate RecoveryPlus Plan are expected to benefit: mental sharpness, productivity, behavior regulation, energy, emotional stability, physical health, and sleep quality. These are intentionally broad because research shows that this level of inquiry can be effective at getting a genuine overview of this domain. Use the 1 to 7 scale to assess each variable, 1 as the lowest score and 7 as the highest score; again, be sure to use the whole range of the scale.

Here is a short description of each variable for you to keep in mind:

*Mental sharpness:* How well could you focus your attention today? Were you forgetting or remembering things? Did you make fewer or more mistakes than usual? How did you feel about your ability to make decisions? How creative did you feel?

*Productivity:* How much did you get done today? Were you able to close loops and cross things off your list? How easy or difficult was it for you to move from moment to moment? Did you feel a sense of accomplishment at the end of the day?

"Shhh. Don't speak ill of your body; your cells are listening." And if you need a little motivational pick-me-up, reflect on your BIG WHY, your long-term goals, and on your internal strengths that got you through the last challenge. Dig deep and bring all your resources to bear on this critically important cause: Your Life.

*Behavior regulation:* How well did you regulate your urges? Were you able to see when you'd 'had enough' (sweets, alcohol, food, social media)? How much did you pay attention to what you were doing? How mindful were you about the goals you set for yourself (e.g., workout, healthy eating, doom scrolling)?

*Energy:* How energetic or sluggish did you feel today? Were you able to push yourself during your workout or did you need to take it easy? How much energy did you have for your work life AND your personal life?

*Emotional stability:* How much were you able to understand your feelings today? Did your feelings overwhelm you or did you let them move through you without resistance? Were you calm and in touch with your emotions or did you feel ill-tempered or reactive and didn't know why?

*Physical health:* Were you in good physical health or under the weather today? Did you have regular bowel movements? Were you sweating a lot? Dizzy? Did you have cold hands or feet?

*Sleep quality:* Did you fall asleep easily last night or was it difficult? How refreshed do you feel this morning? Was your sleep deep enough? Was it long enough? If you dreamed, how did your dreams affect you?

*Plan adherence:* How much did you stick to your action items over the last 24 hours?

# Everything You Always Wanted to Know About the Future of the Downstate (but Were Afraid to Ask)

⸺ • ⸺

R eady to take a walk on the wild side? Right now, we are traveling into a world that, though evidence-based, is highly experimental, somewhat controversial, and may not yet be FDA-approved. In the spirit of venturing beyond the Downstate tools that you were born with, I've put together some commonly asked questions about the latest scientific *innovations*, interventions (e.g., integrative medicine practices, electrical stimulators, and pharmaceuticals), and gadgets, all of which hope to push the boundaries of human excellence.

## Can We Get Smarter/Stronger/Faster?

That is the fundamental question asked by anyone interested in the pursuit of human excellence. And in our most optimistic, unscientific moments, most of us are convinced the answer is: YES, WE CAN! The hope is that our systems can be infiltrated and amplified to superhuman capabilities by enhancing naturally occurring processes—RecoveryPlus on steroids—and it has driven innovations in technology, mechanical and computational engineering, and information and medical sciences, advancing many areas of human functioning including sports and nutrition, military and intelligence, medicine, and neuroscience. Our discoveries are sending humans to Mars and Teslas into space.[1] We run faster, hit harder, spy sneakier, and multitask excellenter.

They say scientists gravitate toward fields of study that personally trigger them. For example, a jittery person might study anxiety disorder; a person who fears aging might investigate telomeres; or someone who has known or loved a person suffering from a mental disorder might gravitate toward researching schizophrenia, which was my dad's story. So, what does it say about me that I have been obsessed with knowing if humans can get smarter throughout my entire scientific career?

On second thought, don't answer that.

The truth is that I've doggedly pursued this question since my grad school days when I discovered that you can get two days out of one, cognitively speaking, by taking a nap. With funding from the National Institutes of Health (NIH), the National Science Foundation, the Department of Defense (DoD), and the Defense Advanced Research Projects Agency (DARPA), my post-PhD projects investigated all manner of tactics designed to improve human cognitive function. (All Institutional Review Board–approved, of course.) On one DARPA project, my collaborators built a brain stimulator that sent electrical signals into the sleeping brain. I used this in my sleep lab to induce greater slow waves in hopes of improving spatial memory. In an NIH project, I gave consenting adults Ambien while they slept in my lab to see whether it would boost their sleep spindles and increase their verbal memory. In yet another DARPA project, I compared a nap with a dose of caffeine to see which was more effective at improving memory. Then, in a DoD project designed to determine whether an agent more powerful than caffeine might do the trick, I administered dexamphetamine, a drug typically prescribed for attention-deficit disorder but widely used as a so-called "smart pill," to healthy, well-rested people in hopes that it would improve cognition.

This list of my former projects is my way of telling you that I have enough research experience in this field of "better" to have formed an evidence-based answer to the question "Can we get smarter/stronger/faster?" And my answer is: sometimes. Interventions generally help you the most when you are at your worst—basically, when you're sleep-deprived, overwhelmed by stress, or at a physical or mental deficit. They don't help when you don't need help.

Think about that Yerkes-Dodson law I mentioned in Chapter 5, which plots an upside-down, U-shaped curve with your arousal or excitement level on the X-axis and your performance on the Y-axis. When you have low arousal (e.g., tired, unmotivated, low energy), you can't get out of the starting gate, resulting in a poor performance. At a moderate level of arousal (e.g., well rested, focused, and stable energy) you hit the "juuuuuust right" eustress state, making your performance as good as it's gonna get. But with too much arousal, you're a hyperexcited dork who can't tell his ass from his elbow, scientifically speaking.

Stimulation, whether it be from drugs, electrodes, sound, or magnets, can shift you to the left or right on that arousal X-axis. When you're drowsy, adding a little excitatory stimulation via caffeine or Adderall can push you into the eustress sweet spot, but too much stimulation can push you into the hyperactive condition where you run around like a headless chicken. If you are already at the sweet spot of alertness, you can't get much better, so any amount of excitatory stimulation will turn you into the aforementioned *poulet* and titrating yourself back down to the right dose can be tricky.

How do you know if you are in the sweet spot? You are the person at the top of your game with a dynamite Upstate fully supported by a strong Downstate connection between your vagus nerve and Central Command; a powerful circadian rhythm; bold slow waves; an active lifestyle; a metabolism that won't quit; and plenty of friendly hugs or thumpin' sex. When your brain and body are operating at this upper limit, the interventions I'll describe in this chapter probably won't push you any higher, and they may even hurt your performance. The simplest, safest, and cheapest route to your best self involves committing to a robust Downstate practice across every area of life.

Of course, you can't always be at your best. For instance, your sleep might suffer occasionally due to a small child tossing cookies into your hair all night, allergies, or some troubled thoughts keeping your mind REVVING when it should be RESTORING. An injury might immobilize you, keeping you from your daily workout. The holidays or vacation may divert your perfectly organized eating plan. In these cases, getting to your best Downstate self might be easier with a little help. They're no substitute for the real thing—your core Downstate practices—but they can pinch hit until you have the Downstate fundamentals working for you again.

Okay, enough soap-boxing . . . let's get to those devilish details.

## Directly Stimulating the Vagus Nerve

You now know all there is to know about the vagus nerve and RESTORE. They like deep breathing, long, romantic walks in the forest, and spending time upside down recirculating and reducing blood pressure.

But did you know that the vagus nerve can be directly activated with a little electric shock? Since electrical impulses are the language of cell-to-cell communication, a common way to speak to neurons is by placing electrodes directly on a nerve itself and sending electrical stimulation down its fibers. A pacemaker is a good example of this intervention.

We know that the vagus nerve is a critical pathway for brain-body communication and cognition. Building on this fact, researchers implanted electrical stimulators directly on the vagus nerve.[2] They discovered that supercharging vagal activity improved memories both in animals and humans.[3] Due to the vagus's wide influence, vagal nerve stimulation benefits many medical conditions as well, including epilepsy, chronic heart failure, rheumatoid arthritis, inflammatory bowel disease, chronic pain, and clinical depression.[4]

These findings were interesting at a scientific level, as they demonstrated the critical role of vagal activity for the brain and body and offered an exciting treatment strategy for people with significant medical conditions, such as epilepsy and depression, who could have an electrical stimulator surgically implanted. But for most people, vagal nerve stimulation was out of reach. Another breakthrough happened recently when scientists invented a way for transcutaneous (through the skin) stimulation along the vagus's branches through the ear.[5] A specially designed earbud electrode was created to send electrical pulses through the skin that directly stimulated the vagus nerve. Although not yet widely available, transcutaneous vagal nerve stimulation (tVNS) technology is a burgeoning new field, offering at-home, FDA-approved treatment for depression and epilepsy, among other conditions. tVNS also shows the same enhancements to cognition as direct stimulation of the nerve, including improved long-term memory and working memory and enhanced emotional processing.[6] Generally, the findings point to a promising future for tVNS in helping people with a wide range of medical and psychological conditions.

## Tapping the Slow Wave

Turning to the edges of sleep science, let's explore one of the longest-held and most audacious questions asked by quacks and rigorous scientists alike: *Can we learn while we sleep?* This idea has circulated throughout the history of psychology, penetrated culture via sci-fi movies, and inspired the invention of devices that claim to teach foreign languages, promote fact memorization, and even help people quit smoking by simply listening to audio recordings during sleep. We now know that there are, in fact, many ways that we can infiltrate the memory process and either improve specific memories or even delete some unwanted memories.[7]

But for the purposes of this book, I'm going to focus on research that directly targets the star of the Downstate: the slow wave. Remember, slow waves are the deepest point of Downstate decompression, where toxins are flushed from the brain, protein synthesis is catalyzed, growth hormone is released, muscle and tissue are repaired, and memories are secured in that glorious library of your brain. But they are also the first sleep feature you lose when you don't get to bed early enough, have trouble sleeping, are too REVVED up, don't exercise enough, have any type of sleep disorder, or eat foods that increase inflammation and oxidative stress. It's the most important character in the Downstate play of your night and yet the most vulnerable to being killed off. If scientists could find a way to noninvasively increase slow waves, they would hit the jackpot.

A group of German researchers discovered that slow waves could be increased by using both auditory and electrical stimulation. In one study, they devised a real-time slow wave detector that identified slow waves in the EEG of sleeping people and instantly triggered a short burst of beeps to be played through headphones worn by the sleeper. When the beeps occurred right at the end of the slow wave, the brain responded by making more slow waves.[8] Researchers think this has to do with the fact that one purpose of slow waves is to keep you in deep sleep, so any noise will cause your brain to ramp up slow wave production to try to keep you from waking up. And because slow waves are also essential for memory consolidation, a secondary benefit to annoying the brain with beeps all night is that it increases memory consolidation. The researchers had subjects learn a set of word pairs before sleep and then sent beeps perfectly timed to coincide with their natural slow waves. The result: more slow waves and, upon waking, better memory recall than the control conditions. These findings blew up the skirt of every sleep scientist, as they introduced a potential way to help people with weak slow waves—which is basically most people aged forty and older—experience deeper sleep and better memory to boot. It may sound sci-fi, but the research showed that hands-on access to your greatest Downstate entry point, the slow wave, may actually be just a beep away.

Electrical stimulation can also be used to increase slow waves. Again, the Germans take the Downstate prize here, as they showed that the brain could be forced to make more slow waves by stimulating it with an electrical current that mimicked the characteristics of the slow wave (e.g., the same frequency, amplitude, duration, etc.) via scalp electrodes placed over the frontal cortex. As with auditory stimulation, the electrical slow wave enhancement produced bigger and more frequent slow waves, as if the brain was responding to the stimulation by upping the ante. And again, the more the electrical stimulation increased slow waves, the better the subject's memory performance upon waking.[9]

As science opens doors that reveal the power of the Downstate, it's also revealing many possible inroads for entrepreneurs, biotech companies, app developers, and wearable technologies. Think of all the possible at-home and wearable devices that could be outfitted with additional stimulation features, such as smells, sounds, vibration, or stimulation via magnets, electricity, or light, to change behavior. If these wearables included brain electrodes, could the auditory or electrical stimulations be synced up to specific parts of sleep, such as natural slow waves, thereby deepening Downstate sleep in, say, older people with the result of improving their memory? Given the strong links between poor slow waves and dementia and Alzheimer's disease, could we start sleeping with devices that will help us generate more and deeper slow waves at home and stave off the onset of these conditions?

One promising wearable device is PeakSleep, developed by my colleagues at Teledyne on a DARPA-funded project in which I was a collaborator (I have no financial interest). PeakSleep wirelessly delivers transcranial electrical stimulation through electrodes located on a headband. The headband can be worn before sleep to shorten the time it takes to fall asleep or during sleep to increase slow waves. I'll bet those research subjects didn't want to give back those PeakSleep devices at the end of the study!

As brain or vagal stimulation devices become as popular as audiobooks, the speed with which they come to market will inevitably outpace researchers' abilities to evaluate their reliability and safety. A similar problem already exists in the wearable sleep trackers corner of the market, where few of the promises match the actual results.[10] This disconnect between commercialization and scientific validation brings up some legal and ethical considerations. Beyond overpromising results, modulation of the sleeping brain is a potentially dangerous skill to put in the hands of strangers, and brings up a lot of questions, such as "Can it be used without a person's consent?" Can robot roommates—Alexa, Siri, and nest, for instance—also be programmed to surreptitiously feed us information while we sleep without our knowledge? Could the learning-while-asleep phenomenon be used on the sly for financial, political, or other nefarious outcomes? And then there's the question of self-experimentation, which may not be too dangerous if we're just talking about beeps and squeaks but could be risky if everyday folks are zapping their brain and vagus nerves like a rat with a cocaine lever. When does the desire to be faster, smarter, and stronger send you up and over the Yerkes-Dodson upside-down U, where better does indeed become the enemy of good?

## From Hipster Alternative to Mainstream Integrative Medicine

In the '80s, the word *alternative* was the antiestablishment hipsters' password for what was cool, as opposed to what was commercial and popular. Postpunk alternative music—X, the Pixies, R.E.M.—was only played on radio stations at the far end of the dial and came to define the character of myself and my fellow Gen Xers.

As with most cultural movements pushing the boundaries of the zeitgeist, alternative music is now just another mainstream music genre. The same can be said for an assortment of medical therapies that began to gain traction in the Western medical world in the '70s, including acupuncture, massage, chiropractic treatment, and osteopathic therapy. For decades, a lack of solid evidence to support the claims of these therapies produced a lot of negative press (just search *craniosacral therapy* on Wikipedia). However, the recent emergence of clinical trials yielding positive results combined with growing patient demand has shifted these therapies from the edge to the center of the recently coined *integrative medicine* approach, now mainstream enough that much of it is covered by insurance plans.

One of these approaches, craniosacral therapy, was developed to treat compression in the skull and spinal cord thought to be caused by blockages in the flow of cerebral spinal fluid that practitioners believe are caused by physical or psychological stress. Anatomically speaking, the craniosacral system includes the skull and cranial sutures (bands of tissue holding the skull together), cerebrospinal fluid, and the membranes of the brain and the spinal cord. In this gentle, hands-on treatment, a practitioner uses subtle manual palpations along with energy work to open passages throughout the body and coax greater movement of fluid. The intention is to restore balance to the many systems of the body supported by the central nervous system, including the musculoskeletal, vascular, and endocrine systems, as well as to the REV and RESTORE systems. Randomized clinical trial studies of craniosacral therapy report significant improvement in chronic pain, fibromyalgia, and infantile colic.[11] (Yes, babies can and do get craniosacral therapy.) In one study, twenty-five weeks of craniosacral therapy showed significant benefits to anxiety, pain, quality of life, and sleep both immediately after treatment and at the six-month follow-up compared with placebo, suggesting this modality may be a valuable supplementary treatment for improving anxiety and quality of life.[12]

I asked Jennifer Fox, PhD, LMT, a certified craniosacral therapist in the Hudson Valley, about how the objective techniques of working with connective tissue and the subjective energy work aspect of the practice come together to benefit her clients.[13] She describes getting in touch with an inherent rhythm in the body, called the craniosacral rhythm or the cranial rhythmic impulse, that can be pushed out of balance due to illness, stress, or maintaining poor posture at the computer or in the car, as well as tapping into deeper rhythms that are more subjective and "not necessarily measurable by any medical instrument. But when you are in it, you know it," she says. "This energetic field that the therapist and client can drop into is the domain of the deeper, broader, more spiritual, if you will, rhythms. That's where the real healing takes place."

For Dr. Fox, a strong connection exists between her practice and the RESTORE system. She has seen particularly "stunning results" in women diagnosed with fibromyalgia, who she treats by directly working with the vagus nerve. "I've found that fibromyalgia and other autoimmune diseases often have a bunched up and bulging hernia of the organs right where the chest and stomach meet, which can cause anything from heart palpitations to body-wide inflammatory states." In these cases, she uses manual palpitations and energy as a way to soften and release adhesions in the abdominal and pelvic cavities that can often start a process of reversing symptoms and tamping down inflammatory states.

One of the biggest distinguishing factors between typical Western medicine approaches and craniosacral therapy, and indeed the entire field of osteopathy (a form of manipulative medicine based on the notion that all of the body's systems are interrelated), is that these alternative therapies embrace the "whole person" approach to treatment.[14] "Many holistic practitioners recognize that imbalance sits at the heart of so many of the health issues we see in our practices," Dr. Fox says. "People are stressed out, disembodied, disconnected from the Earth, and freakishly driven. My clients are either in a state of 'freeze' or 'shutdown,' so my job is to help their system remember its own resilience and innate capacity to achieve dynamic equilibrium." Sounds pretty Downstate, if you ask me.

## Popping Addy like Tic Tacs

Along with social and financial pressures and an increasingly competitive academic environment, college students are under the pressure to choose between taking a little pill that will make them "awesome at everything," or eschewing the temptation and relying on the standard practice of study, sleep, repeat.[15] They've been called #GenerationAdderall, the ADHD-adjacent folks who grew up within the diagnosis boom and thus have unlimited access to the stimulants traditionally used to treat children with the disorder.[16] Nonmedical use (NMU) of prescription drugs includes the opioid crisis currently ravaging America, with such stimulants as Adderall coming in a close second for young people. Unlike opioids, the motivation to misuse stimulants is not to check out; rather, to check in . . . at super-hero scale. Stimulants keep your eyes propped open round the clock; it's a 24-hour Upstate party. After college, young adults continue to use stimulants to keep Doozering round the clock at work, leading to increased addiction and overdose. But to what end?

While some studies show small, short-term increases in attention, working memory, and information processing when the drug is active, other studies report no benefit.[17] But for more complex tasks, such as memory and decision-making, the drugs have the same old inverted U shape in which people with lower baseline performance (without the drug) show the greatest benefits from stimulants; those who function at lower levels of creativity or flexibility show improvements; and individuals who are more creative or have greater cognitive flexibility will see their performance worsened.[18]

The worst part of all this pill spiral is the damage it does to your Downstate. My lab has shown that even a morning dose (nine a.m.) of a stimulant reduces Downstate slow-wave sleep (SWS) by at least an hour, and blocks improvement on cognitive tasks that benefit from overnight sleep.[19] Therefore, even when stimulants are taken earlier in the day, they disrupt nighttime sleep and subsequent cognitive performance.

So, before engaging in casual stimulant use, ask yourself the following questions: Does the marginal cognitive enhancement of stimulants exceed the significant long-term toll on such Downstate domains as sleep and on the cognitive and health processes that rely on sleep? Is the risk of increased substance abuse that comes with misuse of stimulants tolerable? Is it better to be a superhero by taking a pill to stay awake and a pill to go to sleep than to simply work your Downstate Plan of bright morning light, exercise, eating within a reasonable window, and getting to bed early with limited screen time? Only you know the answers for yourself.

## Mother's Little Helpers or Downstate Hurters?

And what about all these herbs and spices making their way into mainstream medicine cabinets? Let's first take a look at cannabis, which has undergone a truly impressive image makeover. Back in my *high* school daze, my friends and I could buy a dime bag of dusty skunk weed illegally procured from a dude who would invite us to sit on his threadbare couch in our school uniforms and smoke a bowl with him before we headed back to class. Oy. Today, it's a multibillion-dollar industry, legal in a growing number of states and sold in brightly lit dispensaries that feel like Apple stores where eager budtenders serve up a tailor-made eighth of Frooty Loopys or whatever strain will provide the nuanced high you are seeking.

Most people think pot is a self-medicator's Downstate dream. But despite the lingering hippy-dippy mellow vibe that has draped its reputation since the '60s, tetrahydrocannabinol (THC, the principle psychoactive constituent of cannabis) is actually a pretty big Upstate agonist, elevating heart rate and blood pressure by stimulating REV and inhibiting RESTORE.[20] A meta-analysis of cannabis's impact on cardiovascular conditions reported that regular use was associated with increased risk of both acute coronary syndrome and chronic cardiovascular disease.[21] The relation between cannabis and sleep is quite controversial with users convinced that their sleep improves with the drug, while data show that this may be a false chimera driven by physical addiction to the substance. THC appears to reduce the time it takes to fall asleep, but these effects are outweighed by the rapid habituation to these sleep-enhancing qualities: with continued use, meaning the more you partake, the more you build up a tolerance.[22] We also know that cannabis use can disturb the circadian rhythm, as measured by increased core body temperature during the night when it should naturally be low.[23] In fact, disturbed sleep is a hallmark withdrawal symptom that can last months after a person stops using, and sleep problems are a risk factor for going back on the drug.[24] This vicious cycle can be mistaken for that Dank Sinatra improving your sleep, when it's merely reducing your withdrawal symptoms.

The cannabis flower comprises over one hundred different cannabinoids, active compounds that can interact with receptors in the brain and body.[25] Cannabinoids work on the endocannabinoid system with two popular plant-based phytocannabinoids: THC and CBD (cannabidiol). The former produces the well-known "high," whereas the latter is growing in popularity as a cure-all, but in truth has few bona fide randomized control trials to its name. CBD does appear to improve pain management, reduce psychotic symptoms in people with schizophrenia, and counter the effects of the THC, as well as offer some other therapeutic effects.[26] CBD may be more promising as a sleep aid, as it doesn't appear to have the same addiction profile and studies indicate that it may help with sleep onset.[27] However, combining CBD with THC appears to disturb deep SWS, definitely something to avoid.[28]

It may also surprise you to learn that popping a few magic mushrooms or a hit of ecstasy, though potentially mind-altering and helpful for disentangling emotional traumas, are not exactly Downstate Express trains either. Ecstasy produces large elevations in the stress hormone cortisol, and both ecstasy and psilocybin (the psychoactive compound in magic mushrooms) drive up heart rate and blood pressure.[29] Given the legalities, there are few studies on Schedule 1 drugs, so caution should be taken in interpreting their results. One study of psilocybin indicated that the drug may suppress slow waves during the first part of the night and delay REM sleep, suggesting that your trip will not be to Downstateville.[30]

But not all hallucinogens give you the Upstate jitters. Ayahuasca, for example, is a highly potent brew made from the leaves of the *Psychotria viridis* shrub along with the stalks of the *Banisteriopsis caapi* vine that can take users on a journey through altered states of consciousness, complete with out-of-body experiences and hallucinations. It was a central feature of ancient Amazonian religious ceremonies and has recently migrated north as the drug of choice for many spiritual-sweat-lodge-vision-questy-type gatherings and young professional organization retreats. Given the wild hallucinatory nature of the journey, it may surprise you to learn about one study reporting that ayahuasca enhanced Downstate slow waves during SWS.[31] The study also showed that the drug curtailed REM sleep.

The reduction in REM sleep from ayahuasca and psilocybin is interesting as this property is also found in the antidepressant family of serotonin reuptake inhibitors (SSRIs), prompting some scientists to propose that REM suppression may have therapeutic benefits for emotional well-being.[32] People with depression are often evening types who sleep late into the morning, increasing their chances of lingering too long in the REM pool.[33] A lot more research is needed in this intriguing and promising field.

Whatever your drug-taking goals are, be it a mellow night enjoying the synchronicity between Pink Floyd's *Dark Side of the Moon* and the *Wizard of Oz*, spelunking emotional depths with a few good friends, or dancing your buns off in a sweaty club, getting a clear picture about each drug's effect on your Downstate is important for maintaining your REV/RESTORE ratios. For example, knowing how jacked REV is going to get by a particular drug can help you prepare for the comedown, and beefing up your Downstate practices can smooth your transition back into the "real world."

## The Downstate Is Essential for Elite Athletic Training: Just Ask an MMA Coach!

The autonomic nervous system is one of the newest elements being used to track athletes' fitness. Specifically, how well are REV and RESTORE playing together during and after exercise? Is there adequate RESTORE on board to match the REV hurricane that comes from a hard workout? How much overtraining is healthy and when does it send you straight into the downward spiral of stress and injury?

These questions are at the top of the list of priorities for Duncan French, PhD, vice president of performance at the UFC (Ultimate Fighting Championship) Performance Institute, a company that trains elite MMA world champions in Las Vegas, Nevada. I was interested in learning about their multidisciplinary, evidence-based, technologically enriched approach because of their specific and unique focus on autonomic recovery as a critical factor in an athlete's success. This Downstate-oriented approach is revolutionary and has brought up a slew of world champion MMA fighters, including rescuing Glover Teixeira from the brink of a downhill career brought on by his burn-twice-as-bright-half-as-long approach of his youth.

The UFC Performance Institute has its work cut out for it, as the typical fighter is used to pushing every boundary to the absolute limit—all crashing Upstate waves, no replenishing Downstate time. The sport itself is a "decathlon of combat components," Dr. French says, requiring the fighter to excel in boxing, wrestling, Muay Thai, Brazilian jujitsu, and more.[34] They need strength and stamina, but also coordination and discipline. The team that typically supports each fighter usually consists of coaches from each discipline who work with the fighter on a daily basis to separately train each skill. Any one of these training sessions would destroy most human beings for weeks; MMA athletes can have three or four trainings a day.

Dr. French describes this situation as "a melting pot of overtraining where they are essentially going off the cliff and their autonomic measurements now show signals of overtraining rather than signs of regeneration and restoration. MMA fighters are predisposed to high training loads and high sympathetic drive (REV), which often overpowers parasympathetic recovery (RESTORE). When it does, it fries them and then they flip the switch, become parasympathetically shut down, and can't recover. This level of overtraining suppresses metabolism, making weight cuts harder. It's a slippery slope in terms of their health and well-being and then, obviously, their performance."

The unique challenge that French and his team see in this work is how to support RESTORE processes in a person who maximally ramps up REV several times a day. Their goal is to bring the science of the autonomic nervous system, sleep, nutrition—basically everything known about Downstate recovery—to bear on training such that they can train wiser, rather than just harder.

One of the biggest areas of growth in the fitness industry involves the rapid development of new technologies designed to give detailed, moment-to-moment accounting of an athlete's physiological status along with specific feedback on how to move closer to a personalized goal. Examples include wrist-worn activity monitors, chest straps, or even devices that simultaneously measure EEG and ECG. Each device is fitted with a different combination of trackers aiming to sell the user on the promise that this company above all others has the secret recipe for getting you stronger, faster, fitter. Since the UFC Performance Institute is a decentralized system working with professional athletes all over the world, wearable technology is one of its solutions for staying on top of athletes' physiology and psychology. However, most devices have not been battle-tested to any satisfying extent, so before adopting any device, Dr. French and his colleagues conduct their own validation study on each one against a gold standard in the field, as well as test the feasibility of incorporating each device into a fighter's daily life. "What we always say is: If you not assessing, you're guessing, and it's hard to win a world championship by guessing your way there," he says. "So, we want to be intentional with our performance behaviors."

One of the devices Dr. French and his team tested was an at-home device combining ECG and EEG that claimed to be able to gather buckets of disparate physiological data and produce a simple green light/red light indicator when the athlete was ready for a hard workout versus needing more recovery time. A device that actually lived up to its promises would be a big win for remote monitoring between athletes and coaches. The team tested the consistency and reliability of the device's readings across days and assessed the device's red light/green light algorithm's ability to predict how well the fighters would perform under hard and easy training conditions.[35] Reality Check Number One was that the device gave inconsistent values when it was tested in the same subject across different days, suggesting that even the device's baseline readings were unreliable. Reality Check Number Two was that the light indicator was not a good predictor of the athletes' readiness. It was even worse at predicting readiness than just asking the athletes whether they felt ready using a simple subjective questionnaire. Another tracker bites the dust!

Athletic training is a multifactorial equation composed of physiological, psychological, social, and emotional factors. In light of the grandiose promises from an ever-expanding field of wearable technology, I asked Dr. French whether he thinks he will ever be able to rely on a device to make training decisions. His answer? "I don't think we'll ever get to a point where a device can replace the coach." For example, he says the coaches use heart rate variability (HRV) for making informed decisions about load management, a.k.a. whether an athlete is ready to go hard or needs more rest, which can lower the frequency of poor decisions to potentially overload and injure the athlete. "If there's typically twenty overtraining exposures without considering HRV, maybe we could reduce that to five overtraining exposures by incorporating HRV information." But he doesn't believe devices can be used deterministically to make nuanced decisions, such as whether an athlete is ready to train for power versus endurance. He does think that when HRV data is combined with a coach's intimate knowledge of his or her athlete's needs, abilities, and training schedule, these devices, and the autonomic information especially, hold some promise.

The bottom line is that if top-tier professional athletes program their training, performance, and recovery to incorporate the Downstate and ensure that REV and RESTORE are in the right ratio, maybe you ought to too.

# CHAPTER TEN

# Becoming a
# Downstate Maven

—————— • ——————

A re you chomping at the bit to dive into your Downstate or do you still need a little more of a motivational boost? This final chapter is the answer to both of these needs, and the message is critical for everyone to hear.

## One Downstate at a Time

The way of the Downstate Maven is a daily practice, requiring an honest look at the choices you make each moment that either helps your zigzagging trajectory toward RecoveryPlus, or veers you off. When you start on this path, the first things to consider are the lifestyle choices that directly undermine your progress with the Plan. Examine each aspect of your life that you habitually accept, yet suspect is not in line with your Downstate goals. Ask yourself whether this behavior is promoting or destroying your REV/RESTORE ratio.

*Two roads diverged in a wood:* Robert Frost's poem depicts the moment when you decide to make a choice that isn't typical, "the one less traveled by."[1] We make these choices every day, in every moment. In fact, it's these little moments that are most important because together, they are the threads of integrity of your own Downstate practice. Think of each choice as a "little w (why) practice" that scaffolds your goals and lofty aspirations and can help in curbing your late-night sweets habit or indulging in a second splash of gin. Start by mentally asking yourself—literally, as your hands are reaching for the dark chocolate–covered cherries—"Why am I eating these right now if I know they're going to jump-start REV and hinder my sleep?"

Just bringing that little bit of consciousness into the moment works eight times out of ten. As Frost concludes, each little w "makes all the difference."

## Making an Upstate Inventory

Nothing happens in a bubble. Our body and mind are one whole organism, despite Descartes's grumblings. So, along with working on the positive behaviors in the Plan that will stabilize the foundation for your Downstate dream home, you will also want to take an inventory of Upstate Party coping mechanisms that undermine your efforts, such as smoking; excessive alcohol consumption; late-night bedtime procrastination activities; or junk food availability. Also consider your lifestyle circumstances and choices that let REV degrade your day-to-day well-being, including stress from work; troubling relationships; unsafety in the home; noise where you sleep; lack of clothes, time, or space for exercise. Here are some specific suggestions for combatting the internal and external Upstate parties conspiring against your Downstate:

- Clear the psychological decks with the help of a therapist, social worker, friend, or support group (such as peer-to-peer fellowships, religious or spiritual community), or self-development course.
- Set limits on electronic interruptions by permanently turning off all beeps and banners or setting up a long Do-Not-Disturb window on your phone. Restrict the number of times you check on comments and Likes to a limited period each day. Disable the AutoPlay function in your streaming settings. Evict the computer, phone, and TV from your bedroom. Get your analog life back!
- My friend gave me a fridge magnet that says, "Eat organic food, or as your grandparents called it: FOOD." Before the days of convenience and preservatives, diets contained whole grains, omega-3s, more fish and colorful fruit and veggies, and less red meat. As Michael Pollan advises, if you can, spend more for food; buy fresh produce; shop at farmers' markets; know where your food comes from and when it came out of the ground; eat seasonally as much as possible; and don't consume anything your great-great-great grandmother wouldn't recognize as food.[2]

- Address the avalanche of stress-induced dysfunction in your life by first admitting that you are stressed and then taking specific actions to deal with it. (See the next section, "The Healing Practice of Naming It.") Join a mindfulness class, avoid triggers for stress or drug and alcohol abuse (people; places; activities), and engage in practices that give you a practical handle on the To-Do list in your head.

## The Healing Practice of Naming It

We have all lived through a recent global trauma, with some individuals feeling the tragedy, pain, and loss of the pandemic more acutely than others. Millions have died, but it is an unequal opportunity virus, one that disproportionately affects poor people and people of color due to longstanding health disparities and systemic inequities, as well as elders and those with preexisting medical conditions. Of course, the pandemic is not the only trauma befalling humanity. We helplessly watch as the Earth burns and floods; children shoot children in classrooms; innocent lives are ended by police violence; displaced refugees live in squalor; women are controlled by and subjected to patriarchal abuse of power; and domestic and global terrorism reigns. The question we need to ask ourselves individually and as a community is: "How do we heal from these devastating experiences?"

Christine Runyan, PhD, is a clinical psychologist and cofounder of Tend Health. She says that trauma engages a whopping Upstate stress response, with our panicked brains putting General REV at the helm and our amygdala running intelligence. Their first order of coup business is to shut Central Command and its analytical thinking up in a tower. Dr. Runyan's technique, called Naming It, is a simple strategy rooted in cognitive behavior therapy that you can use at any time and in any situation to gently reinstate RESTORE functioning and intentionally put Central Command back online and in charge.[3] "It sends the message to the nervous system that it can downregulate, like putting a dimmer switch on the sympathetic response," she says. "It helps calm what's happening beneath the skin."

**Step One:** Do an internal weather check. Ask yourself: *What's my internal weather? Am I feeling a rainstorm? Is it hailing in here, a little bit cloudy, or is the sun peeking through?*

**Step Two:** Do a three-pointed check-in: *How's the weather in my mind? My heart? My body?*

Step One helps acknowledge and honor the feelings inside and subtly underscores the fact that, just like the weather, it can and will change. Step Two develops your ability to occasionally check in with yourself as you move through your day, bringing an awareness that can tame REV, especially during high-stress situations. The practice also helps bring an understanding of how your personal feelings (e.g., irritability, anxiety, frustration, sadness, anger) may be coloring your attitude, which can decrease the likelihood that your responses will be tinged with your own negative feelings.

Dr. Runyan believes that we, as individuals, are only as effective as our community and workplaces allow us to be. Unfortunately, it is exactly these larger social structures, educational systems, healthcare industries, and corporate world dynamics that she says are "driven by revenue and productivity—the Upstate stuff—at the expense of peoples' Downstate needs. And the 24/7 news and social media cycles haven't gotten the memo about the importance of Downstates and recovery either.

"It's incumbent upon companies, bosses, and management to grant autonomy and choice to their employees to access these Downstates," says Dr. Runyan. "Empowerment and psychological safety are critical. When people feel safe and not so constrained and conflicted, that's the place where our nervous system will hum along and unquestionably deliver our best work."

Up to 40 percent of early deaths are caused by lifestyle related factors, such as addiction, poor diet, and lack of exercise, and these preventable health problems cost employers a lot of money.[4] On the one hand, when businesses incentivize workers to commit to their Downstate Plan, both sides of the equation benefit. Some forward-thinking companies are already making strides by offering cash incentives for daily steps, reimbursing workers for gym memberships, offering insurance-premium discounts to those who meet health standards—and surcharges to those who don't. Along with boosting the bottom line, promoting self-care drives loyalty to the job. This win-win solution means that your Downstate is not just in your own hands, but also in the hands of policy makers and business leaders. Let's not let them drop that ball.

## You'll Only Be as Good in Your Upstate
## as You Are in Your Downstate

That oft-repeated adage used throughout this book is the mantra that you'll obsessively whisper to yourself on your path to becoming a Downstate Maven, in both moments of ease and of challenge. The root cause of disease and aging beyond your years is inaction—the failure to seize life's organic opportunities for Downstate rejuvenation. I'm sure you have heard of the mythical "self-cleaning oven." Well, just like there ain't no oven that's gonna clean itself, an Upstate stress response that is not met with an equal and opposite Downstate recovery ain't gonna reach RecoveryPlus by itself either. Downstate Mavens are not looking for one more hour in the day to make up for all the stress and its ensuing trickle-down effects. Downstate Mavens are committed, to the best of their abilities, to living every moment in harmony with the moment that came before and the one that will come next. This is accomplished by prioritizing, planning for, and uplifting the Downstate to the level of equal partnership with the Upstate in the lucky job of living your life.

It's not selfish to prioritize time and space for your Downstate. You are not being lazy when you focus on recovery. Rather, having a Downstate practice will support your inner Doozer, if that is what you are seeking, and it will also make you a better thinker, better giver, better you. The way through is by setting up your own personal Downstate boundaries and gently yet firmly maintaining them, even in the face of the aforementioned 24-hour *Carnaval do Upstate*. This undoubtedly means setting limits with friends, family, and work, and facing your own inner gargoyles that frantically set up internal roadblocks and pitfalls around every corner to "help" you avoid the possibility of something new, even when that new thing can save your life. By sticking with your Downstate health boundaries for a short time, you won't even need the Plan to tap into your Downstate, as you'll be able to read your own body's messages. ("Yikes, I've been procrastinating on work for two days now. Maybe I'm pushing myself too hard and need to get back to my deep breathing/go on a walk in nature to refocus my energy/[insert Downstate action here].") This is the way of the Downstate Maven.

## How to Talk to Gargoyles

The biggest roadblock to transforming your life lives deep down inside of you. Shining a light down into that darkness is a necessary step to breaking through your own resistance. When I first contemplated writing this book, I spoke with my therapist about my resistance to all the self-promotion that authors need to do these days to grow their audience. I considered myself a private person, a focused scientist who rarely visited social media. So, I was particularly unhappy about having to build up my online social media presence, as I believed it would suck up any remaining precious time that I'd rather devote to my research, family, friends, and self-care. Who are all these online strangers anyway, and why should I care what they think?

With my therapist's help I probed this sore spot a little deeper and discovered that social media reminded me of popularity contests in junior high and high school that I always felt I was going to lose. Then, I reached an even earlier hurt that formed when I learned that sharing information about myself wasn't always safe. I found that this feeling lived in my solar plexus as a hard, dark mass with sharp contours that was constantly and defensively changing shape. Did it have a name? Yes: Max, the child inside me who protected me from harm, who always said "NO!" to any potential threat and shut down any chance that I could be manipulated or judged, who kept me safe by never letting me put myself out there. Though sad and scary, it was really helpful to meet the child inside me who I was letting run my whole adult show. Max was holding me back from entering a space that held the possibility of rejection, true, but also of connection to the world.

You have a little Max inside of you, with a different name and shape, living in a different corporeal cave. This child has been protecting you by saying no to anything new, anything that might put you in an uncomfortable, foreign position. Sometimes Max is right, but more often Max is holding adult-you back due to the fears of a small child. This child is stopping you "from stepping into the light of your own self," as Sufi mystic Llewellyn Vaughan-Lee puts it.[5] "People are not so much afraid of the darkness," he says, "as of their own light, of their own power, of their own potential."

A crucial step in saying yes to new experiences that bring you closer to your inner light involves identifying, recognizing, and giving attention to your own little Max. Identify what/who is making you uncomfortable.

Where does this feeling live in your body? How did it get there? Recognize the situations that trigger these feelings. Give your inner Max attention by listening to his concerns, and then let him know that you are safe and that adult-you is making the decisions. Through this process, you are consciously putting Central Command in the driver's seat and buckling up little Max in the car seat behind you where he belongs and will feel calm. It's a deep process and a valuable one that will help you move forward in every domain of your life that you want to upgrade, most importantly your Downstate health boundaries.

## Your Daily Downstate Check-In

Sometimes you will wake up and feel, well, shitty. There's no other way to say it. Your bad mood might be from something specific happening in your life or it might bubble up from a nether world of suffering that we, as humans, have an all-access pass to whether we want it or not. Ignoring your Downstate restorative processes can contribute to this emotional dumpster fire or may even be the culprit. So, regardless of the reason for your crap mood, I've made a Daily Downstate Checklist to provide a quick scan through your natural, renewable resources that will fill up your tanks and get you as ready as possible for the Upstate day that awaits. This is not to say that the Downstate will necessarily wipe away all your woes, but Downstate depletion can cause immediate and acute emotional, physical, and cognitive problems that walk and talk just like a bad mood. So, before you start thinking that your life is a total disaster, do yourself a favor and go through this Checklist to make sure your desire to quit your job, break up with your partner, or post some angry retort online isn't your depleted Downstate talking.

Get into the habit of mentally marking off each item on good days, so that when the bad days hit you are already in the habit of checking your Downstate levels and replenishing the domains in need of support.

Now, here's your checklist:

1. **Have you hugged a tree today?** I mean this seriously. Taking your troubles to nature in the form of a good walk in a park or forest, or along a beach will put you in touch with something bigger and more

stable than your day-to-day thoughts and feelings. When describing the origins of her work, *Lake Lament*, tapestry artist Liv Aanrud explained how she relied on nature to hold and witness her feelings during a spell of family hardship. "I would go down to the lake behind our house to escape a bit—maybe this old friend knew what to do? The lake was unchanged, steadfast, and ready to absorb my tears."[6] Be in nature, get untamed.

2. **How well did you sleep last night?** I'm constantly amazed by the importance of sleep for day-to-day functioning and well-being. For example, a study from my lab showed that a single bad night of sleep can often lead to increased feelings of depression and overwhelm the following day.[7] If you didn't sleep well last night, can you take a nap today? Can you make time for a vigorous walk? Can you go to sleep early tonight? Treat yourself like someone who is not all there, because you aren't. And know that the remedy is on your pillow, like a hotel room sweet left during turndown service.

3. **Did you sit in the sunshine this morning?** Your circadian rhythm isn't just here to keep you awake during the day; it also has a big effect on your psychological well-being. Feelings of happiness follow a circadian rhythm, with peak joy occurring in the Upstate day and peak sadness manifesting in the middle of the night.[8] Harmonizing with that rhythm depends on the right kind of exposure to light. Spending fifteen minutes in the morning sunshine or in front of an all-spectrum light box will get you in sync with the sun and moon and optimize your potential for positive feelings.

4. **How deep is your breath?** If you heard the Bee Gees' "How Deep is Your Love" when you read that line, you are on the right track. A deep belly breath is the same as love, sending a message of safety that stimulates RESTORE and tells REV to stand down. When you are upset, shut down, or angry, give yourself the gift of a slow inhale and exhale through your nose, or take a ten-minute meditation break. Now, ask yourself: How deep is your Downstate?

5. **What's on your plate?** First, did you eat breakfast? Eating a morning meal improves cognitive performance, mood, and alertness.[9] And though it might seem like a candy bar is just the right treat to bridge this chasm you're stuck in, the momentary euphoria will only

last as long as it takes for the chocolate to slide down your throat. How about putting effort into the self-care and mindfulness of making yourself a salad for lunch, and save that treat for later? You are worth the effort.

6. **Who have you talked with today?** When you are down, REV is on alert, so even if the last thing you feel like doing is communicating with another human being, doing so will comfort and calm you, and remind you that there are people who care whether you live or die. A conversation will suffice, but even better would be a hand on your back, a warm hug, snuggling up like puppies, or a pants-off dance-off with your beloved.

## The Downstate Is a Basic Need

Do you ever wonder what keeps you and 7.6 billion other people showing up every day? Beyond the rising sun, your warming body, and that cheerleader, cortisol, flooding your brain, you also have a running list of Upstate activities that get you out of bed in the morning. Psychologists believe that we are driven to Doozer, dance, and defend ourselves in order to get our needs met. Legendary psychologist Abraham Maslow, PhD, organized our universal needs into a five-tiered pyramid with the physiological requirements at its base (air, food, drink, shelter, clothing, warmth, sex, sleep). In the next layer you have the need for safety (security, order, law, stability, freedom from fear), followed by the need for love and belonging (friendship, intimacy, trust, acceptance, the receiving and giving of affection and love, community). Tier four of the pyramid is the need for esteem and respect for oneself (dignity, achievement, independence, mastery) and from others.

A fundamental principle here is that these first four levels have to be satisfied to some extent before a person can move on to the top tier: Growth and Self-actualization. This is an obvious concept when you think about the basic needs that support life: clean air, healthy food, uncontaminated water, restorative sleep. But you also need safety and freedom from fear before you can rise to the level of trust, love, real intimacy, and friendship. We live in a world where these first four tiers of necessity are far from secure for too many people. But once you secure this foundation, you gain the ability, resources, and mojo to move on to Growth and Self-actualization, where you manifest your full potential, your mission in life, your calling. Up here, in the lofty land of the crown chakra, you are motivated by becoming and being, with the luxury to ask yourself the quiet, subtle question of your soul's calling.

As the author of *The Power of the Downstate*, my goal is to introduce you to the natural framework of Upstates and Downstates that govern every aspect of your life. I am making the strong assertion that activating your Downstate is THE WAY to secure all your basic needs, including rest and leisure; sleep and safety; nutrition and exercise; self-respect and healthy boundaries. The Downstate is fundamental for your survival and the foundation for your greatness. From this solid, grounded, personal land of plenty, with your Downstate tanks filled, you have the peace of body and mind to tune into your highest and best self, the part of you in touch with something beyond daily toils and troubles, something as old and as wise as time, something infinite. You can ask: Now that I am the master of my Downstate, what do I really want?

# Epilogue

━━━━━━━ • ━━━━━━━

I wrote this book in a 10 × 12-foot wooden hut situated in a small village on the Hudson River. Although the idea for the book began to take
shape in late 2019, the writing in earnest commenced as the tendrils of the
COVID-19 virus began their mysterious and deadly creep across the globe.
At the pandemic's opening salvo, I was living in San Diego with my two
kids who were suddenly home from elementary school in need of support
and education, while my lab at UC Irvine needed leadership and compassion, and the students in my college zoom classes needed calm and nor-
mality. My then-fiancée, Emily, and I were separated by three thousand
miles, without any notion of how, or even if, we would meet again.

If I had thought that the world could use some Downstate in 2019, by
spring 2020, the necessity for restorative work was reaching unimaginable
proportions. On a daily basis, we were forced to contend with absurdly
high levels of potential physical threat, misinformation, and uncertainty
about every aspect of our lives. The only thing one could count on was the
very present moment, and even that felt precarious. My life was whittled
down to its essentials: isolation, fear, death—mixed in with the need to
keep up some semblance of a school schedule, lower my expectations on
every front, practice gratitude, and love on my kids. All the light, hope,
and feeling of safety went out of me when my house became a repeat target for petty criminals during the first month of the shutdown. It felt as if
the world had suddenly become a much more dangerous place and that I
couldn't protect my home or my family.

In spite of (or because of) the constant fear, pain, and loneliness, the
book gushed out of me. Tibetan Buddhist nun Pema Chödrön teaches
the alchemical transformation of suffering via Tonglen meditation: you

breathe in pain and send out relief.[1] I breathed in terror and sent out sci-ence; I breathed in death and sent out creation.

During a little window of hope in early summer, my kids and I dressed in full-coverage hazmat suits and flew to New York to spend a couple of months with Emily in the woods. But this window closed shortly there-after as the curtains fell on California, compelling us to stay in New York because it had become the safest place in the country. We were pan-demic refugees in paradise, living together as a family in this very present moment. Emily and I got married in a small civil ceremony at a spot on the Hudson River that locals call the "party dock"; she built me a hut so I could write; and we preemptively started couples therapy to help us cope with the turbulence of our insta-family. We joined a pod with neighbors and found a wonderful teacher for the kids. Our lives settled into an unex-pectedly simple and fulfilling rhythm.

And while we were at home counting each and every breath as a bless-ing, a man lost his life under the knee of a police officer in Minneapolis. The world bore witness to the history of America enacted in nine minutes and twenty-nine seconds. This deadly silence was followed by a rush of sound that meant the world had had enough. People wearing masks took to their streets across the globe. And just as quickly as we had erected slogans of Oneness and Boats, we erected divisions and walls, with us over here and y'all over there. Online hatred and fear manifested in small town parades of pickup trucks brandishing gigantic flags and big-city clashes with police. And then came the election, followed by a brief and reluctant armistice. Finally, terrorism at the nation's capital formed the bloody cherry on top of this horrendous year.

I'm writing this Epilogue in the springtime of new beginnings, listen-ing to newborn birds practicing their native tongue, witnessing the vibrant colors of east coast flowers and trees, and observing humans emerge, some cautiously, some raucously, from their sequestered hovels. With these changes, I am aware that we, the Global We, have lived through a trauma, and though there is a quick return of rush-hour traffic, busy sidewalks, and picnics in the park, there is also a pain and a sadness and a fear that will not go away on its own.

*The Power of the Downstate* is my prayer of healing to each and every human being on the planet. We need our Downstates now more than any time in recent history. I have heard it said that a person writes the book s/he needs to read. Well, that is true for me too. It's the best answer I can give for how we can live better than just surviving; it teaches us how we can thrive.

With love,

Sara

# Domains of Action Items

## DOMAIN 1: Vagus, Baby

Action Item #1: Practice slow, deep nasal breathing.

Action Item #2: Practice HRV biofeedback.

Action Item #3: Connect with nature once or twice a week.

Action Item #4: Practice meditation three times a week.

Action Item #5: Do twenty minutes of inversion poses three times a week.

Action Item #6: Engage in consensual physical connection as much as possible.

Action Item #7: Practice autogenic training daily.

## DOMAIN 2: Sleep Your Way to the Bottom (of the Downstate)

Action Item #1: Early to bed, every night.

Action Item #2: Take naps three times a week between one p.m. and three p.m.

Action Item #3: Stop caffeine early in the day and all liquids three hours before bed. (Yes, that includes alcohol.)

Action Item #4: Take a nightly dose of melatonin.

Action Item #5: Control your light exposure.

Action Item #6: Keep a consistent bedtime and wake time schedule.

## DOMAIN 3: Exercise Your Right to Recovery

Action Item #1: Exercise for thirty minutes at least three times a week.

Action Item #2: Exercise in the morning for weight control and in the late afternoon for muscle building.

Action Item #3: Use your autonomic system to inform your workout schedule.

Action Item #4: Practice nasal breathing throughout your entire workout.

Action Item #5: Exercise in nature whenever possible, ideally with a friend, family member, or pet, at least three times a week.

Action Item #6: Exercise at a consistent time each day.

### DOMAIN 4: You Are What and When You Eat

Action Item #1: Eat breakfast every day.

Action Item #2: Eat good-for-you foods throughout the day, every day.

Action Item #3: Practice intermittent fasting.

Action Item #4: Schedule your meals to occur within a twelve-, ten-, or eight-hour window.

Action Item #5: Set consistent mealtimes.

Action Item #6: Buy your food at farmers' markets once a week, join a CSA (community-supported agriculture), or plant your own vegetable garden.

# RecoveryPlus Daily Journal

DATE: _____

ACTION ITEM(S): _____

RESPONSES:

| 1 | 2 | 3 | 4 | 5 | 6 | 7 |
|---|---|---|---|---|---|---|
| WORST EVER | BAD | SLIGHT BAD | NO CHANGE | SLIGHT GOOD | GOOD | BEST EVER |

| OUTCOME VARIABLE | DAY 1 | DAY 2 | DAY 3 | DAY 4 | DAY 5 | DAY 6 | DAY 7 | AVERAGE |
|---|---|---|---|---|---|---|---|---|
| MENTAL SHARPNESS | | | | | | | | |
| PRODUCTIVITY | | | | | | | | |
| BEHAVIOR REGULATION | | | | | | | | |
| ENERGY | | | | | | | | |
| EMOTIONAL STABILITY | | | | | | | | |
| PHYSICAL HEALTH | | | | | | | | |
| SLEEP QUALITY | | | | | | | | |
| PLAN ADHERENCE | | | | | | | | |

# Acknowledgments

*The Power of the Downstate* would not be possible without my brilliant team: Laura Nolan, my guide and protector; Leslie Goldman, my collaborator and editor, a creative and hilarious force of nature; and Angela Baggetta, my champion; and the amazing team at Hachette Go led by the inimitable Renée Sedliar. Thank you, dedicated readers, who lovingly stripped this book down to its best self, Lisa Schwarzbaum, Constantine Caramanis, Bill Maurer, Melora Kuhn, and Lauren Whitehurst. Thank you for your hard work and dedication, you all deserve a ginormous Downstate!

My science lab is family. We, the Sleep and Cognition (SaC) Lab, have seen each other through all of life's greatest rewards and devastating challenges. Throughout these ups and downs, we work, bringing our focus back to a common set of questions that haunt us, motivate us, and unite us. The graduate school experience and the launch of a career is a difficult journey. Thank you for the honor of helping you on your way and for making such exciting and mind-blowing scientific discoveries together. This book is yours too. Denise Cai, Elizabeth McDevitt, Katherine Duggan, Lauren Whitehurst, Ben Yetton, Negin Satari, Pin-Chun Chen, Tenzin Tselha, Frida Corona, Jing Zhang, Alessandra Shuster, Abhishek Dave, Jen Kanady, Kate Simon, Mohsen Naji, Nicola Cellini, Hamid and Mohammad Niknazar, Maryam Ahmadi, and the indomitable Paola Malerba. Thank you to all of the dedicated undergraduate research assistants who have come through the lab; you are the backbone of all the research we do. Thanks especially to the lab members that helped assemble the references for this book, Laura May Warren, Karla Vinces, Nicole Delano, Ashley Chen, Kevin Sam, and Shreya Cho. Enormous gratitude goes to my mentors, Robert Stickgold, Ken Nakayama, Sean Drummond, and Geoffrey Boynton, and science comrades, too many to name here from the fields of sleep, vision, memory, autonomic systems. I hope you know that I am grateful for your inspiring work and your friendship. Thank you, UC Irvine School of Social

Sciences and the Department of Cognitive Sciences, for your support and promotion of the SaCLab.

My friends are family. Oh, how much fun we have, how many long conversations, how many milestones we share, how many times have I been a lost and drifting satellite, and my friends have been my tether and anchor. Thank you all for being such generous, honest, brilliant humans, who know how to laugh and cry and be in awe about it all with me, Karen, Lorella, Emily, Hamsa, Julie Amriti, Corey, Constantine, Roman, Meryl, Denise, Lilah, Susan, Melora, the best little neighborhood in San Diego and my wonderful neighbors Wayland and Carie, my ABC&V crew Paola, Carlos, Carolina, Andrea, Gaby, Ryan, and my kids' besties Inés, Ana Sofia, Belen, Tomás, and Santiago. Thank you, village on the Hudson River that adopted us, Joel, Michele, Lisa, Susan, Mikee, Jon, Theo, Mike, Lily, Elias, Gabi, Tilly, Deborah, Laura Gail, Sydney and Clara, Pete, Ann, Pamela and Steve. I am grateful to the people I interviewed for this book for sharing your stories. Your truths brought these academic concepts to life, Glover, Jon, Mikee, Jordan, Lauren, Carlos, Emily, Bill, and many others. Thank you to Jacqui for keeping my head and heart open, and to HasFit.com for keeping me physically fit throughout this writing process. I light candles to my pantheon of inspiring legends, chief among them Eleanor Roosevelt, Joan Jett, and Janelle Monáe.

My family is the greatest-of-all-family (GOAF). What would I do without my sisters, Amy and Lisa, and my cousin, Signe? I would be lost. I can't thank you three enough for your love and support. Thank you to the best *onkel og tante* in the world, Stor Jesper and Marianne, and all the rest of the Danish contingent, Matthias, Anton, Naja, Mads, Mia, Victor, Maria and company. The American flock, my sisters, Joel, Kip, Sam, Katie, Sophie, Nancy, Will, Diane, Carrie, Elena, Oliver, Emily, Phoebe, Finn, and Bo. The late Birgitte, Sarnoff, and Uncle Ed. You are all who I call home.

Finally, My Turkeys, how can I express what is in my heart for you three (plus Mama, Homer, Roux, and Downstater King Shaffer)? It isn't possible. Violet, my daughter; Jesper, my son—you are both the best of everything your ancestors had to offer, I know you will use these gifts wisely. I'm so proud of you and love you endlessly. Emily, my wife, my constant, my love, my elver, you are brilliant, gorgeous, tantalizing, talented, compassionate, Doozerific, romantic, and ridiculously fun. I am the luckiest woman on the planet.

# Notes

## Introduction

1. Sara C. Mednick et al., "The Restorative Effect of Naps on Perceptual Deterioration," *Nature Neuroscience* 5, no. 7 (July 2002): 677–681, https://doi.org/10.1038/nn864.

2. Sara Mednick, Ken Nakayama, and Robert Stickgold, "Sleep-Dependent Learning: A Nap Is as Good as a Night," *Nature Neuroscience* 6, no. 7 (July 2003): 697–698, https://doi.org/10.1038/nn1078.

3. "Doozers," wiki, Muppet Wiki Fandom, accessed September 8, 2021, https://muppet.fandom.com/wiki/Doozers.

4. Lauren N. Whitehurst, Mohsen Naji, and Sara C. Mednick, "Comparing the Cardiac Autonomic Activity Profile of Daytime Naps and Nighttime Sleep," *Neurobiology of Sleep and Circadian Rhythms* 5 (March 15, 2018): 52–57, https://doi.org/10.1016/j.nbscr.2018.03.001.

5. Lauren N. Whitehurst et al., "Autonomic Activity During Sleep Predicts Memory Consolidation in Humans," *Proceedings of the National Academy of Sciences of the United States of America* 113, no. 26 (June 28, 2016): 7272–7277, https://doi.org/10.1073/pnas.1518202113.

6. Jennifer Moss, "When Passion Leads to Burnout," *Harvard Business Review*, July 1, 2019, https://hbr.org/2019/07/when-passion-leads-to-burnout; John Crowley, "Work Until You Drop: How the Long-Hours Culture Is Killing Us," *People HR*, October 17, 2018, https://www.peoplehr.com/blog/2018/10/17/work-drop-long-hours-culture-killing-us/.

## Chapter One. Everything You Know About Balance Needs an Upgrade

1. D. O. Hebb, *The Organization of Behavior: A Neuropsychological Theory* (Mahwah, NJ: Psychology Press, 2002).

2. Bo Wang et al., "Firing Frequency Maxima of Fast-Spiking Neurons in Human, Monkey, and Mouse Neocortex," *Frontiers in Cellular Neuroscience* 10 (October 18, 2016): 239, https://doi.org/10.3389/fncel.2016.00239.

3. Kenneth R. Turley and David L. Rowland, "Evolving Ideas About the Male Refractory Period: Male Refractory Period," *BJU International* 112, no. 4 (August 2013): 442–452, https://doi.org/10.1111/bju.12011.

4. Prince, "Let's Go Crazy," *Purple Rain*, Warner Bros., 1984, compact disc.

5. Walter B. Cannon, *The Wisdom of the Body* (New York: W. W. Norton, 1932).

6. Riley Sebers, "What's Your Temperament: The Humoral Theory's Influence on Medicine in Ancient Greece," *PDXScholar* (April 2016), https://pdxscholar.library.pdx.edu/younghistorians/2016/oralpres/12.

7. Claude Bernard, *Leçons sur les Phenomenes de la Vie Communs aux Animaux et aux Vegetaux* (Paris: J. B. Baillière et fil, 1878).

8. Terry Real, *Fierce Intimacy*, read by author (Boulder: Sounds True, 2018), Audible Audiobook.

9. Jen Sincero, *You Are a Badass: How to Stop Doubting Your Greatness and Start Living an Awesome Life* (Philadelphia: Perseus Books, 2013), 15.

10. Nir Eyal, *Indistractable: How to Control Your Attention and Choose Your Life* (Dallas: BenBella Books, Inc., 2019).

11. Karin Roelofs, "Freeze for Action: Neurobiological Mechanisms in Animal and Human Freezing," *Philosophical Transactions of the Royal Society B: Biological Sciences* 372, no. 1718 (April 19, 2017): 20160206, https://doi.org/10.1098/rstb.2016.0206; Bernadette von Dawans et al., "The Social Dimension of Stress Reactivity: Acute Stress Increases Pro-social Behavior in Humans," *Psychological Science* 23, no. 6 (June 2012): 651–660, https://doi.org/10.1177/0956797611431576.

12. Karen Kangas Dwyer and Marlina M. Davidson, "Is Public Speaking Really More Feared Than Death?" *Communication Research Reports* 29, no. 2 (April 2012): 99–107, https://doi.org/10.1080/08824096.2012.667772.

13. Susan David, *Emotional Agility: Get Unstuck, Embrace Change, and Thrive in Work and Life* (New York: Penguin, 2016), 127.

14. Christine Runyan, author in conversation with, May 31, 2021.

15. Benno Roozendaal, "Glucocorticoids and the Regulation of Memory Consolidation," *Psychoneuroendocrinology* 25, no. 3 (April 2000): 213–238, https://doi.org/10.1016/S0306-4530(99)00058-X; Bruce S. McEwen, "Structural Plasticity of the Adult Brain: How Animal Models Help Us Understand Brain Changes in Depression and Systemic Disorders Related to Depression," *Dialogues in Clinical Neuroscience* 6, no. 2 (June 2004): 119–133, https://doi.org/10.31887/DCNS.2004.6.2/bmcewen.

16. Firdaus S. Dhabhar and Bruce S. McEwen, "Enhancing Versus Suppressive Effects of Stress Hormones on Skin Immune Function," *Proceedings of the National Academy of Sciences* 96, no. 3 (February 2, 1999): 1059–1064, https://doi.org/10.1073/pnas.96.3.1059.

17. Ziad Boulos and Alan M. Rosenwasser, "A Chronobiological Perspective on Allostasis and Its Application to Shift Work," in *Allostasis, Homeostasis, and the Costs of Physiological Adaptation*, ed. Jay Schulkin, 1st ed. (Cambridge: Cambridge University Press, 2004), 228–301; Björn Folkow and Eric Neil, *Circulation* (London: Oxford University Press, 1971).

18. Claudio Franceschi et al., "Inflammaging: A New Immune–Metabolic Viewpoint for Age-Related Diseases," *Nature Reviews Endocrinology* 14, no. 10 (October 2018): 576–590, https://doi.org/10.1038/s41574-018-0059-4.

19. Sarah F. Leibowitz and Bartley G. Hoebel, "Behavioral Neuroscience and Obesity," in *Handbook of Obesity*, ed. George A. Bray, Claude Bouchard, and W. P. T. James, 1st ed. (New York: CRC Press, 1997).

20. David N. Brindley and Yves Rolland, "Possible Connections between Stress, Diabetes, Obesity, Hypertension and Altered Lipoprotein Metabolism That May Result in Atherosclerosis," *Clinical Science* 77, no. 5 (November 1, 1989): 453–461, https://doi.org/10.1042/cs0770453.

21. Casey Schwartz, "Global, Regional, and National Age–Sex Specific All-Cause and Cause-Specific Mortality for 240 Causes of Death, 1990–2013: A Systematic Analysis for the Global Burden of Disease Study 2013," *Lancet* 385, no. 9963 (January 2015): 117–171, https://doi.org/10.1016/S0140-6736(14)61682-2; Christine Perret-Guillaume, Laure Joly, and Athanase Benetos, "Heart Rate as a Risk Factor for Cardiovascular Disease," *Progress in Cardiovascular Diseases* 52, no. 1 (July 2009): 6–10, https://doi.org/10.1016/j.pcad.2009.05.003; Xavier Jouven et al., "Heart Rate and Risk of Cancer Death in Healthy Men," ed.

Julian Little, *PLOS ONE* 6, no. 8 (August 3, 2011): e21310, https://doi.org/10.1371/journal .pone.0021310.

22. Christine Perret-Guillaume, Laure Joly, and Athanase Benetos, "Heart Rate as a Risk Factor for Cardiovascular Disease," *Progress in Cardiovascular Diseases* 52, no. 1 (July 2009): 6–10, https://doi.org/10.1016/j.pcad.2009.05.003.

23. Silvia Stringhini et al., "Socioeconomic Status and the 25 × 25 Risk Factors as Determinants of Premature Mortality: A Multicohort Study and Meta-Analysis of 1.7 Million Men and Women," *Lancet* 389, no. 10075 (March 2017): 1229–1237, https://doi.org/10 .1016/S0140-6736(16)32380-7; Johan P. Mackenbach et al., "Socioeconomic Inequalities in Health in 22 European Countries," *New England Journal of Medicine* 358, no. 23 (June 5, 2008): 2468–2481, https://doi.org/10.1056/NEJMsa0707519.

24. Ronald C. Kessler, Kristin D. Mickelson, and David R. Williams, "The Prevalence, Distribution, and Mental Health Correlates of Perceived Discrimination in the United States," *Journal of Health and Social Behavior* 40, no. 3 (September 1999): 208, https://doi.org /10.2307/2676349; Thomas E. Fuller-Rowell, Gary W. Evans, and Anthony D. Ong, "Poverty and Health: The Mediating Role of Perceived Discrimination," *Psychological Science* 23, no. 7 (July 2012): 734–739, https://doi.org/10.1177/0956797612439720.

25. Robert S. Stawski et al., "Associations Among Daily Stressors and Salivary Cortisol: Findings from the National Study of Daily Experiences," *Psychoneuroendocrinology* 38, no. 11 (November 2013): 2654–2665, https://doi.org/10.1016/j.psyneuen.2013.06.023.

26. Lisa L. Barnes et al., "Perceived Discrimination and Mortality in a Population-Based Study of Older Adults," *American Journal of Public Health* 98, no. 7 (July 2008): 1241–1247, https://doi.org/10.2105/AJPH.2007.114397; David R. Williams et al., "Racial Differences in Physical and Mental Health: Socio-Economic Status, Stress and Discrimination," *Journal of Health Psychology* 2, no. 3 (July 1997): 335–351, https://doi.org/10.1177 /135910539700200305.

27. Derald Wing Sue et al., "Racial Microaggressions in Everyday Life: Implications for Clinical Practice," *American Psychologist* 62, no. 4 (2007): 271–286, https://doi.org/10 .1037/0003-066X.62.4.271.

28. Sarah L. Szanton et al., "Racial Discrimination Is Associated with a Measure of Red Blood Cell Oxidative Stress: A Potential Pathway for Racial Health Disparities," *International Journal of Behavioral Medicine* 19, no. 4 (December 2012): 489–495, https://doi.org /10.1007/s12529-011-9188-z; Samantha G. Bromfield et al., "Race and Gender Differences in the Association Between Experiences of Everyday Discrimination and Arterial Stiffness Among Patients With Coronary Heart Disease," *Annals of Behavioral Medicine* 54, no. 10 (October 1, 2020): 761–770, https://doi.org/10.1093/abm/kaaa015; Eli Michaels et al., "Coding the Everyday Discrimination Scale: Implications for Exposure Assessment and Associations with Hypertension and Depression Among a Cross Section of Midlife African American Women," *Journal of Epidemiology and Community Health* 73, no. 6 (June 2019): 577–584, https://doi.org/10.1136/jech-2018-211230; Laura B. Zahodne et al., "Inflammatory Mechanisms Underlying the Effects of Everyday Discrimination on Age-Related Memory Decline," *Brain, Behavior, and Immunity* 75 (January 2019): 149–154, https://doi.org/10.1016/j.bbi.2018.10.002.

29. Logan S. Casey et al., "Discrimination in the United States: Experiences of Lesbian, Gay, Bisexual, Transgender, and Queer Americans," *Health Services Research* 54, suppl. 2 (December 2019): 1454–1466, https://doi.org/10.1111/1475-6773.13229.

30. Tyler B. Mason and Robin J. Lewis, "Clustered Patterns of Behavioral and Health-Related Variables Among Young Lesbian Women," *Behavior Therapy* 50, no. 4

(July 2019): 683–695, https://doi.org/10.1016/j.beth.2018.10.006; Robin J. Lewis et al., "Health Disparities Among Exclusively Lesbian, Mostly Lesbian, and Bisexual Young Women," *LGBT Health* 6, no. 8 (December 1, 2019): 400–408, https://doi.org/10.1089/lgbt.2019.0055; Alexis Dewaele, Mieke Van Houtte, and John Vincke, "Visibility and Coping with Minority Stress: A Gender-Specific Analysis Among Lesbians, Gay Men, and Bisexuals in Flanders," *Archives of Sexual Behavior* 43, no. 8 (November 2014): 1601–1614, https://doi.org/10.1007/s10508-014-0380-5.

31. Fausta Rosati et al., "The Cardiovascular Conundrum in Ethnic and Sexual Minorities: A Potential Biomarker of Constant Coping With Discrimination," *Frontiers in Neuroscience* 15 (May 19, 2021): 619171, https://doi.org/10.3389/fnins.2021.619171.

32. "AMA: Racism Is a Threat to Public Health," American Medical Association, accessed November 18, 2020, https://www.ama-assn.org/delivering-care/health-equity /ama-racism-threat-public-health.

33. Maximus Berger and Zoltán Sarnyai, "'More than Skin Deep': Stress Neurobiology and Mental Health Consequences of Racial Discrimination," *Stress* 18, no. 1 (January 2, 2015): 1–10, https://doi.org/10.3109/10253890.2014.989204; Elizabeth Brondolo et al., "Dimensions of Perceived Racism and Self-Reported Health: Examination of Racial/ Ethnic Differences and Potential Mediators," *Annals of Behavioral Medicine: A Publication of the Society of Behavioral Medicine* 42, no. 1 (August 2011): 14–28, https://doi.org/10.1007 /s12160-011-9265-1; Elizabeth A. Pascoe and Laura Smart Richman, "Perceived Discrimination and Health: A Meta-Analytic Review," *Psychological Bulletin* 135, no. 4 (July 2009): 531–554, https://doi.org/10.1037/a0016059; Haslyn E. R. Hunte and David R. Williams, "The Association Between Perceived Discrimination and Obesity in a Population-Based Multiracial and Multiethnic Adult Sample," *American Journal of Public Health* 99, no. 7 (July 2009): 1285–1292, https://doi.org/10.2105/AJPH.2007.128090; Rebecca Din-Dzietham et al., "Perceived Stress Following Race-Based Discrimination at Work Is Associated with Hypertension in African-Americans. The Metro Atlanta Heart Disease Study, 1999–2001," *Social Science & Medicine (1982)* 58, no. 3 (February 2004): 449–461, https://doi .org/10.1016/s0277-9536(03)00211-9; Tené T. Lewis et al., "Self-Reported Experiences of Discrimination and Cardiovascular Disease," *Current Cardiovascular Risk Reports* 8, no. 1 (January 1, 2014): 365, https://doi.org/10.1007/s12170-013-0365-2; Eileen M. Crimmins et al., "Hispanic Paradox in Biological Risk Profiles," *American Journal of Public Health* 97, no. 7 (July 2007): 1305–1310, https://doi.org/10.2105/AJPH.2006.091892.

34. Yuichiro Yano et al., "Racial Differences in Associations of Blood Pressure Components in Young Adulthood With Incident Cardiovascular Disease by Middle Age: Coronary Artery Risk Development in Young Adults (CARDIA) Study," *JAMA Cardiology* 2, no. 4 (April 1, 2017): 381–389, https://doi.org/10.1001/jamacardio.2016.5678; George A. Mensah et al., "State of Disparities in Cardiovascular Health in the United States," *Circulation* 111, no. 10 (March 15, 2005): 1233–1241, https://doi.org/10.1161/01.CIR .0000158136.76824.04.

35. LaBarron K. Hill et al., "Examining the Association Between Perceived Discrimination and Heart Rate Variability in African Americans," *Cultural Diversity & Ethnic Minority Psychology* 23, no. 1 (January 2017): 5–14, https://doi.org/10.1037/cdp0000076.

36. Virginia W. Huynh and Cari Gillen-O'Neel, "Discrimination and Sleep: The Protective Role of School Belonging," *Youth & Society* 48, no. 5 (September 1, 2016): 649–672, https://doi.org/10.1177/0044118X13506720; Thomas E. Fuller-Rowell et al., "Racial Disparities in Sleep: The Role of Neighborhood Disadvantage," *Sleep Medicine* 27–28 (November 1, 2016): 1–8, https://doi.org/10.1016/j.sleep.2016.10.008; "What's the Connection Between Race and Sleep Disorders?" Sleep Foundation, accessed

April 11, 2021, https://www.sleepfoundation.org/how-sleep-works/whats-connection
-between-race-and-sleep-disorders.

## Chapter Two. Get in Sync with Your Inherent Rhythm

1. "Universal Declaration of Human Rights," United Nations, accessed April 11, 2021,
https://www.un.org/en/about-us/universal-declaration-of-human-rights.

2. "Universal Declaration of Human Rights."

3. "Universal Declaration of Human Rights."

4. Pallab Ghosh, "'First Human' Discovered in Ethiopia," BBC News, March 4, 2015,
https://www.bbc.com/news/science-environment-31718336.

5. Meiyu Ke et al., "Auxin Controls Circadian Flower Opening and Closure in the
Waterlily," *BMC Plant Biology* 18, no. 1 (December 2018): 143, https://doi.org/10.1186/
s12870-018-1357-7; Peter K. Jonason, Amy Jones, and Minna Lyons, "Creatures of the
Night: Chronotypes and the Dark Triad Traits," *Personality and Individual Differences* 55, no.
5 (September 2013): 538–541, https://doi.org/10.1016/j.paid.2013.05.001.

6. "Circadian Rhythms," National Institute of General Medical Sciences, accessed April
11, 2021, https://www.nigms.nih.gov/education/fact-sheets/Pages/circadian-rhythms
.aspx.

7. Lars Peter Holst Andersen et al., "The Safety of Melatonin in Humans," *Clinical Drug
Investigation* 36, no. 3 (March 2016): 169–175, https://doi.org/10.1007/s40261-015-0368-5;
Fedor Simko and Ludovit Paulis, "Melatonin as a Potential Antihypertensive Treatment,"
*Journal of Pineal Research* 42, no. 4 (April 2007): 319–322, https://doi.org/10.1111/j.1600
-079X.2007.00436.x; Angelo Cagnacci et al., "Prolonged Melatonin Administration
Decreases Nocturnal Blood Pressure in Women," *American Journal of Hypertension* 18, no.
12 pt. 1 (December 2005): 1614–1618, https://doi.org/10.1016/j.amjhyper.2005.05.008.

8. Juliane Richter et al., "Twice as High Diet-Induced Thermogenesis After Breakfast
vs Dinner on High-Calorie as Well as Low-Calorie Meals," *Journal of Clinical Endocrinology & Metabolism* 105, no. 3 (March 1, 2020): e211–e221, https://doi.org/10.1210/clinem
/dgz311; "People Who Eat a Big Breakfast May Burn Twice as Many Calories: Study Finds
Eating More at Breakfast Instead of Dinner Could Prevent Obesity," ScienceDaily, February 19, 2020, https://www.sciencedaily.com/releases/2020/02/200219092539.htm.

9. Susan Kohl Malone, Maria A. Mendoza, and Freda Patterson, "Social Jetlag, Circadian Disruption, and Cardiometabolic Disease Risk," in *Sleep and Health*, 227–240, https://
doi.org/10.1016/B978-0-12-815373-4.00018-6.

10. Malone, Mendoza, and Patterson, "Social Jetlag, Circadian Disruption, and Cardiometabolic Disease Risk."

11. Malone, Mendoza, and Patterson, "Social Jetlag, Circadian Disruption, and Cardiometabolic Disease Risk."

12. Li-Qiang Qin et al., "The Effects of Nocturnal Life on Endocrine Circadian Patterns in Healthy Adults," *Life Sciences* 73, no. 19 (September 2003): 2467–2475, https://
doi.org/10.1016/S0024-3205(03)00628-3.

13. Pablo Valdez, "Circadian Rhythms in Attention," *Yale Journal of Biology and Medicine* 92, no. 1 (March 2019): 81–92.

14. Yadan Li et al., "Night or Darkness, Which Intensifies the Feeling of Fear?" *International Journal of Psychophysiology* 97, no. 1 (July 2015): 46–57, https://doi.org/10.1016/j
.ijpsycho.2015.04.021.

15. N. Arias et al., "How Demanding Is the Brain on a Reversal Task Under Day and
Night Conditions?" *Neuroscience Letters* 600 (July 2015): 153–157, https://doi.org/10.1016

/j.neulet.2015.06.014; C. Cajochen et al., "Separation of Circadian and Wake Duration-Dependent Modulation of EEG Activation During Wakefulness," *Neuroscience* 114, no. 4 (November 2002): 1047–1060, https://doi.org/10.1016/S0306-4522(02)00209-9.

16. Ron Sender, Shai Fuchs, and Ron Milo, "Revised Estimates for the Number of Human and Bacteria Cells in the Body," *PLOS Biology* 14, no. 8 (August 19, 2016): e1002533, https://doi.org/10.1371/journal.pbio.1002533.

17. Marilyn Hair and Jon Sharpe, "Fast Facts About the Human Microbiome," Center for Ecogenetics & Environmental Health, accessed April 11, 2021, https://depts.washington.edu/ceeh/downloads/FF_Microbiome.pdf.

18. Tomasz Szeligowski et al., "The Gut Microbiome and Schizophrenia: The Current State of the Field and Clinical Applications," *Frontiers in Psychiatry* 11 (March 12, 2020): 156, https://doi.org/10.3389/fpsyt.2020.00156.

19. Hyun Ho Choi and Young-Seok Cho, "Fecal Microbiota Transplantation: Current Applications, Effectiveness, and Future Perspectives," *Clinical Endoscopy* 49, no. 3 (May 30, 2016): 257–265, https://doi.org/10.5946/ce.2015.117.

20. Elaine O. Petrof et al., "Stool Substitute Transplant Therapy for the Eradication of Clostridium Difficile Infection: 'RePOOPulating' the Gut," *Microbiome* 1, no. 1 (December 2013): 3, https://doi.org/10.1186/2049-2618-1-3.

21. Christoph A. Thaiss et al., "Transkingdom Control of Microbiota Diurnal Oscillations Promotes Metabolic Homeostasis," *Cell* 159, no. 3 (October 2014): 514–529, https://doi.org/10.1016/j.cell.2014.09.048.

22. Richard A. Bryant et al., "A Multisite Study of Initial Respiration Rate and Heart Rate as Predictors of Posttraumatic Stress Disorder," *Journal of Clinical Psychiatry* 69, no. 11 (November 30, 2008): 1694–1701, https://doi.org/10.4088/JCP.v69n1104.

23. Thomas M. Penders et al., "Bright Light Therapy as Augmentation of Pharmacotherapy for Treatment of Depression: A Systematic Review and Meta-analysis," *The Primary Care Companion for CNS Disorders*, October 20, 2016, https://doi.org/10.4088/PCC.15r01906.

24. Brant P. Hasler et al., "An Altered Neural Response to Reward May Contribute to Alcohol Problems Among Late Adolescents with an Evening Chronotype," *Psychiatry Research: Neuroimaging* 214, no. 3 (December 2013): 357–364, https://doi.org/10.1016/j.pscychresns.2013.08.005; Meredith E. Rumble et al., "The Relationship of Person-Specific Eveningness Chronotype, Greater Seasonality, and Less Rhythmicity to Suicidal Behavior: A Literature Review," *Journal of Affective Disorders* 227 (February 2018): 721–730, https://doi.org/10.1016/j.jad.2017.11.078.

25. Jade M. Murray et al., "Prevalence of Circadian Misalignment and Its Association with Depressive Symptoms in Delayed Sleep Phase Disorder," *Sleep* 40, no. 1 (January 1, 2017), https://doi.org/10.1093/sleep/zsw002.

26. Neta Ram-Vlasov et al., "Creativity and Habitual Sleep Patterns Among Art and Social Sciences Undergraduate Students," *Psychology of Aesthetics, Creativity, and the Arts* 10, no. 3 (August 2016): 270–777, https://doi.org/10.1037/aca0000062.

27. "Sleeping with the Muse: The Relation Between a Musical Life and Sleep," *Record Union Blog* (blog), March 31, 2020, https://blog.recordunion.com/the-wellness-starter-pack-sleeping-with-the-muse-the-relation-between-a-musical-life-and-sleep.

28. Leandro P. Casiraghi et al., "Access to Electric Light Is Associated with Delays of the Dim-Light Melatonin Onset in a Traditionally Hunter-Gatherer Toba/Qom Community," *Journal of Pineal Research* 69, no. 4 (November 2020), https://doi.org/10.1111/jpi.12689.

29. Ellen R. Stothard et al., "Circadian Entrainment to the Natural Light-Dark Cycle Across Seasons and the Weekend," *Current Biology: CB* 27, no. 4 (February 20, 2017): 508–513, https://doi.org/10.1016/j.cub.2016.12.041.

30. María Juliana Leone, Mariano Sigman, and Diego Andrés Golombek, "Effects of Lockdown on Human Sleep and Chronotype During the COVID-19 Pandemic," *Current Biology: CB* 30, no. 16 (August 17, 2020): R930–R931, https://doi.org/10.1016/j.cub.2020.07.015.

31. Shigehiro Ohdo, Satoru Koyanagi, and Naoya Matsunaga, "Chronopharmacological Strategies Focused on Chrono-Drug Discovery," *Pharmacology & Therapeutics* 202 (October 2019): 72–90, https://doi.org/10.1016/j.pharmthera.2019.05.018.

32. Christoph Scheiermann, Yuya Kunisaki, and Paul S. Frenette, "Circadian Control of the Immune System," *Nature Reviews Immunology* 13, no. 3 (March 2013): 190–198, https://doi.org/10.1038/nri3386.

33. "Time-Sensitive Clues about Cardiovascular Risk," Harvard Health, March 1, 2019, https://www.health.harvard.edu/heart-health/time-sensitive-clues-about-cardio vascular-risk; Lihong Chen and Guangrui Yang, "Recent Advances in Circadian Rhythms in Cardiovascular System," *Frontiers in Pharmacology* 6 (April 1, 2015), https://doi.org /10.3389/fphar.2015.00071.

34. D. Pincus, T. Humeston, and R. Martin, "Further Studies on the Chronotherapy of Asthma with Inhaled Steroids: The Effect of Dosage Timing on Drug Efficacy," *Journal of Allergy and Clinical Immunology* 100, no. 6 (December 1997): 771–774, https://doi.org /10.1016/S0091-6749(97)70272-0; Laxminarayana Bairy, "Chronotherapeutics: A Hype or Future of Chronopharmacology?," *Indian Journal of Pharmacology* 45, no. 6 (2013): 545, https://doi.org/10.4103/0253-7613.121265.

35. Francis Lévi et al., "Implications of Circadian Clocks for the Rhythmic Delivery of Cancer Therapeutics," *Advanced Drug Delivery Reviews* 59, no. 9–10 (August 2007): 1015–1035, https://doi.org/10.1016/j.addr.2006.11.001.

36. Nathaniel P. Hoyle et al., "Circadian Actin Dynamics Drive Rhythmic Fibroblast Mobilization During Wound Healing," *Science Translational Medicine* 9, no. 415 (November 8, 2017): eaal2774, https://doi.org/10.1126/scitranslmed.aal2774.

37. "The Nielsen Total Audience Report: August 2020," Nielsen, August 13, 2020, https://www.nielsen.com/us/en/insights/report/2020/the-nielsen-total-audience-report -august-2020.

38. Susan Kohl Malone, Maria A. Mendoza, and Freda Patterson, "Social Jetlag, Circadian Disruption, and Cardiometabolic Disease Risk," in *Sleep and Health* (Elsevier, 2019), 227–240, https://doi.org/10.1016/B978-0-12-815373-4.00018-6.

39. Norifumi Tsuno, Alain Besset, and Karen Ritchie, "Sleep and Depression," *Journal of Clinical Psychiatry* 66, no. 10 (October 15, 2005): 1254–1269, https://doi.org/10.4088 /JCP.v66n1008.

40. Anitra D. M. Koopman et al., "The Association Between Social Jetlag, the Metabolic Syndrome, and Type 2 Diabetes Mellitus in the General Population: The New Hoorn Study," *Journal of Biological Rhythms* 32, no. 4 (August 2017): 359–368, https://doi.org /10.1177/0748730417713572.

41. Patricia M. Wong et al., "Social Jetlag, Chronotype, and Cardiometabolic Risk," *Journal of Clinical Endocrinology & Metabolism* 100, no. 12 (December 1, 2015): 4612–4620, https://doi.org/10.1210/jc.2015-2923.

42. "UA Research: 'Social Jetlag' Measured by Differences in Sleep Patterns on Days Off vs. Work Days, Associated with Poor Overall Health," UAHS Office of Public Affairs, accessed April 12, 2021, https://opa.uahs.arizona.edu/newsroom/news/2017/ua -research-social-jetlag-measured-differences-sleep-patterns-days-vs-work-days.

43. T. A. Bedrosian and R. J. Nelson, "Influence of the Modern Light Environment on Mood," *Molecular Psychiatry* 18, no. 7 (July 2013): 751–757, https://doi.org/10.1038 /mp.2013.70; X.-S. Wang et al., "Shift Work and Chronic Disease: The Epidemiological

Evidence," *Occupational Medicine* 61, no. 2 (March 1, 2011): 78–89, https://doi.org/10.1093 /occmed/kqr001; E. McFadden et al., "The Relationship Between Obesity and Exposure to Light at Night: Cross-Sectional Analyses of Over 100,000 Women in the Breakthrough Generations Study," *American Journal of Epidemiology* 180, no. 3 (August 1, 2014): 245–250, https://doi.org/10.1093/aje/kwu117; S. Sookoian et al., "Effects of Rotating Shift Work on Biomarkers of Metabolic Syndrome and Inflammation," *Journal of Internal Medicine* 261, no. 3 (March 2007): 285–292, https://doi.org/10.1111/j.1365-2796.2007.01766.x.

44. R. G. Stevens et al., "Considerations of Circadian Impact for Defining 'Shift Work' in Cancer Studies: IARC Working Group Report," *Occupational and Environmental Medicine* 68, no. 2 (February 1, 2011): 154–162, https://doi.org/10.1136/oem.2009.053512; P. Noone, "Nightshift Breast Cancer, Flour Dust and Blue-Light Risk," *Occupational Medicine* 60, no. 6 (September 1, 2010): 499, https://doi.org/10.1093/occmed/kqq096.

45. Heather Dunn, Mary Ann Anderson, and Pamela D. Hill, "Nighttime Lighting in Intensive Care Units," *Critical Care Nurse* 30, no. 3 (June 1, 2010): 31–37, https://doi.org /10.4037/ccn2010342; Laura K. Fonken et al., "Dim Light at Night Impairs Recovery from Global Cerebral Ischemia," *Experimental Neurology* 317 (July 2019): 100–109, https://doi .org/10.1016/j.expneurol.2019.02.008; Esther I. Bernhofer et al., "Hospital Lighting and Its Association with Sleep, Mood and Pain in Medical Inpatients," *Journal of Advanced Nursing* 70, no. 5 (May 2014): 1164–1173, https://doi.org/10.1111/jan.12282.

46. Judith A. Westman et al., "Low Cancer Incidence Rates in Ohio Amish," *Cancer Causes & Control* 21, no. 1 (January 2010): 69–75, https://doi.org/10.1007/s10552-009 -9435-7; Janice A. Egeland and Abram M. Hostetter, "Amish Study, I: Affective Disorders Among the Amish, 1976–1980," *American Journal of Psychiatry* 140, no. 1 (January 1983): 56–61, https://doi.org/10.1176/ajp.140.1.56.

47. C. L. Guarana, C. M. Barnes, and W. J. Ong, "The Effects of Blue-Light Filtration on Sleep and Work Outcomes," *Journal of Applied Psychology* 106, 5 (2021): 784–796.

48. Alix Strauss, "How Kate Pierson, of the B-52s, and Monica Coleman, Spend Their Sundays," *New York Times*, August 14, 2020, sec. New York, https://www.nytimes.com /2020/08/14/nyregion/coronavirus-kate-pierson-b-52s.html.

49. Karin S. Björkstén, Daniel F. Kripke, and Peter Bjerregaard, "Accentuation of Suicides but Not Homicides with Rising Latitudes of Greenland in the Sunny Months," *BMC Psychiatry* 9, no. 20 (2009), https://doi.org/10.1186/1471-244X-9-20.

50. Kari Leibowitz, "The Norwegian Town Where the Sun Doesn't Rise," *Atlantic*, July 1, 2015, https://www.theatlantic.com/health/archive/2015/07/the-norwegian-town-where -the-sun-doesnt-rise/396746/.

51. Weiqun Lu et al., "A Circadian Clock Is Not Required in an Arctic Mammal," *Current Biology* 20, no. 6 (March 2010): 533–537, https://doi.org/10.1016/j.cub.2010.01.042.

52. Liza H. Ashbrook et al., "Genetics of the Human Circadian Clock and Sleep Homeostat," *Neuropsychopharmacology* 45, no. 1 (January 2020): 45–54, https://doi.org/10.1038 /s41386-019-0476-7.

53. Christine M. Walsh et al., "Weaker Circadian Activity Rhythms Are Associated with Poorer Executive Function in Older Women," *Sleep* 37, no. 12 (December 1, 2014): 2009–2016, https://doi.org/10.5665/sleep.4260; Gregory J. Tranah et al., "Circadian Activity Rhythms and Risk of Incident Dementia and Mild Cognitive Impairment in Older Women," *Annals of Neurology* 70, no. 5 (November 2011): 722–732, https://doi.org /10.1002/ana.22468.

54. Adam Mansbach and Ricardo Cortés, eds., *Go the F**k to Sleep* (Edinburgh: Canongate, 2011).

55. A. Roger Ekirch, *At Day's Close: Night in Times Past* (New York: W. W. Norton, 2006).

56. Amy R. Wolfson and Mary A. Carskadon, "Understanding Adolescents' Sleep Patterns and School Performance: A Critical Appraisal," *Sleep Medicine Reviews* 7, no. 6 (January 2003): 491–506, https://doi.org/10.1016/S1087-0792(03)90003-7.

57. Gahan Fallone et al., "Experimental Restriction of Sleep Opportunity in Children: Effects on Teacher Ratings," *Sleep* 28, no. 12 (December 2005): 1561–1567, https://doi.org/10.1093/sleep/28.12.1561; Avi Sadeh, Reut Gruber, and Amiram Raviv, "The Effects of Sleep Restriction and Extension on School-Age Children: What a Difference an Hour Makes," *Child Development* 74, no. 2 (March 2003): 444–455, https://doi.org/10.1111/1467-8624.7402008.

58. Valentina Alfonsi et al., "The Association Between School Start Time and Sleep Duration, Sustained Attention, and Academic Performance," *Nature and Science of Sleep* 12 (December 2020): 1161–1172, https://doi.org/10.2147/NSS.S273875.

59. Matthew Krongsberg, "Why Farms Want Cold Winters," Grist, February 16, 2012, https://grist.org/sustainable-farming/why-farms-want-cold-winters/.

60. Rebecca Ray and John Schmitt, "The Right to Vacation: An International Perspective," *International Journal of Health Services* 38, no. 1 (January 2008): 21–45, https://doi.org/10.2190/HS.38.1.b; Jennifer Moss, "Beyond Burned Out," Physician Leadership, accessed April 19, 2021, https://www.physicianleaders.org/news/beyond-burned-out.

## Chapter Three. Replenish, Revitalize, Rebuild, RESTORE!

1. Kate Teffer and Katerina Semendeferi, "Human Prefrontal Cortex: Evolution, Development, and Pathology," *Progress in Brain Research* 195 (2012): 191–218, https://doi.org/10.1016/B978-0-444-53860-4.00009-X.

2. T. H. Svensson and P. Thorén, "Brain Noradrenergic Neurons in the Locus Coeruleus: Inhibition by Blood Volume Load through Vagal Afferents," *Brain Research* 172, no. 1 (August 17, 1979): 174–178, https://doi.org/10.1016/0006-8993(79)90908-9.

3. Alan W. C. Yuen and Josemir W. Sander, "Can Natural Ways to Stimulate the Vagus Nerve Improve Seizure Control?" *Epilepsy & Behavior: E&B* 67 (February 2017): 105–110, https://doi.org/10.1016/j.yebeh.2016.10.039.

4. Jennifer A. Clancy, Susan A. Deuchars, and Jim Deuchars, "The Wonders of the Wanderer," *Experimental Physiology* 98, no. 1 (January 2013): 38–45, https://doi.org/10.1113/expphysiol.2012.064543.

5. Julian F. Thayer and Richard D. Lane, "Claude Bernard and the Heart-Brain Connection: Further Elaboration of a Model of Neurovisceral Integration," *Neuroscience and Biobehavioral Reviews* 33, no. 2 (February 2009): 81–88, https://doi.org/10.1016/j.neubiorev.2008.08.004.

6. György Buzsáki, Kai Kaila, and Marcus Raichle, "Inhibition and Brain Work," *Neuron* 56, no. 5 (December 6, 2007): 771–783, https://doi.org/10.1016/j.neuron.2007.11.008.

7. Fred Shaffer and J. P. Ginsberg, "An Overview of Heart Rate Variability Metrics and Norms," *Frontiers in Public Health* 5 (2017): 258, https://doi.org/10.3389/fpubh.2017.00258.

8. Marc A. Russo, Danielle M. Santarelli, and Dean O'Rourke, "The Physiological Effects of Slow Breathing in the Healthy Human," *Breathe* 13, no. 4 (2017): 298–309, https://doi.org/10.1183/20734735.009817.

9. Patrick R. Steffen et al., "The Impact of Resonance Frequency Breathing on Measures of Heart Rate Variability, Blood Pressure, and Mood," *Frontiers in Public Health* 5 (2017): 222, https://doi.org/10.3389/fpubh.2017.00222.

10. Swami Muktibodhananda, *Hatha Yoga Pradipika: Light on Hatha Yoga*, 2nd ed. (Bihar: Yoga Publication Trust, 2002).

11. "The Hippies Were Right: It's All About Vibrations, Man!" Scientific American Blog Network, accessed September 5, 2021, https://blogs.scientificamerican.com/observations /the-hippies-were-right-its-all-about-vibrations-man/.

12. Evgeny Vaschillo et al., "Heart Rate Variability Biofeedback as a Method for Assessing Baroreflex Function: A Preliminary Study of Resonance in the Cardiovascular System," *Applied Psychophysiology and Biofeedback* 27, no. 1 (March 2002): 1–27, https://doi.org/10 .1023/a:1014587304314.

13. Patrick R. Steffen et al., "The Impact of Resonance Frequency Breathing on Measures of Heart Rate Variability, Blood Pressure, and Mood," *Frontiers in Public Health* 5 (2017): 222, https://doi.org/10.3389/fpubh.2017.00222.

14. Detlef H. Heck, Robert Kozma, and Leslie M. Kay, "The Rhythm of Memory: How Breathing Shapes Memory Function," *Journal of Neurophysiology* 122, no. 2 (August 1, 2019): 563–571, https://doi.org/10.1152/jn.00200.2019.

15. "Does Breathing Through My Mouth Affect My Dental Health?" Harvard Health, August 6, 2015, https://www.health.harvard.edu/newsletter_article/does-breathing -through-my-mouth-affect-my-dental-health.

16. B. K. S. Iyengar, *Light on Prāṇāyāma : The Yogic Art of Breathing* (New York: Crossroad, 2011).

17. James Nestor, "An Excerpt from Breath," PenguinRandomhouse.com, accessed April 13, 2021, https://www.penguinrandomhouse.com/articles/breath-excerpt.

18. D. Liao et al., "Association of Cardiac Autonomic Function and the Development of Hypertension: The ARIC Study," *American Journal of Hypertension* 9, no. 12 pt. 1 (December 1996): 1147–1156, https://doi.org/10.1016/s0895-7061(96)00249-x.

19. Paolo Palatini et al., "Evolution of Blood Pressure and Cholesterol in Stage 1 Hypertension: Role of Autonomic Nervous System Activity," *Journal of Hypertension* 24, no. 7 (July 2006): 1375–1381, https://doi.org/10.1097/01.hjh.0000234118.25401.1c.

20. Abel Plaza-Florido et al., "The Role of Heart Rate on the Associations Between Body Composition and Heart Rate Variability in Children with Overweight/Obesity: The ActiveBrains Project," *Frontiers in Physiology* 10 (2019): 895, https://doi.org/10.3389/fphys .2019.00895; B. Gwen Windham et al., "The Relationship between Heart Rate Variability and Adiposity Differs for Central and Overall Adiposity," ed. Carl J. Lavie, *Journal of Obesity* 2012 (May 9, 2012): 149516, https://doi.org/10.1155/2012/149516.

21. Sol Rodríguez-Colón et al., "The Circadian Pattern of Cardiac Autonomic Modulation and Obesity in Adolescents," *Clinical Autonomic Research: Official Journal of the Clinical Autonomic Research Society* 24, no. 6 (December 2014): 265–273, https://doi.org/10.1007 /s10286-014-0257-7.

22. Hayley A. Young and David Benton, "Heart-Rate Variability: A Biomarker to Study the Influence of Nutrition on Physiological and Psychological Health?" *Behavioural Pharmacology* 29, nos. 2 and 3 (April 2018): 140–151, https://doi.org/10.1097/FBP .0000000000000383.

23. Julia Silva-e-Oliveira et al., "Heart Rate Variability Based on Risk Stratification for Type 2 *Diabetes Mellitus*," *Einstein* (São Paulo) 15 (June 2017): 141–147, https://doi.org /10.1590/S1679-45082017AO3888; D. Liao et al., "Age, Race, and Sex Differences in Autonomic Cardiac Function Measured by Spectral Analysis of Heart Rate Variability— the ARIC Study. Atherosclerosis Risk in Communities," *American Journal of Cardiology* 76, no. 12 (November 1, 1995): 906–912, https://doi.org/10.1016/s0002-9149(99)80260-4.

24. "ENDO 2018: Wearable Heart Rate Monitor Could Signal Low Blood Sugar in Type 1 Diabetes," Endocrine News, March 22, 2018, https://endocrinenews.endocrine.org/endo -2018-wearable-heart-rate-monitor-could-signal-low-blood-sugar-in-type-1-diabetes/.

25. C. Brock et al., "Cardiac Vagal Tone, a Non-Invasive Measure of Parasympathetic Tone, Is a Clinically Relevant Tool in Type 1 Diabetes Mellitus," *Diabetic Medicine: A Journal of the British Diabetic Association* 34, no. 10 (October 2017): 1428–1434, https://doi.org /10.1111/dme.13421.

26. Julian F. Thayer et al., "Heart Rate Variability, Prefrontal Neural Function, and Cognitive Performance: The Neurovisceral Integration Perspective on Self-Regulation, Adaptation, and Health," *Annals of Behavioral Medicine: A Publication of the Society of Behavioral Medicine* 37, no. 2 (April 2009): 141–153, https://doi.org/10.1007/s12160-009 -9101-z.

27. Suzanne Segerstrom and Lise Solberg Nes, "Heart Rate Variability Reflects Self-Regulatory Strength, Effort, and Fatigue," *Psychological Science* 18 (April 1, 2007): 275–281, https://doi.org/10.1111/j.1467-9280.2007.01888.x; Julian F. Thayer and Richard D. Lane, "A Model of Neurovisceral Integration in Emotion Regulation and Dysregulation," *Journal of Affective Disorders*, 61, no. 3 (December 2, 2000): 201–216, https://doi .org/10.1016/S0165-0327(00)00338-4; Thayer et al., "Heart Rate Variability, Prefrontal Neural Function, and Cognitive Performance."

28. Anita Lill Hansen, Bjørn Helge Johnsen, and Julian F. Thayer, "Vagal Influence on Working Memory and Attention," *International Journal of Psychophysiology: Official Journal of the International Organization of Psychophysiology* 48, no. 3 (June 2003): 263–274, https://doi.org/10.1016/s0167-8760(03)00073-4.

29. Alison Reynard et al., "Heart Rate Variability as a Marker of Self-Regulation," *Applied Psychophysiology and Biofeedback* 36, no. 3 (September 2011): 209–215, https://doi .org/10.1007/s10484-011-9162-1.

30. Raymond Trevor Bradley et al., "Emotion Self-Regulation, Psychophysiological Coherence, and Test Anxiety: Results from an Experiment Using Electrophysiological Measures," *Applied Psychophysiology and Biofeedback* 35, no. 4 (2010): 261–283, https://doi .org/10.1007/s10484-010-9134-x.

31. Peter Koval et al., "Affective Instability in Daily Life Is Predicted by Resting Heart Rate Variability," *PLOS ONE* 8, no. 11 (November 29, 2013): e81536, https://doi .org/10.1371/journal.pone.0081536; Richard P. Sloan et al., "Vagally-Mediated Heart Rate Variability and Indices of Well-Being: Results of a Nationally Representative Study," *Health Psychology: Official Journal of the Division of Health Psychology, American Psychological Association* 36, no. 1 (January 2017): 73–81, https://doi.org/10.1037/hea0000397; Cristina Ottaviani et al., "Physiological Concomitants of Perseverative Cognition: A Systematic Review and Meta-Analysis," *Psychological Bulletin* 142, no. 3 (March 2016): 231–259, https://doi.org/10.1037/bul0000036.

32. Andrew H. Kemp, Julian Koenig, and Julian F. Thayer, "From Psychological Moments to Mortality: A Multidisciplinary Synthesis on Heart Rate Variability Spanning the Continuum of Time," *Neuroscience and Biobehavioral Reviews* 83 (December 2017): 547–567, https://doi.org/10.1016/j.neubiorev.2017.09.006; Gabriel Tan et al., "Heart Rate Variability (HRV) and Posttraumatic Stress Disorder (PTSD): A Pilot Study," *Applied Psychophysiology and Biofeedback* 36, no. 1 (March 1, 2011): 27–35, https://doi.org/10.1007 /s10484-010-9141-y.

33. Ralf Hartmann et al., "Heart Rate Variability as Indicator of Clinical State in Depression," *Frontiers in Psychiatry* 9 (2019): 735, https://doi.org/10.3389/fpsyt .2018.00735.

34. Elisa C. K. Steinfurth et al., "Resting State Vagally-Mediated Heart Rate Variability Is Associated with Neural Activity During Explicit Emotion Regulation," *Frontiers in Neuroscience* 12 (2018): 794, https://doi.org/10.3389/fnins.2018.00794.

35. Jos F. Brosschot, Bart Verkuil, and Julian F. Thayer, "Generalized Unsafety Theory of Stress: Unsafe Environments and Conditions, and the Default Stress Response," *International Journal of Environmental Research and Public Health* 15, no. 3 (March 2018): 464, https://doi.org/10.3390/ijerph15030464.

36. Vladimir Miskovic et al., "Stability of Resting Frontal Electroencephalogram (EEG) Asymmetry and Cardiac Vagal Tone in Adolescent Females Exposed to Child Maltreatment," *Developmental Psychobiology* 51, no. 6 (September 2009): 474–487, https://doi.org/10.1002/dev.20387; Anne T. Park et al., "Amygdala–Medial Prefrontal Cortex Connectivity Relates to Stress and Mental Health in Early Childhood," *Social Cognitive and Affective Neuroscience* 13, no. 4 (April 1, 2018): 430–439, https://doi.org/10.1093/scan/nsy017.

37. James A. Coan and David A. Sbarra, "Social Baseline Theory: The Social Regulation of Risk and Effort," *Current Opinion in Psychology* 1 (February 2015): 87–91, https://doi.org/10.1016/j.copsyc.2014.12.021.

38. Annaliese K. Beery and Daniela Kaufer, "Stress, Social Behavior, and Resilience: Insights from Rodents," *Neurobiology of Stress* (January 1, 2015): 116–127, https://doi.org/10.1016/j.ynstr.2014.10.004.

39. Ethan Kross et al., "Facebook Use Predicts Declines in Subjective Well-Being in Young Adults," *PLOS ONE* 8, no. 8 (2013): e69841, https://doi.org/10.1371/journal.pone.0069841; N. Xia and H. Li, "Loneliness, Social Isolation, and Cardiovascular Health," *Antioxidants & Redox Signaling*, 28, no. 9 (2018): 837–851, doi:10.1089/ars.2017.7312.

40. Stephen W. Porges, "The Polyvagal Perspective," *Biological Psychology* 74, no. 2 (February 2007): 116–43, https://doi.org/10.1016/j.biopsycho.2006.06.009; John T. Cacioppo et al., "The Neuroendocrinology of Social Isolation," *Annual Review of Psychology* 66 (January 3, 2015): 733–767, https://doi.org/10.1146/annurev-psych-010814-015240.

41. Cacioppo et al., "The Neuroendocrinology of Social Isolation."

42. Jos F. Brosschot, Bart Verkuil, and Julian F. Thayer, "Generalized Unsafety Theory of Stress: Unsafe Environments and Conditions, and the Default Stress Response."

43. Phil Jackson, *Sacred Hoops: Spiritual Lessons of a Hardwood Warrior* (New York: Hyperion, 1995); Relu Cernes and Reuven Zimlichman, "Role of Paced Breathing for Treatment of Hypertension," *Current Hypertension Reports* 19, no. 6 (June 2017): 45, https://doi.org/10.1007/s11906-017-0742-1; Andrea Zaccaro et al., "How Breath-Control Can Change Your Life: A Systematic Review on Psycho-Physiological Correlates of Slow Breathing," *Frontiers in Human Neuroscience* 12 (2018): 353, https://doi.org/10.3389/fnhum.2018.00353.

44. James Nestor, *Breath: The New Science of a Lost Art* (New York: Penguin Publishing Group, 2020).

45. H. Benson et al., "Body Temperature Changes During the Practice of g Tum-Mo Yoga," *Nature* 295, no. 5846 (January 21, 1982): 234–236, https://doi.org/10.1038/295234a0.

46. Mehdi Harorani et al., "The Effect of Benson's Relaxation Response on Sleep Quality and Anorexia in Cancer Patients Undergoing Chemotherapy: A Randomized Controlled Trial," *Complementary Therapies in Medicine* 50 (May 1, 2020): 102344, https://doi.org/10.1016/j.ctim.2020.102344.

47. "Biofeedback Therapy for Raynaud's Disease Symptoms," *Raynaud's Association* (blog), August 30, 2010, https://www.raynauds.org/2010/08/30/biofeedback-helps-alleviate-raynauds-disease-symptoms/; Amelia M. Stanton et al., "Heart Rate Variability Biofeedback Increases Sexual Arousal Among Women with Female Sexual Arousal Disorder:

Results from a Randomized-Controlled Trial," *Behaviour Research and Therapy*, Contemporary Issues in Behavioral Medicine, 115 (April 1, 2019): 90–102, https://doi.org/10.1016/j.brat.2018.10.016; "Biofeedback & Relaxation Training for Headache | AMF," American Migraine Foundation, accessed September 7, 2021, https://americanmigrainefoundation.org/resource-library/biofeedback-and-relaxation-training/.

48. B. Rael Cahn and John Polich, "Meditation States and Traits: EEG, ERP, and Neuroimaging Studies," *Psychological Bulletin* 132, no. 2 (March 2006): 180–211, https://doi.org/10.1037/0033-2909.132.2.180.

49. Li-Ching Yu et al., "One-Year Cardiovascular Prognosis of the Randomized, Controlled, Short-Term Heart Rate Variability Biofeedback Among Patients with Coronary Artery Disease," *International Journal of Behavioral Medicine* 25, no. 3 (June 2018): 271–282, https://doi.org/10.1007/s12529-017-9707-7; Martin Siepmann et al., "A Pilot Study on the Effects of Heart Rate Variability Biofeedback in Patients with Depression and in Healthy Subjects," *Applied Psychophysiology and Biofeedback* 33, no. 4 (December 2008): 195–201, https://doi.org/10.1007/s10484-008-9064-z; Inga Dziembowska et al., "Effects of Heart Rate Variability Biofeedback on EEG Alpha Asymmetry and Anxiety Symptoms in Male Athletes: A Pilot Study," *Applied Psychophysiology and Biofeedback* 41, no. 2 (June 2016): 141–150, https://doi.org/10.1007/s10484-015-9319-4.

50. Auditya Purwandini Sutarto, Muhammad Nubli Abdul Wahab, and Nora Mat Zin, "Resonant Breathing Biofeedback Training for Stress Reduction Among Manufacturing Operators," *International Journal of Occupational Safety and Ergonomics: JOSE* 18, no. 4 (2012): 549–561, https://doi.org/10.1080/10803548.2012.11076959.

51. Dziembowska et al., "Effects of Heart Rate Variability Biofeedback."

52. Paramahansa Yogananda, *Autobiography of a Yogi* (Self-Realization Fellowship, 1998).

53. Fu-Jung Huang, Ding-Kuo Chien, and Ue-Lin Chung, "Effects of Hatha Yoga on Stress in Middle-Aged Women," *Journal of Nursing Research: JNR* 21, no. 1 (March 2013): 59–66, https://doi.org/10.1097/jnr.0b013e3182829d6d; A. J. Bowman et al., "Effects of Aerobic Exercise Training and Yoga on the Baroreflex in Healthy Elderly Persons," *European Journal of Clinical Investigation* 27, no. 5 (1997): 443–449, https://doi.org/10.1046/j.1365-2362.1997.1340681.x; Neha Gothe et al., "The Acute Effects of Yoga on Executive Function," *Journal of Physical Activity & Health* 10, no. 4 (May 2013): 488–495, https://doi.org/10.1123/jpah.10.4.488; Savita Singh et al., "Influence of Pranayamas and Yoga-Asanas on Serum Insulin, Blood Glucose and Lipid Profile in Type 2 Diabetes," *Indian Journal of Clinical Biochemistry: IJCB* 23, no. 4 (October 2008): 365–368, https://doi.org/10.1007/s12291-008-0080-9; Caroline A. Smith et al., "Relaxation Techniques for Pain Management in Labour," *Cochrane Database of Systematic Reviews* 3 (March 28, 2018): CD009514, https://doi.org/10.1002/14651858.CD009514.pub2; Ghafoureh Ghaffarilaleh et al., "Effects of Yoga on Quality of Sleep of Women with Premenstrual Syndrome," *Alternative Therapies in Health and Medicine* 25, no. 5 (September 2019): 40–47, https://pubmed.ncbi.nlm.nih.gov/31221931/.

54. Brett Froeliger, Eric L. Garland, and F. Joseph McClernon, "Yoga Meditation Practitioners Exhibit Greater Gray Matter Volume and Fewer Reported Cognitive Failures: Results of a Preliminary Voxel-Based Morphometric Analysis," *Evidence-Based Complementary and Alternative Medicine: ECAM* 2012 (2012): 821307, https://doi.org/10.1155/2012/821307; G. H. Naveen et al., "Serum Cortisol and BDNF in Patients with Major Depression-Effect of Yoga," *International Review of Psychiatry* (Abingdon, England) 28, no. 3 (June 2016): 273–278, https://doi.org/10.1080/09540261.2016.1175419.

55. Rameswar Pal et al., "Age-Related Changes in Cardiovascular System, Autonomic Functions, and Levels of BDNF of Healthy Active Males: Role of Yogic Practice," *Age* (Dordrecht, Netherlands) 36, no. 4 (2014): 9683, https://doi.org/10.1007/s11357-014-9683-7.

56. Julia Frank et al., "Yoga in School Sports Improves Functioning of Autonomic Nervous System in Young Adults: A Non-randomized Controlled Pilot Study," *PLOS ONE* 15, no. 4 (April 13, 2020): e0231299, https://doi.org/10.1371/journal.pone.0231299.

57. Marian E. Papp et al., "Increased Heart Rate Variability but No Effect on Blood Pressure from 8 Weeks of Hatha Yoga—A Pilot Study," *BMC Research Notes* 6, no. 1 (February 11, 2013): 59, https://doi.org/10.1186/1756-0500-6-59.

58. Chandra Patel and W. R. S. North, "Randomised Controlled Trial of Yoga and Bio-Feedback in Management of Hypertension," *Lancet*, originally published as vol. 1, no. 7925, 306 (July 19, 1975): 93–95, https://doi.org/10.1016/S0140-6736(75)90002-1.

59. Rocco S. Calabrò et al., "Neuroanatomy and Function of Human Sexual Behavior: A Neglected or Unknown Issue?" *Brain and Behavior* 9, no. 12 (2019): e01389, https://doi.org/10.1002/brb3.1389.

60. Sophia Mitrokostas, "12 Things That Happen in Your Brain When You Have an Orgasm," Business Insider, accessed April 13, 2021, https://www.businessinsider.com/what-happens-to-your-brain-during-orgasm-2019-1.

61. Rui Miguel Costa and Stuart Brody, "Greater Resting Heart Rate Variability is Associated with Orgasms Through Penile-Vaginal Intercourse, but Not with Orgasms from Other Sources," *Journal of Sexual Medicine* 9, no. 1 (2012): 188–197, https://doi.org/10.1111/j.1743-6109.2011.02541.x.

62. Sigrid Breit et al., "Vagus Nerve as Modulator of the Brain-Gut Axis in Psychiatric and Inflammatory Disorders," *Frontiers in Psychiatry* 9 (March 13, 2018): 44, https://doi.org/10.3389/fpsyt.2018.00044.

63. Willem J. Kop et al., "Autonomic Nervous System Reactivity to Positive and Negative Mood Induction: The Role of Acute Psychological Responses and Frontal Electrocortical Activity," *Biological Psychology* 86, no. 3 (March 2011): 230–238, https://doi.org/10.1016/j.biopsycho.2010.12.003.

64. Amelia M. Stanton et al., "One Session of Autogenic Training Increases Acute Subjective Sexual Arousal in Premenopausal Women Reporting Sexual Arousal Problems," *Journal of Sexual Medicine* 15, no. 1 (January 1, 2018): 64–76, https://doi.org/10.1016/j.jsxm.2017.11.012.

65. S. Brody, R. Veit, and H. Rau, "A Preliminary Report Relating Frequency of Vaginal Intercourse to Heart Rate Variability, Valsalva Ratio, Blood Pressure, and Cohabitation Status," *Biological Psychology* 52, no. 3 (April 2000): 251–257, https://doi.org/10.1016/s0301-0511(99)00048-4; Stuart Brody and Ragnar Preut, "Vaginal Intercourse Frequency and Heart Rate Variability," *Journal of Sex & Marital Therapy* 29, no. 5 (2003): 371–380, https://doi.org/10.1080/00926230390224747.

66. Melissa Febos, "I Spent My Life Consenting to Touch I Didn't Want," *New York Times*, March 31, 2021, sec. Magazine, https://www.nytimes.com/2021/03/31/magazine/consent.html.

67. L. F. Berkman, "The Role of Social Relations in Health Promotion," *Psychosomatic Medicine* 57, no. 3 (June 1995): 245–254, https://doi.org/10.1097/00006842-199505000-00006.

68. Kory Floyd, "Relational and Health Correlates of Affection Deprivation," *Western Journal of Communication* 78, no. 4 (July 1, 2014): 383–403, https://doi.org/10.1080/10570314.2014.927071.

69. Brant R. Burleson, "Emotional Support Skills," in *Handbook of Communication and Social Interaction Skills* (Routledge Handbooks Online, 2003), https://doi.org/10.4324 /9781410607133.ch14.

70. Brittany K. Jakubiak and Brooke C. Feeney, "Keep in Touch: The Effects of Imagined Touch Support on Stress and Exploration," *Journal of Experimental Social Psychology* 65 (July 1, 2016): 59–67, https://doi.org/10.1016/j.jesp.2016.04.001.

71. James A. Coan, Hillary S. Schaefer, and Richard J. Davidson, "Lending a Hand: Social Regulation of the Neural Response to Threat," *Psychological Science* 17, no. 12 (December 2006): 1032–1039, https://doi.org/10.1111/j.1467-9280.2006.01832.x.

72. Ruth Feldman, Zehava Rosenthal, and Arthur I. Eidelman, "Maternal-Preterm Skin-to-Skin Contact Enhances Child Physiologic Organization and Cognitive Control Across the First 10 Years of Life," *Biological Psychiatry* 75, no. 1 (January 1, 2014): 56–64, https://doi.org/10.1016/j.biopsych.2013.08.012.

73. Kathleen C. Light, Karen M. Grewen, and Janet A. Amico, "More Frequent Partner Hugs and Higher Oxytocin Levels Are Linked to Lower Blood Pressure and Heart Rate in Premenopausal Women," *Biological Psychology* 69, no. 1 (April 2005): 5–21, https:// doi.org/10.1016/j.biopsycho.2004.11.002; Gertraud Stadler et al., "Close Relationships and Health in Daily Life: A Review and Empirical Data on Intimacy and Somatic Symptoms," *Psychosomatic Medicine* 74, no. 4 (May 2012): 398–409, https://doi.org/10.1097 /PSY.0b013e31825473b8.

74. Glennon Doyle, *Untamed* (New York: Dial Press, 2020).

75. Neil E. Klepeis et al., "The National Human Activity Pattern Survey (NHAPS): A Resource for Assessing Exposure to Environmental Pollutants," *Journal of Exposure Science & Environmental Epidemiology* 11, no. 3 (July 2001): 231–252, https://doi.org/10.1038/sj.jea .7500165; United Nations, Department of Economic and Social Affairs, Population Division (2014), *World Urbanization Prospects: The 2014 Revision, Highlights* (*ST/ESA/SER.A/352*).

76. Bum Jin Park et al., "The Physiological Effects of Shinrin-Yoku (Taking in the Forest Atmosphere or Forest Bathing): Evidence from Field Experiments in 24 Forests Across Japan," *Environmental Health and Preventive Medicine* 15, no. 1 (January 2010): 18–26, https://doi.org/10.1007/s12199-009-0086-9; Qing Li et al., "Acute Effects of Walking in Forest Environments on Cardiovascular and Metabolic Parameters," *European Journal of Applied Physiology* 111, no. 11 (November 1, 2011): 2845–2853, https://doi.org/10.1007 /s00421-011-1918-z.

77. Chia-Pin Yu et al., "Effects of Short Forest Bathing Program on Autonomic Nervous System Activity and Mood States in Middle-Aged and Elderly Individuals," *International Journal of Environmental Research and Public Health* 14, no. 8 (August 2017): 897, https://doi.org/10.3390/ijerph14080897.

78. Q. Li et al., "Effect of Phytoncide from Trees on Human Natural Killer Cell Function," *International Journal of Immunopathology and Pharmacology* 22, no. 4 (October 1, 2009): 951–959, https://doi.org/10.1177/039463200902200410.

79. Qing Li et al., "A Day Trip to a Forest Park Increases Human Natural Killer Activity and the Expression of Anti-Cancer Proteins in Male Subjects," *Journal of Biological Regulators and Homeostatic Agents* 24, no. 2 (June 2010): 157–165, https://pubmed.ncbi.nlm.nih .gov/20487629/.

80. Misha Ross and Georgia J. Mason, "The Effects of Preferred Natural Stimuli on Humans' Affective States, Physiological Stress and Mental Health, and the Potential Implications for Well-Being in Captive Animals," *Neuroscience and Biobehavioral Reviews* 83 (December 2017): 46–62, https://doi.org/10.1016/j.neubiorev.2017.09.012.

81. Jacqueline Kerr et al., "Outdoor Physical Activity and Self Rated Health in Older Adults Living in Two Regions of the U.S.," *International Journal of Behavioral Nutrition and Physical Activity* 9, no. 1 (July 30, 2012), https://doi.org/10.1186/1479-5868-9-89.

82. Chia-Pin Yu et al., "Effects of Short Forest Bathing Program."

83. Valerie F. Gladwell et al., "A Lunchtime Walk in Nature Enhances Restoration of Autonomic Control During Night-Time Sleep: Results from a Preliminary Study," *International Journal of Environmental Research and Public Health* 13, no. 3 (March 2016): 280, https://doi.org/10.3390/ijerph13030280.

84. Margaret M. Hansen, Reo Jones, and Kirsten Tocchini, "Shinrin-Yoku (Forest Bathing) and Nature Therapy: A State-of-the-Art Review," *International Journal of Environmental Research and Public Health* 14, no. 8 (August 2017): 851, https://doi.org/10.3390/ijerph14080851.

85. Hansen, Jones, and Tocchini, "Shinrin-Yoku (Forest Bathing) and Nature Therapy."

86. "Autogenic Training—Whole Health Library," General Information, accessed September 22, 2021, https://www.va.gov/WHOLEHEALTHLIBRARY/tools/autogenic-training.asp.

87. Andrei C. Miu, Renata M. Heilman, and Mircea Miclea, "Reduced Heart Rate Variability and Vagal Tone in Anxiety: Trait versus State, and the Effects of Autogenic Training," *Autonomic Neuroscience: Basic & Clinical* 145, no. 1–2 (January 28, 2009): 99–103, https://doi.org/10.1016/j.autneu.2008.11.010; Friedhelm Stetter and Sirko Kupper, "Autogenic Training: A Meta-Analysis of Clinical Outcome Studies," *Applied Psychophysiology and Biofeedback* 27, no. 1 (March 2002): 45–98, https://doi.org/10.1023/a:1014576505223; Masae Shinozaki et al., "Effect of Autogenic Training on General Improvement in Patients with Irritable Bowel Syndrome: A Randomized Controlled Trial," *Applied Psychophysiology and Biofeedback* 35, no. 3 (September 2010): 189–198, https://doi.org/10.1007/s10484-009-9125-y; Amelia Stanton and Cindy Meston, "A Single Session of Autogenic Training Increases Acute Subjective and Physiological Sexual Arousal in Sexually Functional Women," *Journal of Sex & Marital Therapy* 43, no. 7 (October 3, 2017): 601–617, https://doi.org/10.1080/0092623X.2016.1211206.

88. Stanton and Meston, "A Single Session of Autogenic Training," 601–617.

**Chapter Four. Join the Rest-o-lution, Deepen Your Sleep**

1. William Shakespeare, *Macbeth*, act 2, scene 2.

2. "Sleep and Sleep Disorders," Centers for Disease Control and Prevention, February 13, 2019, https://www.cdc.gov/sleep/about_us.html.

3. Jodi A. Mindell et al., "Sleep Education in Medical School Curriculum: A Glimpse Across Countries," *Sleep Medicine* 12, no. 9 (October 2011): 928–931, https://doi.org/10.1016/j.sleep.2011.07.001.

4. Harvey R. Colten and Bruce M. Altevogt, *Sleep Disorders and Sleep Deprivation: An Unmet Public Health Problem* (Washington, DC: National Academies Press, 2006), https://doi.org/10.17226/11617.

5. Sara C. Mednick, *Take a Nap! Change Your Life* (New York: Workman Publishing, 2006).

6. Yu. F. Pastukhov, "Slow-Wave Sleep and Molecular Chaperones," *Journal of Evolutionary Biochemistry and Physiology* 52, no. 1 (January 2016): 87–101, https://doi.org/10.1134/S0022093016010117; Hajime Nakanishi et al., "Positive Correlations Between Cerebral Protein Synthesis Rates and Deep Sleep in Macaca Mulatta," *European Journal of Neuro-*

*science* 9, no. 2 (February 1997): 271–279, https://doi.org/10.1111/j.1460-9568.1997 .tb01397.x.

7. Giulio Tononi and Chiara Cirelli, "Sleep and the Price of Plasticity: from Synaptic and Cellular Homeostasis to Memory Consolidation and Integration," *Neuron* 81, no. 1 (2014), 12–34.

8. A. Korner, "Growth Hormone Control of Biosynthesis of Protein and Ribonucleic Acid" *Recent Progress in Hormone Research* 21 (1965): 205–240; Kirstine Adam and Ian Oswald, "Protein Synthesis, Bodily Renewal and the Sleep-Wake Cycle," *Clinical Science* 65, no. 6 (December 1, 1983): 561–567, https://doi.org/10.1042/cs0650561.

9. Lauren N. Whitehurst et al., "Autonomic Activity during Sleep Predicts Memory Consolidation in Humans," *Proceedings of the National Academy of Sciences of the United States of America* 113, no. 26 (June 28, 2016): 7272–7277, https://doi.org/10.1073/pnas .1518202113; Mohsen Naji et al., "Coupling of Autonomic and Central Events during Sleep Benefits Declarative Memory Consolidation," *Neurobiology of Learning and Memory* 157 (January 2019): 139–150, https://doi.org/10.1016/j.nlm.2018.12.008; Mohsen Naji et al., "Timing between Cortical Slow Oscillations and Heart Rate Bursts During Sleep Predicts Temporal Processing Speed, but Not Offline Consolidation," *Journal of Cognitive Neuroscience* 31, no. 10 (October 1, 2019): 1484–1490, https://doi.org/10.1162/jocn_a_01432; Pin-Chun Chen et al., "Autonomic Activity During a Daytime Nap Facilitates Working Memory Improvement," *Journal of Cognitive Neuroscience* 32, no. 10 (October 2020): 1963–1974, https://doi.org/10.1162/jocn_a_01588; Lauren Whitehurst et al., "New Directions in Sleep and Memory Research: The Role of Autonomic Activity," *Current Opinion in Behavioral Sciences* 33 (December 1, 2019), https://doi.org/10.1016/j.cobeha.2019.11.001; Pin-Chun Chen et al., "Autonomic/Central Coupling Boosts Working Memory in Healthy Young Adults," *Neurobiology of Learning and Memory* 173 (September 2020), https://doi .org/10.1101/2020.04.22.056481.

10. J. Trinder et al., "Autonomic Activity During Human Sleep as a Function of Time and Sleep Stage," *Journal of Sleep Research* 10, no. 4 (December 2001): 253–264, https://doi .org/10.1046/j.1365-2869.2001.00263.x.

11. J. Trinder et al., "Autonomic Activity During Human Sleep," 253–264.

12. Julian F. Thayer, Shelby S. Yamamoto, and Jos F. Brosschot, "The Relationship of Autonomic Imbalance, Heart Rate Variability and Cardiovascular Disease Risk Factors," *International Journal of Cardiology* 141, no. 2 (May 28, 2010): 122–131, https://doi .org/10.1016/j.ijcard.2009.09.543; John Trinder et al., "Sleep and Cardiovascular Regulation," *Pflügers Archiv: European Journal of Physiology* 463, no. 1 (January 2012): 161–168, https://doi.org/10.1007/s00424-011-1041-3.

13. Lisa Mednick Powell, *Finding the Azimuth* (Joshua Tree, CA: Cholla Needles Arts & Literary Library, 2018).

14. Roger Bohn and James Short, "Measuring Consumer Information," *International Journal of Communication* 6 (2012): 980–1000. https://ijoc.org/index.php/ijoc/article /viewFile/1566/743.

15. Pete Docter and Ronnie Del Carmen, *Inside Out* (Walt Disney Studios Motion Pictures, 2015).

16. Armando D'Agostino et al., "Efficacy of Triple Chronotherapy in Unipolar and Bipolar Depression: A Systematic Review of the Available Evidence," *Journal of Affective Disorders* 276 (November 1, 2020): 297–304, https://doi.org/10.1016/j.jad.2020.07.026.

17. Per Kristian Eide et al., "Sleep Deprivation Impairs Molecular Clearance from the Human Brain," *Brain: A Journal of Neurology* 144, no. 3 (April 12, 2021): 863–874, https:// doi.org/10.1093/brain/awaa443.

18. Rachel Leproult and Eve Van Cauter, "Role of Sleep and Sleep Loss in Hormonal Release and Metabolism," *Endocrine Development* 17 (2010): 11–21, https://doi.org/10.1159/000262524.

19. Chunyan Hu et al., "Association of Bedtime with the Risk of Non-alcoholic Fatty Liver Disease among Middle-Aged and Elderly Chinese Adults with Pre-diabetes and Diabetes," *Diabetes/Metabolism Research and Reviews* 36, no. 6 (September 2020), https://doi.org/10.1002/dmrr.3322; Eide et al., "Sleep Deprivation Impairs Molecular Clearance."

20. Allen Gannett, *The Creative Curve: How to Develop the Right Idea, at the Right Time*, 1st ed. (New York: Currency, 2018); Sal Cerra, *Destiny Dreams: Discovering the Divine Blueprint for Your Life* (Destiny Fire Ministries, 2020).

21. M. A. Wilson and B. L. McNaughton, "Reactivation of Hippocampal Ensemble Memories During Sleep," *Science* (New York) 265, no. 5172 (July 29, 1994): 676–679, https://doi.org/10.1126/science.8036517.

22. Susanne Diekelmann and Jan Born, "The Memory Function of Sleep," *Nature Reviews. Neuroscience* 11, no. 2 (February 2010): 114–126, https://doi.org/10.1038/nrn2762.

23. Mohammad Niknazar et al., "Coupling of Thalamocortical Sleep Oscillations Are Important for Memory Consolidation in Humans," ed. Vladyslav Vyazovskiy, *PLOS ONE* 10, no. 12 (December 15, 2015): e0144720, https://doi.org/10.1371/journal.pone.0144720.

24. Fabio Ferrarelli et al., "An Increase in Sleep Slow Waves Predicts Better Working Memory Performance in Healthy Individuals," *NeuroImage* 191 (May 2019): 1–9, https://doi.org/10.1016/j.neuroimage.2019.02.020.

25. Benjamin A. Plog and Maiken Nedergaard, "The Glymphatic System in Central Nervous System Health and Disease: Past, Present, and Future," *Annual Review of Pathology: Mechanisms of Disease* 13, no. 1 (January 24, 2018): 379–394, https://doi.org/10.1146/annurev-pathol-051217-111018.

26. Adam P. Spira et al., "Impact of Sleep on the Risk of Cognitive Decline and Dementia," *Current Opinion in Psychiatry* 27, no. 6 (November 2014): 478–483, https://doi.org/10.1097/YCO.0000000000000106.

27. Gabriele Cipriani et al., "Sleep Disturbances and Dementia," *Psychogeriatrics: The Official Journal of the Japanese Psychogeriatric Society* 15, no. 1 (March 2015): 65–74, https://doi.org/10.1111/psyg.12069.

28. "12 Quotes from Famous Authors About Drinking | Penguin Random House," PenguinRandomhouse.com, n.d., https://www.penguinrandomhouse.com/the-read-down/13-quotes-from-famous-authors-about-drinking.

29. Melora Kuhn, author in conversation with, May 12, 2021.

30. Diána Kuperczkó et al., "Late Bedtime Is Associated with Decreased Hippocampal Volume in Young Healthy Subjects: Bedtime and Hippocampus," *Sleep and Biological Rhythms* 13, no. 1 (January 2015): 68–75, https://doi.org/10.1111/sbr.12077.

31. Sun Ju Chung, Hyeyoung An, and Sooyeon Suh, "What Do People Do Before Going to Bed? A Study of Bedtime Procrastination Using Time Use Surveys," *Sleep* 43, no. 4 (April 15, 2020): 267, https://doi.org/10.1093/sleep/zsz267.

32. Chung, An, and Suh, "What Do People Do Before Going to Bed?"

33. Nobuaki Sakamoto et al., "Bedtime and Sleep Duration in Relation to Depressive Symptoms Among Japanese Workers," *Journal of Occupational Health* 55, no. 6 (November 2013): 479–486, https://doi.org/10.1539/joh.13-0074-OA.

34. Kelly G. Baron et al., "Role of Sleep Timing in Caloric Intake and BMI," *Obesity (Silver Spring, MD)* 19, no. 7 (July 2011): 1374–81, https://doi.org/10.1038/oby.2011.100.

35. Sarah E. Anderson, Rebecca Andridge, and Robert C. Whitaker, "Bedtime in Preschool-Aged Children and Risk for Adolescent Obesity," *Journal of Pediatrics* 176 (September 2016): 17–22, https://doi.org/10.1016/j.jpeds.2016.06.005.

36. Kristi B. Adamo, "Later Bedtime Is Associated with Greater Daily Energy Intake and Screen Time in Obese Adolescents Independent of Sleep Duration," *Journal of Sleep Disorders & Therapy* 2, no. 4 (2013), https://doi.org/10.4172/2167-0277.1000126.

37. R. K. Golley et al., "Sleep Duration or Bedtime? Exploring the Association Between Sleep Timing Behaviour, Diet and BMI in Children and Adolescents," *International Journal of Obesity* 37, no. 4 (April 2013): 546–551, https://doi.org/10.1038/ijo.2012.212.

38. Julius Edward Miller Hvidt et al., "Associations of Bedtime, Sleep Duration, and Sleep Quality with Semen Quality in Males Seeking Fertility Treatment: A Preliminary Study," *Basic and Clinical Andrology* 30, no. 1 (December 2020): 5, https://doi.org/10.1186/s12610-020-00103-7.

39. Miller Hvidt et al., "Associations of Bedtime, Sleep Duration, and Sleep Quality."

40. Kneginja Richter et al., "Shiftwork and Alcohol Consumption: A Systematic Review of the Literature," *European Addiction Research* 27, no. 1 (2021): 9–15, https://doi.org/10.1159/000507573.

41. Timothy Roehrs and Thomas Roth, "Insomnia as a Path to Alcoholism: Tolerance Development and Dose Escalation," *Sleep* 41, no. 8 (August 1, 2018), https://doi.org/10.1093/sleep/zsy091.

42. Irshaad O. Ebrahim et al., "Alcohol and Sleep I: Effects on Normal Sleep," *Alcoholism, Clinical and Experimental Research* 37, no. 4 (April 2013): 539–549, https://doi.org/10.1111/acer.12006.

43. Irina V. Zhdanova et al., "Melatonin Treatment for Age-Related Insomnia," *Journal of Clinical Endocrinology & Metabolism* 86, no. 10 (October 2001): 4727–4730, https://doi.org/10.1210/jcem.86.10.7901.

44. Ahmed S. BaHammam, "Sleep from an Islamic Perspective," *Annals of Thoracic Medicine* 6, no. 4 (2011): 187, https://doi.org/10.4103/1817-1737.84771.

45. Hang Sun, Aaron M. Gusdon, and Shen Qu, "Effects of Melatonin on Cardiovascular Diseases: Progress in the Past Year," *Current Opinion in Lipidology* 27, no. 4 (August 2016): 408–413, https://doi.org/10.1097/MOL.0000000000000314; Syed Suhail Andrabi, Suhel Parvez, and Heena Tabassum, "Melatonin and Ischemic Stroke: Mechanistic Roles and Action," *Advances in Pharmacological Sciences* 2015 (2015): 1–11, https://doi.org/10.1155/2015/384750.

46. Patricia Rubio-Sastre et al., "Acute Melatonin Administration in Humans Impairs Glucose Tolerance in Both the Morning and Evening," *Sleep* 37, no. 10 (October 1, 2014): 1715–1719, https://doi.org/10.5665/sleep.4088.

47. BaHammam, "Sleep from an Islamic Perspective.

48. Joseph Millar, *Dark Harvest: New and Selected Poems*, permission by the poet.

49. Annette van Maanen et al., "The Effects of Light Therapy on Sleep Problems: A Systematic Review and Meta-Analysis," *Sleep Medicine Reviews* 29 (October 2016): 52–62, https://doi.org/10.1016/j.smrv.2015.08.009.

50. Lisa M. Wu et al., "The Effect of Systematic Light Exposure on Sleep in a Mixed Group of Fatigued Cancer Survivors," *Journal of Clinical Sleep Medicine: JCSM: Official Publication of the American Academy of Sleep Medicine* 14, no. 1 (January 15, 2018): 31–39, https://doi.org/10.5664/jcsm.6874.

51. Kara M. Duraccio et al., "Does iPhone Night Shift Mitigate Negative Effects of Smartphone Use on Sleep Outcomes in Emerging Adults?" *Sleep Health* 7, no. 4 (August 2021): 478–484, https://doi.org/10.1016/j.sleh.2021.03.005.

52. Jay A. Olson et al., "Developing a Light-Based Intervention to Reduce Fatigue and Improve Sleep in Rapidly Rotating Shift Workers," *Chronobiology International* 37, no. 4 (April 2020): 573–91, https://doi.org/10.1080/07420528.2019.1698591.

53. James Nestor, "An Excerpt from Breath," PenguinRandomhouse.com, accessed April 13, 2021, https://www.penguinrandomhouse.com/articles/breath-excerpt.

54. Krzysztof Krysta et al., "Cognitive Deficits in Adults with Obstructive Sleep Apnea Compared to Children and Adolescents," *Journal of Neural Transmission* 124, no. S1 (February 2017): 187–201, https://doi.org/10.1007/s00702-015-1501-6.

55. Katherine A. Duggan et al., "Personality and Healthy Sleep: The Importance of Conscientiousness and Neuroticism," ed. Oscar Arias-Carrion, *PLOS ONE* 9, no. 3 (March 20, 2014): e90628, https://doi.org/10.1371/journal.pone.0090628.

56. Mason Currey, *Daily Rituals: How Artists Work*, 1st ed. (New York: Knopf, 2013).

57. Heather E. Gunn et al., "Sleep–Wake Concordance in Couples Is Inversely Associated with Cardiovascular Disease Risk Markers," *Sleep* 40, no. 1 (January 1, 2017), https://doi.org/10.1093/sleep/zsw028; Kneginja Richter et al., "Two in a Bed: The Influence of Couple Sleeping and Chronotypes on Relationship and Sleep. An Overview," *Chronobiology International* 33, no. 10 (November 25, 2016): 1464–1472, https://doi.org/10.1080/07420 528.2016.1220388.

58. "Battle of the Bedtimes," The Sleep Judge, June 4, 2019, https://www.thesleep judge.com/battle-of-bedtimes/.

59. "Why Couples Sleep Apart," Better Sleep Council, February 5, 2018, https://better sleep.org/blog/why-couples-sleep-apart/.

## Chapter Five. Exercise Your Right to Recovery

1. Faye S. Routledge et al., "Improvements in Heart Rate Variability with Exercise Therapy," *Canadian Journal of Cardiology* 26, no. 6 (2010): 303–312.

2. Dick H. J. Thijssen et al., "Association of Exercise Preconditioning with Immediate Cardioprotection: A Review," *JAMA Cardiology* 3, no. 2 (February 2018): 169–176, https://doi.org/10.1001/jamacardio.2017.4495.

3. Zurine De Miguel et al., "Exercise Plasma Boosts Memory and Dampens Brain Inflammation via Clusterin," *Nature* 600 (December 8, 2021), https://doi.org/10.1038/s41586-021-04183-x.

4. Sayaka Aritake-Okada et al., "Diurnal Repeated Exercise Promotes Slow-Wave Activity and Fast-Sigma Power During Sleep with Increase in Body Temperature: A Human Crossover Trial," *Journal of Applied Physiology* 127, no. 1 (July 1, 2019): 168–177, https://doi.org/10.1152/japplphysiol.00765.2018.

5. Ana Kovacevic et al., "The Effect of Resistance Exercise on Sleep: A Systematic Review of Randomized Controlled Trials," *Sleep Medicine Reviews* 39 (June 2018): 52–68, https://doi.org/10.1016/j.smrv.2017.07.002.

6. Kathryn J. Reid et al., "Aerobic Exercise Improves Self-Reported Sleep and Quality of Life in Older Adults with Insomnia," *Sleep Medicine* 11, no. 9 (October 2010): 934–940, https://doi.org/10.1016/j.sleep.2010.04.014.

7. "National Sleep Foundation Poll Finds Exercise Key to Good Sleep," Sleep Foundation, October 19, 2018, https://www.sleepfoundation.org/professionals/sleep-americar -polls/2013-exercise-and-sleep.

8. Giselle Soares Passos et al., "Is Exercise an Alternative Treatment for Chronic Insomnia?" *Clinics* 67, no. 6 (June 2012): 653–659, https://doi.org/10.6061/clinics/2012(06)17.

9. Allan Rechtschaffen and Anthony Kales, ed., *A Manual of Standardized Terminology, Techniques and Scoring System for Sleep Stages of Human Subjects*, Publication No. 204 (National Institutes of Health [US]), accessed from https://nla.gov.au/nla.cat-vn823711 (Bethesda, MD: US National Institute of Neurological Diseases and Blindness, Neurological Information Network, 1968).

10. Helen S. Driver and Sheila R. Taylor, "Exercise and Sleep," *Sleep Medicine Reviews* 4, no. 4 (August 2000): 387–402, https://doi.org/10.1053/smrv.2000.0110; Tero Myllymäki et al., "Effects of Vigorous Late-Night Exercise on Sleep Quality and Cardiac Autonomic Activity," *Journal of Sleep Research* 20, no. 1pt2 (2011): 146–153, https://doi.org/10.1111/j.1365-2869.2010.00874.x; D. Menicucci et al., "Brain Connectivity is Altered by Extreme Physical Exercise During Non-REM Sleep and Wakefulness: Indications from EEG and FMRI Studies," *Archives Italiennes de Biologie* 154, no. 4 (December 1, 2016): 103–117, https://doi.org/10.12871/00039829201641.

11. Laís Monteiro Rodrigues Loureiro, Caio Eduardo Gonçalves Reis, and Teresa Helena Macedo da Costa, "Effects of Coffee Components on Muscle Glycogen Recovery: A Systematic Review," *International Journal of Sport Nutrition and Exercise Metabolism* 28, no. 3 (May 1, 2018): 284–293, https://doi.org/10.1123/ijsnem.2017-0342.

12. Veronique J. Deschodt and Laurent M. Arsac, "Morning vs. Evening Maximal Cycle Power and Technical Swimming Ability," *Journal of Strength and Conditioning Research* 18, no. 1 (February 2004): 149–154, https://doi.org/10.1519/1533-4287(2004)018<0149:mvemcp>2.0.co;2; Brendan M. Gabriel and Juleen R. Zierath, "Circadian Rhythms and Exercise—Re-setting the Clock in Metabolic Disease," *National Review of Endocrinology* 15, no. 4 (April 2019): 197–206, https://doi: 10.1038/s41574-018-0150-x.

13. Hamdi Chtourou and Nizar Souissi, "The Effect of Training at a Specific Time of Day: A Review," *Journal of Strength and Conditioning Research* 26, no. 7 (July 2012): 1984–2005, https://doi.org/10.1519/JSC.0b013e31825770a7.

14. Maria Küüsmaa et al., "Effects of Morning Versus Evening Combined Strength and Endurance Training on Physical Performance, Muscle Hypertrophy, and Serum Hormone Concentrations," *Applied Physiology, Nutrition, and Metabolism = Physiologie appliquée, nutrition et metabolisme* 41, no. 12 (December 2016): 1285–1294, https://doi.org/10.1139/apnm-2016-0271.

15. Elise Facer-Childs and Roland Brandstaetter, "The Impact of Circadian Phenotype and Time Since Awakening on Diurnal Performance in Athletes," *Current Biology* 5, no. 4 (February 16, 2015): 518–522, https://doi.org/10.1016/j.cub.2014.12.036.

16. Andrew M. Watson, "Sleep and Athletic Performance," *Current Sports Medicine Reports* 16, no. 6 (December 2017): 413–418, https://doi.org/10.1249/JSR.0000000000000418.

17. Watson, "Sleep and Athletic Performance."

18. John Temesi et al., "Does Central Fatigue Explain Reduced Cycling after Complete Sleep Deprivation?" *Medicine and Science in Sports and Exercise* 45, no. 12 (December 2013): 2243–2253, https://doi.org/10.1249/MSS.0b013e31829ce379.

19. Watson, "Sleep and Athletic Performance," 413–418.

20. J. E. Wright et al., "Effects of Travel Across Time Zones (Jet-Lag) on Exercise Capacity and Performance," *Aviation, Space, and Environmental Medicine* 54, no. 2 (February 1983): 132–137.

21. J. Matthew Thomas et al., "Circadian Rhythm Phase Shifts Caused by Timed Exercise Vary with Chronotype," *JCI Insight* 5, no. 3 (February 13, 2020): 134270, https://doi.org/10.1172/jci.insight.134270.

22. Erin K. Baehr et al., "Circadian Phase-Shifting Effects of Nocturnal Exercise in Older Compared with Young Adults," *American Journal of Physiology. Regulatory, Integrative and Comparative Physiology* 284, no. 6 (June 2003): R1542–R1550, https://doi.org/10.1152/ajpregu.00761.2002.

23. Oliver Soehnlein et al., "Neutrophils as Protagonists and Targets in Chronic Inflammation," *Nature Reviews Immunology* 17, no. 4 (April 2017): 248–261, https://doi.org/10.1038/nri.2017.10.

24. DeWayne P. Williams et al., "Heart Rate Variability and Inflammation: A Meta-Analysis of Human Studies," *Brain, Behavior, and Immunity* 80 (August 1, 2019): 219–226, https://doi.org/10.1016/j.bbi.2019.03.009.

25. Nemat Khansari, Yadollah Shakiba, and Mahdi Mahmoudi, "Chronic Inflammation and Oxidative Stress as a Major Cause of Age-Related Diseases and Cancer," *Recent Patents on Inflammation & Allergy Drug Discovery* 3, no. 1 (January 2009): 73–80, https://doi.org/10.2174/187221309787158371.

26. Sandeep Bansal and Paul M. Ridker, "Comparison of Characteristics of Future Myocardial Infarctions in Women with Baseline High versus Baseline Low Levels of High-Sensitivity C-Reactive Protein," *American Journal of Cardiology* 99, no. 11 (June 1, 2007): 1500–1503, https://doi.org/10.1016/j.amjcard.2007.01.022; T. E. Strandberg and R. S. Tilvis, "C-Reactive Protein, Cardiovascular Risk Factors, and Mortality in a Prospective Study in the Elderly," *Arteriosclerosis, Thrombosis, and Vascular Biology* 20, no. 4 (April 2000): 1057–1060, https://doi.org/10.1161/01.atv.20.4.1057.

27. DeWayne P. Williams et al., "Heart Rate Variability and Inflammation."

28. Kristen M. Beavers, Tina E. Brinkley, and Barbara J. Nicklas, "Effect of Exercise Training on Chronic Inflammation," *Clinica Chimica Acta; International Journal of Clinical Chemistry* 411, nos. 11–12 (June 3, 2010): 785–793, https://doi.org/10.1016/j.cca.2010.02.069.

29. Jerome L. Abramson and Viola Vaccarino, "Relationship between Physical Activity and Inflammation Among Apparently Healthy Middle-Aged and Older US Adults," *Archives of Internal Medicine* 162, no. 11 (June 10, 2002): 1286–1292, https://doi.org/10.1001/archinte.162.11.1286.

30. Beavers, Brinkley, and Nicklas, "Effect of Exercise Training."

31. Matthew M. Schubert et al., "Acute Exercise and Hormones Related to Appetite Regulation: A Meta-Analysis," *Sports Medicine* (Auckland, NZ) 44, no. 3 (March 2014): 387–403, https://doi.org/10.1007/s40279-013-0120-3.

32. Paddy C. Dempsey et al., "Interrupting Prolonged Sitting with Brief Bouts of Light Walking or Simple Resistance Activities Reduces Resting Blood Pressure and Plasma Noradrenaline in Type 2 Diabetes," *Journal of Hypertension* 34, no. 12 (December 2016): 2376–2382, https://doi.org/10.1097/HJH.0000000000001101.

33. Andrew N. Reynolds et al., "Advice to Walk After Meals Is More Effective for Lowering Postprandial Glycaemia in Type 2 Diabetes Mellitus Than Advice That Does Not Specify Timing: A Randomised Crossover Study," *Diabetologia* 59, no. 12 (December 2016): 2572–2578, https://doi.org/10.1007/s00125-016-4085-2.

34. Leslie Goldman, "Work Out, Feel the Joy," *Real Simple Mental Wellbeing Bookazine*, November 2020, 3.

35. Kirk I. Erickson, Regina L. Leckie, and Andrea M. Weinstein, "Physical Activity, Fitness, and Gray Matter Volume," *Neurobiology of Aging* 35, suppl. 2 (September 2014): S20–528, https://doi.org/10.1016/j.neurobiolaging.2014.03.034.

36. Patrick Z. Liu and Robin Nusslock, "Exercise-Mediated Neurogenesis in the Hippocampus via BDNF," *Frontiers in Neuroscience* 12 (2018): 52, https://doi.org/10.3389/fnins.2018.00052.

37. Kristel Knaepen et al., "Neuroplasticity—Exercise-Induced Response of Peripheral Brain-Derived Neurotrophic Factor: A Systematic Review of Experimental Studies in Human Subjects," *Sports Medicine* (Auckland, NZ) 40, no. 9 (September 1, 2010): 765–801, https://doi.org/10.2165/11534530-000000000-00000; Katharina Wittfeld et al., "Cardiorespiratory Fitness and Gray Matter Volume in the Temporal, Frontal, and Cerebellar Regions in the General Population," *Mayo Clinic Proceedings* 95, no. 1 (January 2020): 44–56, https://doi.org/10.1016/j.mayocp.2019.05.030.

38. Janet E. Fulton, "Physical Inactivity Is More Common among Racial and Ethnic Minorities in Most States," Centers for Disease Control and Prevention, accessed September 7, 2021, https://blogs.cdc.gov/healthequity/2020/04/01/physical-inactivity/.

39. Muazzam Nasrullah and Sana Muazzam, "Drowning Mortality in the United States, 1999–2006," *Journal of Community Health* 36, no. 1 (February 2011): 69–75, https://doi.org/10.1007/s10900-010-9281-2.

40. Mitchell S. Jackson, "Twelve Minutes and a Life," Runner's World, June 18, 2020, https://www.runnersworld.com/runners-stories/a32883923/ahmaud-arbery-death-running-and-racism/.

41. Kurt Streeter, "Running While Black: Our Readers Respond," accessed September 7, 2021, https://www.nytimes.com/2020/05/18/sports/running-while-black-ahmaud-arbery.html; Jan Ransom, "Amy Cooper Faces Charges After Calling Police on Black Bird-Watcher," accessed September 7, 2021, https://www.nytimes.com/2020/07/06/nyregion/amy-cooper-false-report-charge.html.

42. K. I. August and D. H. Sorkin, "Racial/Ethnic Disparities in Exercise and Dietary Behaviors of Middle-Aged and Older Adults," *Journal of General Internal Medicine* 26, no. 3 (March 2011): 245–250. https://doi.org: 10.1007/s11606-010-1514-7, Epub September 24, 2010, PMID: 20865342; PMCID: PMC3043172.

43. Eric Adams, *Healthy at Last: A Plant-Based Approach to Preventing and Reversing Diabetes and Other Chronic Illnesses* (California: Hay House, 2020).

44. Jane E. Brody, "An Inspiring Story of Weight Loss and Its Aftermath," *New York Times*, January 2, 2017, accessed September 7, 2021, https://www.nytimes.com/2017/01/02/well/an-inspiring-story-of-weight-loss-and-its-aftermath.html.

45. Brody, "An Inspiring Story of Weight Loss and Its Aftermath."

46. Brody, "An Inspiring Story of Weight Loss and Its Aftermath."

47. Brody, "An Inspiring Story of Weight Loss and Its Aftermath."

48. "Mayor de Blasio Announces Citywide Meatless Mondays," Official website of the City of New York, March 11, 2019, http://www1.nyc.gov/office-of-the-mayor/news/135-19/mayor-de-blasio-chancellor-carranza-brooklyn-borough-president-adams-citywide; Adams, "Healthy at Last," 2.

49. "Brooklyn Borough President Eric Adams Announces Bid for Mayor," *NBC New York* (blog), accessed September 7, 2021, https://www.nbcnewyork.com/news/local/brooklyn-borough-president-eric-adams-announces-bid-for-mayor/2731095/; Adams, "Healthy at Last," 2.

50. "Brooklyn Politician Eric Adams Shares How He Reversed Type 2 Diabetes Through Diet," EverydayHealth.com, accessed September 7, 2021, https://www.everydayhealth.com/type-2-diabetes/living-with/brooklyn-politician-eric-adams-shares-how-he-reversed-type-2-diabetes-through-diet/.

51. Haney Aguirre-Loaiza et al., "Effect of Acute Physical Exercise on Executive Functions and Emotional Recognition: Analysis of Moderate to High Intensity in Young Adults," *Frontiers in Psychology* 10 (2019): 2774, https://doi.org/10.3389/fpsyg.2019.02774.

52. Julia C. Basso and Wendy A. Suzuki, "The Effects of Acute Exercise on Mood, Cognition, Neurophysiology, and Neurochemical Pathways: A Review," *Brain Plasticity* 2, no. 2 (n.d.): 127–152, https://doi.org/10.3233/BPL-160040.

53. Basso and Suzuki, "The Effects of Acute Exercise."

54. James P. Herman et al., "Limbic System Mechanisms of Stress Regulation: Hypothalamo-Pituitary-Adrenocortical Axis," *Progress in Neuro-Psychopharmacology & Biological Psychiatry* 29, no. 8 (December 2005): 1201–1213, https://doi.org/10.1016/j.pnpbp.2005.08.006.

55. Neha P. Gothe, Rahul K. Keswani, and Edward McAuley, "Yoga Practice Improves Executive Function by Attenuating Stress Levels," *Biological Psychology* 121, pt. A (December 2016): 109–116, https://doi.org/10.1016/j.biopsycho.2016.10.010.

56. Gothe, Keswani, and McAuley, "Yoga Practice Improves Executive Function."

57. Laura D. Baker et al., "Effects of Aerobic Exercise on Mild Cognitive Impairment: A Controlled Trial," *Archives of Neurology* 67, no. 1 (January 2010): 71–79, https://doi.org/10.1001/archneurol.2009.307.

58. Christoph Laske et al., "Exercise-Induced Normalization of Decreased BDNF Serum Concentration in Elderly Women with Remitted Major Depression," *International Journal of Neuropsychopharmacology* 13, no. 5 (June 2010): 595–602, https://doi.org/10.1017/S1461145709991234.

59. Stephanie Easton et al., "Young People's Experiences of Viewing the Fitspiration Social Media Trend: Qualitative Study," accessed September 7, 2021, https://www.jmir.org/2018/6/e219/.

60. Jon Nandor, author in conversation with, October 5, 2020.

61. Carol Ewing Garber et al., "American College of Sports Medicine Position Stand. Quantity and Quality of Exercise for Developing and Maintaining Cardiorespiratory, Musculoskeletal, and Neuromotor Fitness in Apparently Healthy Adults: Guidance for Prescribing Exercise," *Medicine and Science in Sports and Exercise* 43, no. 7 (July 2011): 1334–1359, https://doi.org/10.1249/MSS.0b013e318213fefb.

62. Joan A. Grossman, Danielle Arigo, and Jessica L. Bachman, "Meaningful Weight Loss in Obese Postmenopausal Women: A Pilot Study of High-Intensity Interval Training and Wearable Technology," *Menopause* 25, no. 4 (April 2018): 465–470, https://doi.org/10.1097/GME.0000000000001013.

63. Shigenori Ito, "High-Intensity Interval Training for Health Benefits and Care of Cardiac Diseases—The Key to an Efficient Exercise Protocol," *World Journal of Cardiology* 11, no. 7 (July 26, 2019): 171–188, https://doi.org/10.4330/wjc.v11.i7.171.

64. "Target Heart Rates Chart," American Heart Association, March 9, 2021, https://www.heart.org/en/healthy-living/fitness/fitness-basics/target-heart-rates.

65. Serena Williams (u/serenawilliams), "Letter to My Mom," forum, reddit, accessed September 3, 2021, https://www.reddit.com/user/serenawilliams/comments/714c1b/letter_to_my_mom/.

66. David Lange, "Male Grand Slam Winners with Most Titles 2020," database, Statista, March 1, 2021, https://www.statista.com/statistics/263034/male-tennis-players-with-the-most-victories-at-grand-slam-tournaments/.

67. Lange, "Male Grand Slam Winners with Most Titles 2020."

68. Britni de la Cretaz, "Serena Williams Is the GOAT. Why Is That So Hard for Some People to Say?" Refinery29, February 8, 2021, https://www.refinery29.com/en-us/2021/02/10301081/serena-williams-accomplishments-goat-tom-brady-debate.

69. Natalie Morris, "'Racism and Stereotypes' Prevent East Asian Women from Taking Part in Sport," *Metro* (blog), March 4, 2020, https://metro.co.uk/2020/03/04

/racism-damaging-stereotypes-preventing-east-asian-people-taking-part-sport
-12333557/.

70. "Elena Delle Donne: 2019 WNBA Most Valuable Player," WNBA.com—Official Site of the WNBA, accessed September 3, 2021, https://www.wnba.com/elena
-delle-donne-2019-wnba-most-valuable-player/.

71. Martenzie Johnson, "'Get Back into the Kitchen': A WNBA Roundtable on Sexism in Basketball," *The Undefeated* (blog), August 20, 2018, https://theundefeated.com
/features/wnba-roundtable-on-sexism-in-basketball-imani-mcgee-stafford-devereaux
-peters-mistie-bass-elena-delle-donne-aja-wilson-candace-parker/.

72. Joan Steidinger, *Stand Up and Shout Out: Women's Fight for Equal Pay, Equal Rights, and Equal Opportunities in Sports* (Lanham, MD: Rowman & Littlefield, 2020).

73. Nicole Rura, "Close to Half of U.S. Population Projected to Have Obesity by 2030," *Harvard Gazette* (blog), December 18, 2019, https://news.harvard.edu/gazette/story/2019
/12/close-to-half-of-u-s-population-projected-to-have-obesity-by-2030/.

74. Leslie Goldman, "An Open Letter to Anyone Who Feels Like They Don't Belong in the Gym," Shape, January 16, 2019, https://www.shape.com/fitness/tips
/open-letter-women-who-feel-they-dont-belong-gym.

75. Harold W. Goforth Jr. et al., "Effects of Depletion Exercise and Light Training on Muscle Glycogen Supercompensation in Men," *American Journal of Physiology. Endocrinology and Metabolism* 285, no. 6 (December 2003): E1304–E1311, https://doi.org/10.1152
/ajpendo.00209.2003.

76. Takashi Matsui et al., "Brain Glycogen Supercompensation Following Exhaustive Exercise," *Journal of Physiology* 590, no. 3 (2012): 607–616, https://doi.org/10.1113
/jphysiol.2011.217919.

77. Shona L. Halson et al., "Time Course of Performance Changes and Fatigue Markers During Intensified Training in Trained Cyclists," *Journal of Applied Physiology* 93, no. 3 (September 2002): 947–956, https://doi.org/10.1152/japplphysiol.01164.2001.

78. Lindsey Dahl, "Effects of Over-Reaching on Sleep Heart Rate" (Thesis, Winnipeg, Canada: University of Manitoba, 2007), https://mspace.lib.umanitoba.ca/bitstream
/handle/1993/20952/Dahl_Effects_of.pdf?sequence=1&isAllowed=y.

79. M. Kellmann, "Preventing Overtraining in Athletes in High-Intensity Sports and Stress/Recovery Monitoring," *Scandinavian Journal of Medicine & Science in Sports* 20, no. s2 (2010): 95–102, https://doi.org/10.1111/j.1600-0838.2010.01192.x.

80. L. Hermansen, E. Hultman, and B. Saltin, "Muscle Glycogen During Prolonged Severe Exercise," *Acta Physiologica Scandinavica* 71, no. 2 (November 1967): 129–139, https://doi.org/10.1111/j.1748-1716.1967.tb03719.x.

81. P. C. Blom, D. L. Costill, and N. K. Vøllestad, "Exhaustive Running: Inappropriate as a Stimulus of Muscle Glycogen Super-Compensation," *Medicine and Science in Sports and Exercise* 19, no. 4 (August 1987): 398–403.

82. Vladimir M. Zatsiorsky, William J. Kraemer, and Andrew C. Fry, *Science and Practice of Strength Training*, 3rd ed. (Champaign, IL: Human Kinetics, 2020).

83. Rudolph H. Dressendorfer, Charles E. Wade, and Jack H. Scaff, "Increased Morning Heart Rate in Runners: A Valid Sign of Overtraining?" *The Physician and Sportsmedicine* 13, no. 8 (August 1, 1985): 77–86, https://doi.org/10.1080/00913847.1985.11708858.

84. Glover Teixeira, author in conversation with, September 16, 2021.

85. Eckhart Tolle, *The Power of Now: A Guide to Spiritual Enlightenment* (Novato, CA: New World Library, 2004).

86. Deepak Chopra, *The Seven Spiritual Laws of Success* (Novato, CA: New World Library/Amber-Allen Publishing, 1994).

87. Antti M. Kiviniemi et al., "Endurance Training Guided Individually by Daily Heart Rate Variability Measurements," *European Journal of Applied Physiology* 101, no. 6 (December 2007): 743–751, https://doi.org/10.1007/s00421-007-0552-2.

88. Olli-Pekka Nuuttila et al., "Effects of HRV-Guided vs. Predetermined Block Training on Performance, HRV and Serum Hormones," *International Journal of Sports Medicine* 38, no. 12 (November 2017): 909–920, https://doi.org/10.1055/s-0043-115122.

89. Kyle D. Flack et al., "Aging, Resistance Training, and Diabetes Prevention," *Journal of Aging Research* 2011 (December 15, 2010): 127315, https://doi.org/10.4061/2011/127315; Taylor J. Marcell, "Sarcopenia: Causes, Consequences, and Preventions," *Journals of Gerontology. Series A, Biological Sciences and Medical Sciences* 58, no. 10 (October 2003): M911–M916, https://doi.org/10.1093/gerona/58.10.m911.

90. A. Ram Hong and Sang Wan Kim, "Effects of Resistance Exercise on Bone Health," *Endocrinology and Metabolism* (Seoul, Korea) 33, no. 4 (December 2018): 435–444, https://doi.org/10.3803/EnM.2018.33.4.435.

91. Wayne L. Westcott, "Resistance Training Is Medicine: Effects of Strength Training on Health," *Current Sports Medicine Reports* 11, no. 4 (August 2012): 209–216, https://doi.org/10.1249/JSR.0b013e31825dabb8.

92. George Dallam et al., "Effect of Nasal Versus Oral Breathing on $VO_{2max}$ and Physiological Economy in Recreational Runners Following an Extended Period Spent Using Nasally Restricted Breathing," *International Journal of Kinesiology and Sports Science* 6, no. 2 (April 30, 2018): 22, https://doi.org/10.7575/aiac.ijkss.v.6n.2p.22.

93. Giancarlo Ottaviano et al., "Breathing Parameters Associated to Two Different External Nasal Dilator Strips in Endurance Athletes," *Auris, Nasus, Larynx* 44, no. 6 (December 2017): 713–718, https://doi.org/10.1016/j.anl.2017.01.006.

94. Ottaviano et al., "Breathing Parameters Associated."

95. Antti M. Kiviniemi et al., "Daily Exercise Prescription on the Basis of HR Variability Among Men and Women," *Medicine and Science in Sports and Exercise* 42, no. 7 (July 2010): 1355–1363, https://doi.org/10.1249/mss.0b013e3181cd5f39.

96. John O'Leary, *In Awe: Rediscover Your Childlike Wonder to Unleash Inspiration, Meaning, and Joy* (New York: Currency, 2020).

97. Susan Fox Rogers, *My Reach, a Hudson River Memoir* (Ithaca, NY: Cornell University Press, 2011).

98. Martin Niedermeier et al., "Affective Responses in Mountain Hiking—A Randomized Crossover Trial Focusing on Differences Between Indoor and Outdoor Activity," *PLOS ONE* 12, no. 5 (May 16, 2017): e0177719, https://doi.org/10.1371/journal.pone.0177719.

## Chapter Six. You Are What and When You Eat

1. Erez Dror et al., "Postprandial Macrophage-Derived IL-1β Stimulates Insulin, and Both Synergistically Promote Glucose Disposal and Inflammation," *Nature Immunology* 18, no. 3 (March 2017): 283–922, https://doi.org/10.1038/ni.3659.

2. Mike Zimmerman, "Could Decreasing Inflammation Be the Cure for Everything?" January 17, 2020, https://www.aarp.org/health/conditions-treatments/info-2019/lowering-inflammation-to-improve-health.html.

3. Rebecca J. Brown and Kristina I. Rother, "Effects of Beta-Cell Rest on Beta-Cell Function: A Review of Clinical and Preclinical Data," *Pediatric Diabetes* 9, no. 3, pt. 2 (2008): 14–22, https://doi.org/10.1111/j.1399-5448.2007.00272.x.

4. Danina M. Muntean et al., "Modulation of Cancer Metabolism by Phytochemicals—A Brief Overview," *Anti-Cancer Agents in Medicinal Chemistry* 18, no. 5 (2018): 684–

692, https://doi.org/10.2174/1871520617666171114102218; Lara Testai, "Flavonoids and Mitochondrial Pharmacology: A New Paradigm for Cardioprotection," *Life Sciences* 135 (August 15, 2015): 68–76, https://doi.org/10.1016/j.lfs.2015.04.017.

5. Anna Atlante et al., "Functional Foods: An Approach to Modulate Molecular Mechanisms of Alzheimer's Disease," *Cells* 9, no. 11 (October 23, 2020): 2347, https://doi.org/10.3390/cells9112347; Babitha Nugala et al., "Role of Green Tea as an Antioxidant in Periodontal Disease: The Asian Paradox," *Journal of Indian Society of Periodontology* 16, no. 3 (2012): 313–316, https://doi.org/10.4103/0972-124X.100902.

6. "Antioxidants: In Depth," NCCIH, accessed September 7, 2021, https://www.nccih.nih.gov/health/antioxidants-in-depth.

7. Helmut Sies, "Oxidative Eustress: On Constant Alert for Redox Homeostasis," *Redox Biology* 41 (May 2021): 101867, https://doi.org/10.1016/j.redox.2021.101867.

8. "Processed Meat (Sausages, Ham, Bacon, Hot Dogs, Salami)," *American Institute for Cancer Research* (blog), accessed September 7, 2021, https://www.aicr.org/cancer-prevention/food-facts/processed-meat/; "Cancer: Carcinogenicity of the Consumption of Red Meat and Processed Meat," World Health Organization, accessed September 7, 2021, https://www.who.int/news-room/q-a-detail/cancer-carcinogenicity-of-the-consumption-of-red-meat-and-processed-meat.

9. Wendy Bazilian, DrPH, RD, author in conversation with, March 23, 2021.

10. Judith J. Wurtman, *The Serotonin Power Diet: Eat Carbs—Nature's Own Appetite Suppressant—to Stop Emotional Overeating and Halt Antidepressant-Associated Weight Gain* (New York: Rodale, 2006).

11. Shanon L. Casperson et al., "Increasing Chocolate's Sugar Content Enhances Its Psychoactive Effects and Intake," *Nutrients* 11, no. 3 (March 12, 2019): 596, https://doi.org/10.3390/nu11030596.

12. Johan L. Vinther et al., "Marital Transitions and Associated Changes in Fruit and Vegetable Intake: Findings from the Population-Based Prospective EPIC-Norfolk Cohort, UK," *Social Science & Medicine* 157 (May 1, 2016): 120–126, https://doi.org/10.1016/j.socscimed.2016.04.004.

13. James E. Gangwisch et al., "High Glycemic Index Diet as a Risk Factor for Depression: Analyses from the Women's Health Initiative," *American Journal of Clinical Nutrition* 102, no. 2 (August 2015): 454–463, https://doi.org/10.3945/ajcn.114.103846; Tina Ljungberg, Emma Bondza, and Connie Lethin, "Evidence of the Importance of Dietary Habits Regarding Depressive Symptoms and Depression," *International Journal of Environmental Research and Public Health* 17, no. 5 (March 2, 2020): 1616, https://doi.org/10.3390/ijerph17051616.

14. Eva Selhub MD, "Nutritional Psychiatry: Your Brain on Food," Harvard Health, November 16, 2015, https://www.health.harvard.edu/blog/nutritional-psychiatry-your-brain-on-food-201511168626.

15. J. R. Hibbeln, "Fish Consumption and Major Depression," *Lancet* 351, no. 9110 (April 18, 1998): 1213, https://doi.org/10.1016/S0140-6736(05)79168-6.

16. M. Maes et al., "In Humans, Serum Polyunsaturated Fatty Acid Levels Predict the Response of Proinflammatory Cytokines to Psychologic Stress," *Biological Psychiatry* 47, no. 10 (May 15, 2000): 910–920, https://doi.org/10.1016/s0006-3223(99)00268-1.

17. Kuan-Pin Su, Yutaka Matsuoka, and Chi-Un Pae, "Omega-3 Polyunsaturated Fatty Acids in Prevention of Mood and Anxiety Disorders," *Clinical Psychopharmacology and Neuroscience* 13, no. 2 (August 30, 2015): 129–137, https://doi.org/10.9758/cpn.2015.13.2.129.

18. Shinichi Kuriyama et al., "Green Tea Consumption and Cognitive Function: A Cross-Sectional Study from the Tsurugaya Project 1," *American Journal of Clinical Nutrition* 83, no. 2 (February 2006): 355–361, https://doi.org/10.1093/ajcn/83.2.355.

19. D. R. Braun et al., "Early Hominin Diet Included Diverse Terrestrial and Aquatic Animals 1.95 Ma in East Turkana, Kenya," *Proceedings of the National Academy of Sciences* 107, no. 22 (June 1, 2010): 10002–100007, https://doi.org/10.1073/pnas.1002181107.

20. Fernando Gómez-Pinilla, "Brain Foods: The Effects of Nutrients on Brain Function," *Nature Reviews. Neuroscience* 9, no. 7 (July 2008): 568–578, https://doi.org/10.1038/nrn2421.

21. Richard J. Wurtman, "A Nutrient Combination That Can Affect Synapse Formation," *Nutrients* 6, no. 4 (April 23, 2014): 1701–1710, https://doi.org/10.3390/nu6041701.

22. Hooman Allayee, Nitzan Roth, and Howard N. Hodis, "Polyunsaturated Fatty Acids and Cardiovascular Disease: Implications for Nutrigenetics," *Journal of Nutrigenetics and Nutrigenomics* 2, no. 3 (2009): 140–148, https://doi.org/10.1159/000235562.

23. A. P. Simopoulos, "Evolutionary Aspects of Omega-3 Fatty Acids in the Food Supply," *Prostaglandins, Leukotrienes, and Essential Fatty Acids* 60, nos. 5–6 (June 1999): 421–429, https://doi.org/10.1016/s0952-3278(99)80023-4.

24. Michio Hashimoto and Shahdat Hossain, "Neuroprotective and Ameliorative Actions of Polyunsaturated Fatty Acids Against Neuronal Diseases: Beneficial Effect of Docosahexaenoic Acid on Cognitive Decline in Alzheimer's Disease," *Journal of Pharmacological Sciences* 116, no. 2 (2011): 150–162, https://doi.org/10.1254/jphs.10r33fm.

25. Juan Zhou et al., "Effects of Lutein Supplementation on Inflammatory Biomarkers and Metabolic Risk Factors in Adults with Central Obesity: Study Protocol for a Randomised Controlled Study," *Trials* 21, no. 1 (January 6, 2020): 32, https://doi.org/10.1186/s13063-019-3998-8.

26. Julien Bensalem et al., "Polyphenols from Grape and Blueberry Improve Episodic Memory in Healthy Elderly with Lower Level of Memory Performance: A Bicentric Double-Blind, Randomized, Placebo-Controlled Clinical Study," *Journals of Gerontology. Series A, Biological Sciences and Medical Sciences* 74, no. 7 (June 18, 2019): 996–1007, https://doi.org/10.1093/gerona/gly166.

27. Gary W. Small et al., "Memory and Brain Amyloid and Tau Effects of a Bioavailable Form of Curcumin in Non-Demented Adults: A Double-Blind, Placebo-Controlled 18-Month Trial," *American Journal of Geriatric Psychiatry: Official Journal of the American Association for Geriatric Psychiatry* 26, no. 3 (March 2018): 266–277, https://doi.org/10.1016/j.jagp.2017.10.010.

28. Gary W. Small et al., "Memory and Brain Amyloid and Tau Effects."

29. Lee Hooper et al., "Flavonoids, Flavonoid-Rich Foods, and Cardiovascular Risk: A Meta-analysis of Randomized Controlled Trials," *American Journal of Clinical Nutrition* 88, no. 1 (July 2008): 38–50, https://doi.org/10.1093/ajcn/88.1.38.

30. Eleanor Wood et al., "Blueberries and Cardiovascular Disease Prevention," *Food & Function* 10, no. 12 (December 11, 2019): 7621–7633, https://doi.org/10.1039/c9fo02291k.

31. Andrew Steptoe et al., "The Effects of Tea on Psychophysiological Stress Responsivity and Post-Stress Recovery: A Randomised Double-Blind Trial," *Psychopharmacology* 190, no. 1 (January 2007): 81–89, https://doi.org/10.1007/s00213-006-0573-2; Petra H. Wirtz et al., "Dark Chocolate Intake Buffers Stress Reactivity in Humans," *Journal of the American College of Cardiology* 63, no. 21 (June 3, 2014): 2297–2299, https://doi.org/10.1016/j.jacc.2014.02.580; Denise Ruttke Dillenburg et al., "Resveratrol and Grape Juice Differentially Ameliorate Cardiovascular Autonomic Modulation in L-NAME-Treated

Rats," *Autonomic Neuroscience: Basic & Clinical* 179, no. 1–2 (December 2013): 9–13, https://doi.org/10.1016/j.autneu.2013.06.002.

32. Arno Greyling et al., "Effects of Wine and Grape Polyphenols on Blood Pressure, Endothelial Function and Sympathetic Nervous System Activity in Treated Hypertensive Subjects," *Journal of Functional Foods* 27 (December 2016): 448–460, https://doi.org/10.1016/j.jff.2016.10.003.

33. Henriette van Praag et al., "Plant-Derived Flavanol Epicatechin Enhances Angiogenesis and Retention of Spatial Memory in Mice," *Journal of Neuroscience* 27, no. 22 (May 30, 2007): 5869–5678, https://doi.org/10.1523/JNEUROSCI.0914-07.2007.

34. María Angeles Martín, Luis Goya, and Sonia de Pascual-Teresa, "Effect of Cocoa and Cocoa Products on Cognitive Performance in Young Adults," *Nutrients* 12, no. 12 (November 30, 2020): E3691, https://doi.org/10.3390/nu12123691.

35. Edward J. Szczygiel, Sungeun Cho, and Robin M. Tucker, "The Effect of Sleep Curtailment on Hedonic Responses to Liquid and Solid Food," *Foods* 8, no. 10 (October 10, 2019): 465, https://doi.org/10.3390/foods8100465.

36. "Obesity Prevention Source: Sleep," Harvard T.H. Chan School of Public Health, accessed September 7, 2021, https://www.hsph.harvard.edu/obesity-prevention-source/obesity-causes/sleep-and-obesity/.

37. F. Phillips et al., "Isocaloric Diet Changes and Electroencephalographic Sleep," *Lancet* 2, no. 7938 (October 18, 1975): 723–725, https://doi.org/10.1016/s0140-6736(75)90718-7; Katsuhiko Yajima et al., "Effects of Nutrient Composition of Dinner on Sleep Architecture and Energy Metabolism During Sleep," *Journal of Nutritional Science and Vitaminology* 60, no. 2 (2014): 114–121, https://doi.org/10.3177/jnsv.60.114.

38. Katsuhiko Yajima et al., "Effects of Nutrient Composition of Dinner," 114–121.

39. "Mauritius Joint Child Health Project," USC Dana and David Dornsife College of Letters, Arts and Sciences, accessed September 22, 2021, http://dornsife.usc.edu/labs/susan-luczak/mauritius-joint-child-health-project/.

40. Jianghong Liu et al., "Malnutrition at Age 3 Years and Lower Cognitive Ability at Age 11 Years: Independence from Psychosocial Adversity," *Archives of Pediatrics & Adolescent Medicine* 157, no. 6 (June 1, 2003): 593–600, https://doi.org/10.1001/archpedi.157.6.593; Jianghong Liu et al., "Malnutrition at Age 3 Years and Externalizing Behavior Problems at Ages 8, 11, and 17 Years," *American Journal of Psychiatry* 161, no. 11 (November 2004): 2005–2013, https://doi.org/10.1176/appi.ajp.161.11.2005.

41. Louise Bergmann Sørensen et al., "Diet-Induced Changes in Iron and $n$-3 Fatty Acid Status and Associations with Cognitive Performance in 8–11-Year-Old Danish Children: Secondary Analyses of the Optimal Well-Being, Development and Health for Danish Children through a Healthy New Nordic Diet School Meal Study," *British Journal of Nutrition* 114, no. 10 (November 28, 2015): 1623–1637, https://doi.org/10.1017/S0007114515003323.

42. "11 Facts About Food Deserts," DoSomething.org, accessed September 7, 2021, https://www.dosomething.org/us/facts/11-facts-about-food-deserts.

43. Michele Ver Ploeg et al., "Access to Affordable and Nutritious Food: Measuring and Understanding Food Deserts and Their Consequences," accessed September 17, 2021, https://www.ers.usda.gov/webdocs/publications/42711/12716_ap036_1_.pdf?v=41055.

44. Ashanté M. Reese, "Black Food Geographies: Race, Self-Reliance, and Food Access in Washington, D.C.," University of North Carolina Press, accessed September 7, 2021, https://uncpress.org/book/9781469651507/black-food-geographies/; Jerry Shannon, "Dollar Stores, Retailer Redlining, and the Metropolitan Geographies of Precarious Consumption, *Annals of the American Association of Geographers* 111, no. 4, accessed

September 7, 2021, https://www.tandfonline.com/doiabs/10.1080/24694452.2020 .1775544?journalCode=raag21.

45. Anna Brones, "Karen Washington: It's Not a Food Desert, It's Food Apartheid," *Guernica*, May 7, 2018, https://www.guernicamag.com/karen-washington-its-not-a-food -desert-its-food-apartheid/.

46. "Our Story," Black Farmer Fund, accessed September 7, 2021, https://www.black farmerfund.org/.

47. "2012 Census of Agriculture Highlights—Black Farmers," United States Department of Agriculture, September 2014, https://www.nass.usda.gov/Publications/High lights/2014/Highlights_Black_Farmers.pdf.

48. Jordan Thomas, author in conversation with, December 16, 2020.

49. David Yaffe-Bellany and Michael Corkery, "Dumped Milk, Smashed Eggs, Plowed Vegetables: Food Waste of the Pandemic," *New York Times*, accessed September 7, 2021, https://www.nytimes.com/2020/04/11/business/coronavirus-destroying-food.html.

50. The Byrds, "Turn! Turn! Turn!," track 1 on *Turn! Turn! Turn!*, Columbia Records, 1965.

51. Fabien Pifferi et al., "Caloric Restriction Increases Lifespan but Affects Brain Integrity in Grey Mouse Lemur Primates," *Communications Biology* 1, no. 1 (April 5, 2018): 1–8, https://doi.org/10.1038/s42003-018-0024-8; Luigi Fontana, "Interventions to Promote Cardiometabolic Health and Slow Cardiovascular Ageing," *Nature Reviews Cardiology* 15, no. 9 (September 2018): 566–577, https://doi.org/10.1038/s41569-018-0026-8.

52. Emily Kumlien, "Calorie Restriction Lets Monkeys Live Long and Prosper," University of Wisconsin-Madison, January 17, 2017, https://news.wisc.edu/calorie -restriction-lets-monkeys-live-long-and-prosper/; Terry Devitt, "Reduced Diet Thwarts Aging, Disease in Monkeys," University of Wisconsin-Madison, July 9, 2009, https:// news.wisc.edu/reduced-diet-thwarts-aging-disease-in-monkeys/.

53. Ciera L. Bartholomew et al., "Association of Periodic Fasting Lifestyles with Survival and Incident Major Adverse Cardiovascular Events in Patients Undergoing Cardiac Catheterization," *European Journal of Preventive Cardiology*, no. zwaa050 (September 22, 2020), https://doi.org/10.1093/eurjpc/zwaa050.

54. Tiffany A. Dong et al., "Intermittent Fasting: A Heart Healthy Dietary Pattern?" *American Journal of Medicine* 133, no. 8 (August 2020): 901–907, https://doi.org/10.1016/j .amjmed.2020.03.030.

55. Stephen D. Anton et al., "Flipping the Metabolic Switch: Understanding and Applying the Health Benefits of Fasting," *Obesity* 26, no. 2 (February 2018): 254–268, https://doi.org/10.1002/oby.22065.

56. Sebastian Brandhorst et al., "A Periodic Diet That Mimics Fasting Promotes Multi-System Regeneration, Enhanced Cognitive Performance, and Healthspan," *Cell Metabolism* 22, no. 1 (July 7, 2015): 86–99, https://doi.org/10.1016/j.cmet.2015.05.012.

57. Richard Conniff, "The Hunger Gains: Extreme Calorie-Restriction Diet Shows Anti-aging Results," *Scientific American*, accessed September 7, 2021, https://www .scientificamerican.com/article/the-hunger-gains-extreme-calorie-restriction-diet -shows-anti-aging-results/; Min Wei et al., "Fasting-Mimicking Diet and Markers/Risk Factors for Aging, Diabetes, Cancer, and Cardiovascular Disease," *Science Translational Medicine* 9, no. 37 (February 15, 2017), https://doi.org/10.1126/scitranslmed.aai8700.

58. Conniff, "The Hunger Gains."

59. Rima Solianik et al., "Effect of 48 h Fasting on Autonomic Function, Brain Activity, Cognition, and Mood in Amateur Weight Lifters," *BioMed Research International* 2016 (2016): 1503956, https://doi.org/10.1155/2016/1503956.

60. Satchin Panda, *The Circadian Code: Lose Weight, Supercharge Your Energy, and Transform Your Health from Morning to Midnight* (New York: Rodale Books, 2018), 267.

61. Salk Institute, "Clinical Study Finds Eating Within 10-Hour Window May Help Stave off Diabetes, Heart Disease," ScienceDaily, December 5, 2019, https://www.science daily.com/releases/2019/12/191205141731.htm.

62. Lori Zanteson, "Gut Health and Immunity—It's All About the Good Bacteria That Can Help Fight Disease," Today's Dietitian, June 2012, https://www.todaysdietitian.com /newarchives/060112p58.shtml; G. Vighi et al., "Allergy and the Gastrointestinal System," *Clinical and Experimental Immunology* 153, Suppl. 1, (September 2008): 3–6, https:// doi.org/10.1111/j.1365-2249.2008.03713.x.

63. S. M. O'Mahony et al., "Serotonin, Tryptophan Metabolism and the Brain-Gut-Microbiome Axis," *Special Issue: Serotonin* 277 (January 15, 2015): 32–48, https://doi.org /10.1016/j.bbr.2014.07.027.

64. Paula Perez-Pardo et al., "The Gut-Brain Axis in Parkinson's Disease: Possibilities for Food-Based Therapies," *European Journal of Pharmacology* 817 (December 15, 2017): 86–95, https://doi.org/10.1016/j.ejphar.2017.05.042.

65. L. Ohlsson et al., "Leaky Gut Biomarkers in Depression and Suicidal Behavior," *Acta Psychiatrica Scandinavica* 139, no. 2 (February 2019): 185–193, https://doi.org/10.1111 /acps.12978.

66. Jing Li et al., "Gut Microbiota Dysbiosis Contributes to the Development of Hypertension," *Microbiome* 5, no. 1 (February 1, 2017): 14, https://doi.org/10.1186/s40168 -016-0222-x.

67. D. Benton, C. Williams, and A. Brown, "Impact of Consuming a Milk Drink Containing a Probiotic on Mood and Cognition," *European Journal of Clinical Nutrition* 61, no. 3 (March 1, 2007): 355–361, https://doi.org/10.1038/sj.ejcn.1602546.

68. Hassan S. Dashti et al., "Genome-Wide Association Study of Breakfast Skipping Links Clock Regulation with Food Timing," *American Journal of Clinical Nutrition* 110, no. 2 (August 1, 2019): 473–484, https://doi.org/10.1093/ajcn/nqz076.

69. Marie-Pierre St-Onge, Anja Mikic, and Cara E Pietrolungo, "Effects of Diet on Sleep Quality," *Advances in Nutrition* 7, no. 5 (September 15, 2016): 938–949, https://doi .org/10.3945/an.116.012336; Kayo Kurotani et al., "Dietary Patterns and Sleep Symptoms in Japanese Workers: The Furukawa Nutrition and Health Study," *Sleep Medicine* 16, no. 2 (February 1, 2015): 298–304, https://doi.org/10.1016/j.sleep.2014.09.017.

70. "New MIND Diet May Significantly Protect Against Alzheimer's Disease," accessed September 7, 2021, https://www.rush.edu/news/new-mind-diet-may-significantly -protect-against-alzheimers-disease; L Cherian et al., "Mediterranean-Dash Intervention for Neurodegenerative Delay (MIND) Diet Slows Cognitive Decline After Stroke," *Journal of Prevention of Alzheimer's Disease* 6, no. 4 (2019): 267–273, https://doi.org/10.14283 /jpad.2019.28.

71. "New MIND Diet May Significantly Protect Against Alzheimer's Disease," accessed September 7, 2021, https://www.rush.edu/news/new-mind-diet-may-significantly-pro tect-against-alzheimers-disease; Neurology Reviews, "Moderate Adherence to MIND Diet May Protect Against Alzheimer's Disease," MDedge, May 2015, https://www.mdedge.com /neurology/article/99259/alzheimers-cognition/moderate-adherence-mind-diet-may -protect-against.

72. Martha C. Morris et al., "MIND Diet Associated with Reduced Incidence of Alzheimer's Disease," *Alzheimer's & Dementia: The Journal of the Alzheimer's Association* 11, no. 9 (September 2015): 1007–1014, https://doi.org/10.1016/j.jalz.2014.11.009.

73. Jennifer Ventrelle, author in conversation with, February 12, 2021.

74. Ryoko Katagiri et al., "Low Intake of Vegetables, High Intake of Confectionary, and Unhealthy Eating Habits Are Associated with Poor Sleep Quality among Middle-Aged Female Japanese Workers," *Journal of Occupational Health* 56, no. 5 (September 1, 2014): 359–368, https://doi.org/10.1539/joh.14-0051-OA.

## Chapter Seven. Guess What? You Are Aging NOW!

1. Timothy A. Salthouse, "Trajectories of Normal Cognitive Aging," *Psychology and Aging* 34, no. 1 (February 2019): 17–24, https://doi.org/10.1037/pag0000288.

2. Alfonso J. Cruz-Jentoft et al., "Sarcopenia: Revised European Consensus on Definition and Diagnosis," *Age and Ageing* 48, no. 1 (January 1, 2019): 16–31, https://doi.org/10.1093/ageing/afy169.

3. Gary F. Mitchell et al., "Changes in Arterial Stiffness and Wave Reflection with Advancing Age in Healthy Men and Women: The Framingham Heart Study," *Hypertension* (Dallas: 1979) 43, no. 6 (June 2004): 1239–1245, https://doi.org/10.1161/01.HYP.0000128420.01881.aa; Junzhen Wu et al., "The Role of Oxidative Stress and Inflammation in Cardiovascular Aging," *BioMed Research International* 2014 (July 20, 2014): e615312, https://doi.org/10.1155/2014/615312.

4. Séverine Sabia et al., "Association of Sleep Duration in Middle and Old Age with Incidence of Dementia," *Nature Communications* 12, no. 1 (April 20, 2021): 2289, https://doi.org/10.1038/s41467-021-22354-2.

5. Thomas J. LaRocca, Christopher R. Martens, and Douglas R. Seals, "Nutrition and Other Lifestyle Influences on Arterial Aging," *Ageing Research Reviews* 39 (October 1, 2017): 106–119, https://doi.org/10.1016/j.arr.2016.09.002.

6. A. Colosimo et al., "Estimating a Cardiac Age by Means of Heart Rate Variability," *American Journal of Physiology* 273, no. 4 (October 1997): H1841–H1847, https://doi.org/10.1152/ajpheart.1997.273.4.H1841; I. A. D. O'Brien et al., "The Prevalence of Autonomic Neuropathy in Insulin-Dependent Diabetes Mellitus: A Controlled Study Based on Heart Rate Variability," *QJM: An International Journal of Medicine* 61, no. 1 (October 1, 1986): 957–967, https://doi.org/10.1093/oxfordjournals.qjmed.a068054; Andrew H. Kemp, Julian Koenig, and Julian F. Thayer, "From Psychological Moments to Mortality: A Multidisciplinary Synthesis on Heart Rate Variability Spanning the Continuum of Time," *Neuroscience and Biobehavioral Reviews* 83 (December 2017): 547–567, https://doi.org/10.1016/j.neubiorev.2017.09.006.

7. Benjamin D. Yetton et al., "Quantifying Sleep Architecture Dynamics and Individual Differences Using Big Data and Bayesian Networks," *PLOS ONE* 13, no. 4 (2018): e0194604, https://doi.org/10.1371/journal.pone.0194604.

8. Claudio Franceschi et al., "Inflammaging: A New Immune–Metabolic Viewpoint for Age-Related Diseases," *Nature Reviews Endocrinology* 14, no. 10 (October 2018): 576–590, https://doi.org/10.1038/s41574-018-0059-4.

9. Stephanie J Wilson et al., "Loneliness and Telomere Length: Immune and Parasympathetic Function in Associations with Accelerated Aging," *Annals of Behavioral Medicine: A Publication of the Society of Behavioral Medicine* 53, no. 6 (August 13, 2018): 541–550, https://doi.org/10.1093/abm/kay064.

10. Qi Wang et al., "Telomere Length and All-Cause Mortality: A Meta-analysis," *Ageing Research Reviews* 48 (December 2018): 11–20, https://doi.org/10.1016/j.arr.2018.09.002.

11. Nan-ping Weng, "Telomeres and Immune Competency," *Current Opinion in Immunology* 24, no. 4 (August 2012): 470–475, https://doi.org/10.1016/j.coi.2012.05.001.

12. Sarah E. Baker et al., "Aging Alters the Relative Contributions of the Sympathetic and Parasympathetic Nervous System to Blood Pressure Control in Women," *Hypertension* (Dallas: 1979) 72, no. 5 (November 2018): 1236–1242, https://doi.org/10.1161/HYPERTENSIONAHA.118.11550.

13. Yi-Yuan Tang et al., "Long-Term Physical Exercise and Mindfulness Practice in an Aging Population," *Frontiers in Psychology* 11 (2020): 358, https://doi.org/10.3389/fpsyg.2020.00358.

14. Chulee Ublosakka-Jones et al., "Slow Loaded Breathing Training Improves Blood Pressure, Lung Capacity and Arm Exercise Endurance for Older People with Treated and Stable Isolated Systolic Hypertension," *Experimental Gerontology* 108 (July 15, 2018): 48–53, https://doi.org/10.1016/j.exger.2018.03.023.

15. Dylan J. Jester, Ellen K. Rozek, and Ryan A. McKelley, "Heart Rate Variability Biofeedback: Implications for Cognitive and Psychiatric Effects in Older Adults," *Aging & Mental Health* 23, no. 5 (May 2019): 574–580, https://doi.org/10.1080/13607863.2018.1432031.

16. E. Van Cauter, R. Leproult, and L. Plat, "Age-Related Changes in Slow Wave Sleep and REM Sleep and Relationship with Growth Hormone and Cortisol Levels in Healthy Men," *JAMA* 284, no. 7 (August 16, 2000): 861–868, https://doi.org/10.1001/jama.284.7.861.

17. Joseph R. Winer et al., "Sleep as a Potential Biomarker of Tau and β-Amyloid Burden in the Human Brain," *Journal of Neuroscience*, June 17, 2019, https://doi.org/10.1523/JNEUROSCI.0503-19.2019.

18. Shirley Leanos et al., "The Impact of Learning Multiple Real-World Skills on Cognitive Abilities and Functional Independence in Healthy Older Adults," *Journals of Gerontology. Series B, Psychological Sciences and Social Sciences* 75, no. 6 (June 2, 2020): 1155–1169, https://doi.org/10.1093/geronb/gbz084.

19. Recep Or and Asiye Kartal, "Influence of Caregiver Burden on Well-Being of Family Member Caregivers of Older Adults," *Psychogeriatrics* 19, no. 5 (2019): 482–490, https://doi.org/10.1111/psyg.12421.

20. "How the Aging Brain Affects Thinking," National Institute on Aging, accessed April 27, 2021, http://www.nia.nih.gov/health/how-aging-brain-affects-thinking.

21. Erik S. Musiek and David M. Holtzman, "Mechanisms Linking Circadian Clocks, Sleep, and Neurodegeneration," *Science* (New York) 354, no. 6315 (November 25, 2016): 1004–1008, https://doi.org/10.1126/science.aah4968.

22. V. Daneault et al., "Light-Sensitive Brain Pathways and Aging," *Journal of Physiological Anthropology* 35, no. 1 (March 15, 2016): 9, https://doi.org/10.1186/s40101-016-0091-9.

23. R. C. Espiritu et al., "Low Illumination Experienced by San Diego Adults: Association with Atypical Depressive Symptoms," *Biological Psychiatry* 35, no. 6 (March 15, 1994): 403–407, https://doi.org/10.1016/0006-3223(94)90007-8; N. Hanford and M. Figueiro, "Light Therapy and Alzheimer's Disease and Related Dementia: Past, Present, and Future," *Journal of Alzheimer's Disease* 33, no. 4 (2013): 913–922. https://doi.org: 10.3233/JAD-2012-121645, PMID: 23099814; PMCID: PMC3553247.

24. Omonigho M. Bubu et al., "Obstructive Sleep Apnea, Cognition and Alzheimer's Disease: A Systematic Review Integrating Three Decades of Multidisciplinary Research," *Sleep Medicine Reviews* 50 (April 1, 2020): 101250, https://doi.org/10.1016/j.smrv.2019.101250.

25. Patrick Lemoine et al., "Prolonged-Release Melatonin Improves Sleep Quality and Morning Alertness in Insomnia Patients Aged 55 Years and Older and Has No Withdrawal

Effects," *Journal of Sleep Research* 16, no. 4 (December 2007): 372–380, https://doi .org/10.1111/j.1365-2869.2007.00613.x.

26. Sanjib Patra and Shirley Telles, "Positive Impact of Cyclic Meditation on Subsequent Sleep," *Medical Science Monitor: International Medical Journal of Experimental and Clinical Research* 15, no. 7 (July 2009): CR375–C381, https://europepmc.org/article/med /19564829; Sanjib Patra and Shirley Telles, "Heart Rate Variability During Sleep Following the Practice of Cyclic Meditation and Supine Rest," *Applied Psychophysiology and Biofeedback* 35, no. 2 (June 2010): 135–140, https://doi.org/10.1007/s10484-009-9114-1.

27. Sayaka Aritake-Okada et al., "Diurnal Repeated Exercise Promotes Slow-Wave Activity and Fast-Sigma Power During Sleep with Increase in Body Temperature: A Human Crossover Trial," *Journal of Applied Physiology* (Bethesda, MD: 1985) 127, no. 1 (July 1, 2019): 168–177, https://doi.org/10.1152/japplphysiol.00765.2018; Neha Sinha et al., "Increased Dynamic Flexibility in the Medial Temporal Lobe Network Following an Exercise Intervention Mediates Generalization of Prior Learning," *Neurobiology of Learning and Memory* 177 (January 2021): 107340, https://doi.org/10.1016/j.nlm.2020.107340.

28. Mariana G. Figueiro et al., "Tailored Lighting Intervention Improves Measures of Sleep, Depression, and Agitation in Persons with Alzheimer's Disease and Related Dementia Living in Long-Term Care Facilities," *Clinical Interventions in Aging* 9 (September 12, 2014): 1527–1537, https://doi.org/10.2147/CIA.S68557.

29. Figueiro, "Tailored Lighting Intervention."

30. "Adults Need More Physical Activity," Centers for Disease Control and Prevention, June 9, 2021, https://www.cdc.gov/physicalactivity/inactivity-among-adults-50plus/ index.html.

31. Deborah E. Barnes and Kristine Yaffe, "The Projected Effect of Risk Factor Reduction on Alzheimer's Disease Prevalence," *Lancet Neurology* 10, no. 9 (September 2011): 819–828, https://doi.org/10.1016/S1474-4422(11)70072-2; Susan A. Carlson et al., "Percentage of Deaths Associated with Inadequate Physical Activity in the United States," *Preventing Chronic Disease* 15 (March 29, 2018): E38, https://doi.org/10.5888/pcd18.170354.

32. Jeremy D. Walston, "Sarcopenia in Older Adults," *Current Opinion in Rheumatology* 24, no. 6 (November 2012): 623–627, https://doi.org/10.1097/BOR.0b013e328358d59b.

33. Andrew S. Jackson et al., "Longitudinal Changes in Body Composition Associated with Healthy Ageing: Men, Aged 20–96 Years," *British Journal of Nutrition* 107, no. 7 (April 2012): 1085–1091, https://doi.org/10.1017/S0007114511003886; Fulvio Lauretani et al., "Age-Associated Changes in Skeletal Muscles and Their Effect on Mobility: An Operational Diagnosis of Sarcopenia," *Journal of Applied Physiology* (Bethesda, MD: 1985) 95, no. 5 (November 2003): 1851–1860, https://doi.org/10.1152/japplphysiol.00246.2003.

34. Magdalena I. Tolea and James E. Galvin, "Sarcopenia and Impairment in Cognitive and Physical Performance," *Clinical Interventions in Aging* 10 (March 30, 2015): 663–671, https://doi.org/10.2147/CIA.S76275.

35. Consuelo H. Wilkins et al., "Mild Physical Impairment Predicts Future Diagnosis of Dementia of the Alzheimer's Type," *Journal of the American Geriatrics Society* 61, no. 7 (July 2013): 1055–1059, https://doi.org/10.1111/jgs.12255.

36. Gretchen Reynolds, "The Right Kind of Exercise May Boost Memory and Lower Dementia Risk," *New York Times*, November 6, 2019, sec. Well, https://www.nytimes.com /2019/11/06/well/move/exercise-dementia-memory-alzheimers-brain-seniors-middle -age.html.

37. Barnes and Yaffe, "The Projected Effect of Risk Factor Reduction."

38. A. R. Tari et al., "Temporal Changes in Cardiorespiratory Fitness and Risk of Dementia Incidence and Mortality: A Population-Based Prospective Cohort Study," *Lancet*

*Public Health* 4, no. 11 (November 2019): e565–e574, doi: 10.1016/S2468-2667(19)30183-5. PMID: 31677775.

39. Amanda E. Paluch et al., "Steps per Day and All-Cause Mortality in Middle-Aged Adults in the Coronary Artery Risk Development in Young Adults Study," *JAMA Network Open* 4, no. 9 (September 1, 2021): e2124516, https://doi.org/10.1001/jamanetwork open.2021.24516.

40. Peter Schnohr et al., "U-Shaped Association Between Duration of Sports Activities and Mortality: Copenhagen City Heart Study," *Mayo Clinic Proceedings* (August 17, 2021), https://doi.org/10.1016/j.mayocp.2021.05.028.

41. Jérémy Raffin et al., "Exercise Frequency Determines Heart Rate Variability Gains in Older People: A Meta-analysis and Meta-regression," *Sports Medicine* 49, no. 5 (May 2019): 719–729, https://doi.org/10.1007/s40279-019-01097-7.

42. T. Cordes et al., "Multicomponent Exercise to Improve Motor Functions, Cognition and Well-Being for Nursing Home Residents Who Are Unable to Walk: A Randomized Controlled Trial," *Experimental Gerontology* 153, no. 6 (October 1, 2021): 111484, https://doi.org/ 10.1016/j.exger.2021.111484, Epub July 20, 2021, PMID: 34293413.

43. Susan Fox Rogers, *When Birds Are Near: Dispatches from Contemporary Writers* (Ithaca, NY: Comstock Publishing Associates, 2020); Susan Fox Rogers, *Learning the Birds* (Cornell University Press, 2022).

44. Hayley Wright, Rebecca A. Jenks, and Nele Demeyere, "Frequent Sexual Activity Predicts Specific Cognitive Abilities in Older Adults," *Journals of Gerontology. Series B, Psychological Sciences and Social Sciences* 74, no. 1 (January 1, 2019): 47–51, https://doi.org /10.1093/geronb/gbx065.

45. Ravinder Nagpal et al., "Gut Microbiome and Aging: Physiological and Mechanistic Insights," *Nutrition and Healthy Aging* 4, no. 4 (June 15, 2018): 267–285, https://doi.org /10.3233/NHA-170030.

46. Paul W. O'Toole and Ian B. Jeffery, "Gut Microbiota and Aging," *Science* 350, no. 6265 (December 4, 2015): 1214–1215, https://doi.org/10.1126/science.aac8469; Neal S. Fedarko, "The Biology of Aging and Frailty," *Clinics in Geriatric Medicine* 27, no. 1 (February 1, 2011): 27–37, https://doi.org/10.1016/j.cger.2010.08.006.

47. Bamini Gopinath et al., "Association Between Carbohydrate Nutrition and Successful Aging over 10 Years," *Journals of Gerontology: Series A* 71, no. 10 (October 1, 2016): 1335–1340, https://doi.org/10.1093/gerona/glw091.

48. Yufei Cui et al., "Relationship Between Daily Isoflavone Intake and Sleep in Japanese Adults: A Cross-Sectional Study," *Nutrition Journal* 14, no. 1 (December 29, 2015): 127, https://doi.org/10.1186/s12937-015-0117-x.

49. Yasutake Tomata et al., "Dietary Patterns and Incident Dementia in Elderly Japanese: The Ohsaki Cohort 2006 Study," *Journals of Gerontology: Series A* 71, no. 10 (October 1, 2016): 1322–1328, https://doi.org/10.1093/gerona/glw117; "Okinawa, Japan," Blue Zones, accessed January 16, 2021, https://www.bluezones.com/exploration/okinawa-japan/.

50. W. B. Cutler, "Lunar and Menstrual Phase Locking," *American Journal of Obstetrics and Gynecology* 137, no. 7 (August 1, 1980): 834–839, https://doi.org/10.1016/0002 -9378(80)90895-9; I. Ilias et al., "Do Lunar Phases Influence Menstruation? A Year-Long Retrospective Study," *Endocrine Regulations* 47, no. 3 (July 2013): 121–122, https://doi .org/10.4149/endo_2013_03_121.

51. Karyn M. Frick et al., "Sex Steroid Hormones Matter for Learning and Memory: Estrogenic Regulation of Hippocampal Function in Male and Female Rodents," *Learning & Memory* 22, no. 9 (September 2015): 472–493, https://doi.org/10.1101/lm.037267.114; Agneta Herlitz, Eija Airaksinen, Eva Nordström, "Sex Differences in Episodic Memory:

The Impact of Verbal and Visuospatial Ability," *Neuropsychology* 13, no. 4 (1999), https://psycnet.apa.org/doiLanding?doi=10.1037%2F0894-4105.13.4.590.

52. Fiona C. Baker et al., "Impact of Sex Steroids and Reproductive Stage on Sleep-Dependent Memory Consolidation in Women," *Neurobiology of Learning and Memory* 160 (April 2019): 118–131, https://doi.org/10.1016/j.nlm.2018.03.017; Negin Sattari et al., "The Effect of Sex and Menstrual Phase on Memory Formation During a Nap," *Neurobiology of Learning and Memory* 145 (November 2017): 119–128, https://doi.org/10.1016/j.nlm.2017.09.007.

53. A. Ahokas et al., "Estrogen Deficiency in Severe Postpartum Depression: Successful Treatment with Sublingual Physiologic 17beta-Estradiol: A Preliminary Study," *Journal of Clinical Psychiatry* 62, no. 5 (May 2001): 332–336, https://doi.org/10.4088/jcp.v62n0504; Gordon Barraclough Parker and Heather Lorraine Brotchie, "From Diathesis to Dimorphism: The Biology of Gender Differences in Depression," *Journal of Nervous and Mental Disease* 192, no. 3 (March 2004): 210–216, https://doi.org/10.1097/01.nmd.0000116464.60500.6; Matia B. Solomon and James P. Herman, "Sex Differences in Psychopathology: Of Gonads, Adrenals and Mental Illness," *Physiology & Behavior* 97, no. 2 (May 25, 2009): 250–258, https://doi.org/10.1016/j.physbeh.2009.02.033.

54. Fiona C. Baker and Kathryn Aldrich Lee, "Menstrual Cycle Effects on Sleep," *Sleep Medicine Clinics* 13, no. 3 (September 2018): 283–294, https://doi.org/10.1016/j.jsmc.2018.04.002; George M. Slavich and Julia Sacher, "Stress, Sex Hormones, Inflammation, and Major Depressive Disorder: Extending Social Signal Transduction Theory of Depression to Account for Sex Differences in Mood Disorders," *Psychopharmacology* 236, no. 10 (October 2019): 3063–3079, https://doi.org/10.1007/s00213-019-05326-9.

55. Adrienne O'Neil et al., "Gender/Sex as a Social Determinant of Cardiovascular Risk," *Circulation* 137, no. 8 (February 20, 2018): 854–864, https://doi.org/10.1161/CIRCULATIONAHA.117.028595.

56. O'Neil, "Gender/Sex as a Social Determinant," 854–864.

57. Yang Du et al., "Trends in Adherence to the Physical Activity Guidelines for Americans for Aerobic Activity and Time Spent on Sedentary Behavior Among US Adults, 2007 to 2016," *JAMA Network Open* 2, no. 7 (July 26, 2019): e197597, https://doi.org/10.1001/jamanetworkopen.2019.7597.

58. P. Smith, J. Frank, and C. Mustard, "Trends in Educational Inequalities in Smoking and Physical Activity in Canada: 1974–2005," *Journal of Epidemiology & Community Health* 63, no. 4 (April 1, 2009): 317–323, https://doi.org/10.1136/jech.2008.078204.

59. Kimberle Crenshaw, "Demarginalizing the Intersection of Race and Sex: A Black Feminist Critique of Antidiscrimination Doctrine, Feminist Theory and Antiracist Politics," n.d., 31, https://chicagounbound.uchicago.edu/cgi/viewcontent.cgi?article=1052&context=uclf.

60. Hayfa Abichahine and Gerry Veenstra, "Inter-Categorical Intersectionality and Leisure-Based Physical Activity in Canada," *Health Promotion International* 32, no. 4 (August 1, 2017): 691–701, https://doi.org/10.1093/heapro/daw009; Laura H. McArthur and Thomas D. Raedeke, "Race and Sex Differences in College Student Physical Activity Correlates," *American Journal of Health Behavior* 33, no. 1 (February 2009): 80–90, https://doi.org/10.5993/ajhb.33.1.8.

61. Mariane M. Fahlman, Heather L. Hall, and Robyn Lock, "Ethnic and Socioeconomic Comparisons of Fitness, Activity Levels, and Barriers to Exercise in High School Females," *Journal of School Health* 76, no. 1 (January 2006): 12–17, https://doi.org/10.1111/j.1746-1561.2006.00061.x; Gwen M. Felton et al., "Differences in Physical Activity Between Black and White Girls Living in Rural and Urban Areas," *Journal of School*

*Health* 72, no. 6 (2002): 250–255, https://doi.org/10.1111/j.1746-1561.2002.tb07338.x; Laura H. McArthur and Thomas D. Raedeke, "Race and Sex Differences in College Student Physical Activity Correlates," *American Journal of Health Behavior* 33, no. 1 (February 2009): 80–90, https://doi.org/10.5993/ajhb.33.1.8.

62. Audre Lorde, *A Burst of Light* (Ithaca, NY: Firebrand Books, 1988).

63. Nancy Noyola-Martínez, Ali Halhali, and David Barrera, "Steroid Hormones and Pregnancy," *Gynecological Endocrinology* 35, no. 5 (May 4, 2019): 376–384, https://doi.org/10.1080/09513590.2018.1564742.

64. Nicola De Pisapia et al., "Sex Differences in Directional Brain Responses to Infant Hunger Cries," *NeuroReport* 24, no. 3 (February 13, 2013): 142–146, https://doi.org/10.1097/WNR.0b013e32835df4fa.

65. Massimiliano de Zambotti et al., "Acute Stress Alters Autonomic Modulation During Sleep in Women Approaching Menopause," *Psychoneuroendocrinology* 66 (April 2016): 1–10, https://doi.org/10.1016/j.psyneuen.2015.12.017; Lauren L. Drogos et al., "Objective Cognitive Performance Is Related to Subjective Memory Complaints in Midlife Women with Moderate to Severe Vasomotor Symptoms," *Menopause* 20, no. 12 (December 2013): 1236–1242, https://doi.org/10.1097/GME.0b013e318291f5a6.

66. Mihoko Akiyoshi et al., "Relationship Between Estrogen, Vasomotor Symptoms, and Heart Rate Variability in Climacteric Women," *Journal of Medical and Dental Sciences* 58, no. 2 (July 4, 2011): 49–59.

67. Gail A. Greendale, Carol A. Derby, and Pauline M. Maki, "Perimenopause and Cognition," *Obstetrics and Gynecology Clinics of North America* 38, no. 3 (September 2011): 519–535, https://doi.org/10.1016/j.ogc.2011.05.007.

68. Brandalyn C. Riedel, Paul M. Thompson, and Roberta Diaz Brinton, "Age, APOE and Sex: Triad of Risk of Alzheimer's Disease," *Journal of Steroid Biochemistry and Molecular Biology* 160 (June 2016): 134–247, https://doi.org/10.1016/j.jsbmb.2016.03.012.

69. Di Zhao et al., "Endogenous Sex Hormones and Incident Cardiovascular Disease in Post-Menopausal Women," *Journal of the American College of Cardiology* 71, no. 22 (June 5, 2018): 2555–2566, https://doi.org/10.1016/j.jacc.2018.01.083; Ying Zhou et al., "Prevalence and Risk Factors of Hypertension among Pre- and Post-Menopausal Women: A Cross-Sectional Study in a Rural Area of Northeast China," *Maturitas* 80, no. 3 (March 2015): 282–287, https://doi.org/10.1016/j.maturitas.2014.12.001; S. R. Davis et al., "Understanding Weight Gain at Menopause," *Climacteric: The Journal of the International Menopause Society* 15, no. 5 (October 2012): 419–429, https://doi.org/10.3109/13697137.2012.707385.

70. M. Shepherd-Banigan et al., "Improving Vasomotor Symptoms; Psychological Symptoms; and Health-Related Quality of Life in Peri- or Post-Menopausal Women through Yoga: An Umbrella Systematic Review and Meta-analysis," *Complementary Therapies in Medicine* 34 (October 2017): 156–164, https://doi.org/10.1016/j.ctim.2017.08.011.

71. Aarti Nagarkar, Rashmi Gadkari, Snehal Kulkarnia, "Correlates of Functional Limitations in Midlife: A Cross-Sectional Study in Middle-Aged Men (45–59 Years) from Pune," *Journal of Mid-Life Health* 11 (September 29, 2020): 144–148, https://doi.org/10.4103/jmh.JMH_79_19.

72. A. Vermeulen, "Andropause," *Maturitas* 34, no. 1 (January 15, 2000): 5–15, https://doi.org/10.1016/s0378-5122(99)00075-4.

73. Y. Joel Wong et al., "Meta-analyses of the Relationship Between Conformity to Masculine Norms and Mental Health-Related Outcomes," *Journal of Counseling Psychology* 64, no. 1 (2017): 80–93, https://doi.org/10.1037/cou0000176.

74. Kenneth D. Kochanek et al., "Deaths: Final Data for 2002," *National Vital Statistics Reports: From the Centers for Disease Control and Prevention, National Center for Health*

*Statistics, National Vital Statistics System* 53, no. 5 (October 12, 2004): 1–115, https://www.cdc.gov/nchs/data/nvsr/nvsr53/nvsr53_05.pdf.

75. James R. Mahalik, Shaun M. Burns, and Matthew Syzdek, "Masculinity and Perceived Normative Health Behaviors as Predictors of Men's Health Behaviors," *Social Science & Medicine* (1982) 64, no. 11 (June 2007): 2201–2209, https://doi.org/10.1016/j.socscimed.2007.02.035.

76. "Men and Heart Disease," Centers for Disease Control and Prevention, February 3, 2021, https://www.cdc.gov/heartdisease/men.htm.

77. Benjamin D. Yetton et al., "Quantifying Sleep Architecture Dynamics and Individual Differences Using Big Data and Bayesian Networks," *PLOS ONE* 13, no. 4 (2018): e0194604, https://doi.org/10.1371/journal.pone.0194604.

78. Julie Carrier et al., "Sleep Slow Wave Changes during the Middle Years of Life," *European Journal of Neuroscience* 33, no. 4 (February 2011): 758–766, https://doi.org/10.1111/j.1460-9568.2010.07543.x.

79. Marta Jackowska and Dorina Cadar, "The Mediating Role of Low-Grade Inflammation on the Prospective Association Between Sleep and Cognitive Function in Older Men and Women: 8-Year Follow-Up from the English Longitudinal Study of Ageing," *Archives of Gerontology and Geriatrics* 87 (April 2020): 103967, https://doi.org/10.1016/j.archger.2019.103967.

80. Wei Shen et al., "Race and Sex Differences of Long-Term Blood Pressure Profiles from Childhood and Adult Hypertension: The Bogalusa Heart Study," *Hypertension* (Dallas: 1979) 70, no. 1 (July 2017): 66–74, https://doi.org/10.1161/HYPERTENSIONAHA.117.09537.

81. Louise Pilote et al., "A Comprehensive View of Sex-Specific Issues Related to Cardiovascular Disease," *CMAJ: Canadian Medical Association Journal = Journal de l'Association médicale canadienne* 176, no. 6 (March 13, 2007): S1–S44, https://doi.org/10.1503/cmaj.051455.

82. Bijil Simon Arackal and Vivek Benegal, "Prevalence of Sexual Dysfunction in Male Subjects with Alcohol Dependence," *Indian Journal of Psychiatry* 49, no. 2 (April 2007): 109–112, https://doi.org/10.4103/0019-5545.33257; Bang-Ping Jiann, "Effect of Alcohol Consumption on the Risk of Erectile Dysfunction," *Urological Science* 21, no. 4 (December 1, 2010): 163–168, https://doi.org/10.1016/S1879-5226(10)60037-1; Rena R. Wing et al., "Effects of Weight Loss Intervention on Erectile Function in Older Men with Type 2 Diabetes in the Look AHEAD Trial," *Journal of Sexual Medicine* 7, no. 1 (January 2010): 156–165, https://doi.org/10.1111/j.1743-6109.2009.01458.x.

83. Tanjaniina Laukkanen et al., "Sauna Bathing Is Inversely Associated with Dementia and Alzheimer's Disease in Middle-Aged Finnish Men," *Age and Ageing* 46, no. 2 (March 1, 2017): 245–249, https://doi.org/10.1093/ageing/afw212.

84. Lawrence D. Hayes et al., "Exercise-Induced Responses in Salivary Testosterone, Cortisol, and Their Ratios in Men: A Meta-analysis," *Sports Medicine* 45, no. 5 (May 2015): 713–726, https://doi.org/10.1007/s40279-015-0306-y.

85. Danielle S. Berke, Dennis Reidy, and Amos Zeichner, "Masculinity, Emotion Regulation, and Psychopathology: A Critical Review and Integrated Model," *Clinical Psychology Review* 66 (December 2018): 106–116, https://doi.org/10.1016/j.cpr.2018.01.004.

86. Berke, Reidy, and Zeichner, "Masculinity, Emotion Regulation, and Psychopathology."

87. James Mahali, "Incorporating a Gender Role Strain Perspective in Assessing and Treating Men's Cognitive Distortions," *Professional Psychology: Research and Practice* 30 (August 1, 1999): 333–340, https://doi.org/10.1037/0735-7028.30.4.333.

## Part Three. Hitting the Reset Button

1. Janelle Monáe, "Victory," *The Electric Lady*, Wondaland Records, Bad Boy Entertainment, Atlantic Records, 2013, compact disc.

## Chapter Eight. The Downstate RecoveryPlus Plan

1. James H. Fowler and Nicholas A. Christakis, *Connected: The Surprising Power of Our Social Networks and How They Shape Our Lives—How Your Friends' Friends' Friends Affect Everything You Feel, Think, and Do*, illustrated ed. (New York: Little, Brown Spark, 2011).

2. Phillippa Lally et al., "How Are Habits Formed: Modelling Habit Formation in the Real World," *European Journal of Social Psychology* 40, no. 6 (2010): 998–1009, https://doi.org/10.1002/ejsp.674.

3. Qing Li, *Forest Bathing* (New York: Penguin Random House, 2018), https://www.penguinrandomhouse.com/books/579709/forest-bathing-by-dr-qing-li/.

4. Rollin McCraty and Maria A. Zayas, "Cardiac Coherence, Self-Regulation, Autonomic Stability, and Psychosocial Well-Being," *Frontiers in Psychology* 5 (2014): 1090, https://doi.org/10.3389/fpsyg.2014.01090; Noortje H. Rijken et al., "Increasing Performance of Professional Soccer Players and Elite Track and Field Athletes with Peak Performance Training and Biofeedback: A Pilot Study," *Applied Psychophysiology and Biofeedback* 41, no. 4 (December 1, 2016): 421–430, https://doi.org/10.1007/s10484-016-9344-y; James B. Burch et al., "Shift Work and Heart Rate Variability Coherence: Pilot Study Among Nurses," *Applied Psychophysiology and Biofeedback* 44, no. 1 (March 1, 2019): 21–30, https://doi.org/10.1007/s10484-018-9419-z.

5. Cindy Meston and Amelia Stanton, "A Single Session of Autogenic Training Increases Acute Subjective and Physiological Sexual Arousal in Sexually Functional Women," *Journal of Sex & Marital Therapy* 43, no. 7 (October 3, 2017): 601–617, https://doi.org/10.1080/0092623X.2016.1211206.

6. Martha Davis, Elizabeth Robbins Eshelman, and Matthew McKay, *The Relaxation and Stress Reduction Workbook*, 6th ed. (Oakland, CA: New Harbinger Publications, 2008).

7. Danielle Pacheco and Heather Wright, "The Best Temperature for Sleep: Advice & Tips," Sleep Foundation, June 24, 2021, https://www.sleepfoundation.org/bedroom-environment/best-temperature-for-sleep.

8. Pacheco and Wright, "Best Temperature."

9. Lauren Fountain, "Best Earplugs for Sleeping of 2021," Sleep Foundation, August 17, 2021, https://www.sleepfoundation.org/best-earplugs-for-sleep.

10. CDC, "Move More; Sit Less," Centers for Disease Control and Prevention, October 7, 2020, https://www.cdc.gov/physicalactivity/basics/adults/index.htm.

11. Zahra Alizadeh et al., "Acute Effect of Morning and Afternoon Aerobic Exercise on Appetite of Overweight Women," *Asian Journal of Sports Medicine* 6, no. 2 (June 2015): e24222, https://doi.org/10.5812/asjsm.6(2)20156.24222.

12. Valerie F Gladwell et al., "The Great Outdoors: How a Green Exercise Environment Can Benefit All," *Extreme Physiology & Medicine* 2, no. 1 (January 3, 2013): 3, https://doi.org/10.1186/2046-7648-2-3.

13. Leah M. Schumacher et al., "Consistent Morning Exercise May Be Beneficial for Individuals with Obesity," *Exercise and Sport Sciences Reviews* 48, no. 4 (2020), https://journals.lww.com/acsm-essr/Fulltext/2020/10000/Consistent_Morning_Exercise_May_Be_Beneficial_for.7.aspx.

14. A. K. Mohiuddin, "Skipping Breakfast Everyday Keeps Well-Being Away," *Pharmaceutical Sciences* 7, no. 1 (January 18, 2019): 7, https://www.fortunejournals.com/articles /skipping-breakfast-everyday-keeps-wellbeing-away.html.

15. Jennie I. Macdiarmid, "Seasonality and Dietary Requirements: Will Eating Seasonal Food Contribute to Health and Environmental Sustainability?," *Proceedings of the Nutrition Society* 73, no. 3 (2014): 368–375, https://doi.org/10.1017/S0029665113003753; Maria Ibars et al., "Seasonal Consumption of Polyphenol-Rich Fruits Affects the Hypothalamic Leptin Signaling System in a Photoperiod-Dependent Mode," *Scientific Reports* 8, no. 1 (September 11, 2018): 13572, https://doi.org/10.1038/s41598-018-31855-y.

## Chapter Nine. Everything You Always Wanted to Know About the Future of the Downstate (but Were Afraid to Ask)

1. SpaceX, "Live Views of Starman," filmed February 6, 2018, YouTube video, https:// www.youtube.com/watch?v=aBr2kKAHN6M.

2. J. K. Penry and J. C. Dean, "Prevention of Intractable Partial Seizures by Intermittent Vagal Stimulation in Humans: Preliminary Results," *Epilepsia* 31, suppl. 2 (1990): S40–S43, https://doi.org/10.1111/j.1528-1157.1990.tb05848.x.

3. K. B. Clark et al., "Enhanced Recognition Memory Following Vagus Nerve Stimulation in Human Subjects," *Nature Neuroscience* 2, no. 1 (January 1999): 94–98, https://doi .org/10.1038/4600.

4. Hsiangkuo Yuan and Stephen D. Silberstein, "Vagus Nerve and Vagus Nerve Stimulation, a Comprehensive Review: Part II," *Headache: The Journal of Head and Face Pain* 56, no. 2 (February 2016): 259–266, https://doi.org/10.1111/head.12650.

5. Robert H. Howland, "Vagus Nerve Stimulation," *Current Behavioral Neuroscience Reports* 1, no. 2 (June 1, 2014): 64–73, https://doi.org/10.1007/s40473-014-0010-5.

6. Lorenza Colzato and Christian Beste, "A Literature Review on the Neurophysiological Underpinnings and Cognitive Effects of Transcutaneous Vagus Nerve Stimulation: Challenges and Future Directions," *Journal of Neurophysiology* 123, no. 5 (May 1, 2020): 1739–1755, https://doi.org/10.1152/jn.00057.2020.

7. Björn Rasch et al., "Odor Cues During Slow-Wave Sleep Prompt Declarative Memory Consolidation," *Science* 315, no. 5817 (March 9, 2007): 1426–1429, https://doi.org /10.1126/science.1138581; John D. Rudoy et al., "Strengthening Individual Memories by Reactivating Them During Sleep," *Science* 326, no. 5956 (November 20, 2009): 1079, https://doi.org/10.1126/science.1179013; Katharine C. N. S. Simon, Rebecca L. Gómez, and Lynn Nadel, "Losing Memories During Sleep after Targeted Memory Reactivation," *Neurobiology of Learning and Memory* 151 (May 2018): 10–17, https://doi.org/10.1016/j.nlm .2018.03.003.

8. Hong-Viet V. Ngo et al., "Auditory Closed-Loop Stimulation of the Sleep Slow Oscillation Enhances Memory," *Neuron* 78, no. 3 (May 2013): 545–553, https://doi.org/10 .1016/j.neuron.2013.03.006.

9. Lisa Marshall et al., "Boosting Slow Oscillations During Sleep Potentiates Memory," *Nature* 444, no. 7119 (November 2006): 610–613, https://doi.org/10.1038/nature05278.

10. Massimiliano de Zambotti et al., "The Boom in Wearable Technology: Cause for Alarm or Just What Is Needed to Better Understand Sleep?" *Sleep* 39, no. 9 (September 2016): 1761–1762, https://doi.org/10.5665/sleep.6108.

11. Heidemarie Haller et al., "Craniosacral Therapy for Chronic Pain: A Systematic Review and Meta-analysis of Randomized Controlled Trials," *BMC Musculoskeletal Disorders* 21, no. 1 (December 2020): 1, https://doi.org/10.1186/s12891-019-3017-y;

M. Castejón-Castejón et al., "Effectiveness of Craniosacral Therapy in the Treatment of Infantile Colic. A Randomized Controlled Trial," *Complementary Therapies in Medicine* 47 (December 2019): 102164, https://doi.org/10.1016/j.ctim.2019.07.023.

12. Guillermo A. Matarán-Peñarrocha et al., "Influence of Craniosacral Therapy on Anxiety, Depression and Quality of Life in Patients with Fibromyalgia," *Evidence-Based Complementary and Alternative Medicine* 2011 (2011): 1–9, https://doi.org/10.1093/ecam/nep125.

13. Jennifer Fox, author in conversation with, April 23, 2021.

14. "What Is a DO?" American Osteopathic Association, accessed September 3, 2021, https://osteopathic.org/what-is-osteopathic-medicine/what-is-a-do/.

15. *Take Your Pills*, directed by Alison Klayman (Motto Pictures, 2018), https://www.netflix.com/title/80117831.

16. Casey Schwartz, "Generation Adderall," *New York Times*, October 12, 2016, sec. Magazine, https://www.nytimes.com/2016/10/16/magazine/generation-adderall-addiction.html.

17. Tenzin Tselha et al., "Morning Stimulant Administration Reduces Sleep and Overnight Working Memory Improvement," *Behavioural Brain Research* 370 (September 16, 2019): 111940, https://doi.org/10.1016/j.bbr.2019.111940; Lauren N. Whitehurst et al., "The Impact of Psychostimulants on Sustained Attention over a 24-h Period," *Cognition* 193 (December 1, 2019): 104015, https://doi.org/10.1016/j.cognition.2019.104015.

18. Martha J. Farah et al., "When We Enhance Cognition with Adderall, Do We Sacrifice Creativity? A Preliminary Study," *Psychopharmacology* 202, no. 1 (January 1, 2009): 541–547, https://doi.org/10.1007/s00213-008-1369-3; Gregory R. Samanez-Larkin et al., "A Thalamocorticostriatal Dopamine Network for Psychostimulant-Enhanced Human Cognitive Flexibility," *Biological Psychiatry* 74, no. 2 (July 15, 2013): 99–105, https://doi.org/10.1016/j.biopsych.2012.10.032.

19. Lauren N. Whitehurst and Sara C. Mednick, "Psychostimulants May Block Long-Term Memory Formation via Degraded Sleep in Healthy Adults," *Neurobiology of Learning and Memory* 178 (February 2021): 107342, https://doi.org/10.1016/j.nlm.2020.107342; Lauren N. Whitehurst et al., "The Impact of Psychostimulants on Sustained Attention over a 24-h Period," *Cognition* 193 (December 1, 2019): 104015, https://doi.org/10.1016/j.cognition.2019.104015.

20. P. Beaconsfield, J. Ginsburg, and R. Rainsbury, "Marihuana Smoking. Cardiovascular Effects in Man and Possible Mechanisms," *New England Journal of Medicine* 287, no. 5 (August 3, 1972): 209–212, https://doi.org/10.1056/NEJM197208032870501; C. Kanakis, J. M. Pouget, and K. M. Rosen, "The Effects of Delta-9-Tetrahydrocannabinol (Cannabis) on Cardiac Performance with and Without Beta Blockade," *Circulation* 53, no. 4 (April 1976): 703–707, https://doi.org/10.1161/01.cir.53.4.703.

21. John R. Richards et al., "Cannabis Use and Acute Coronary Syndrome," *Clinical Toxicology* 57, no. 10 (October 3, 2019): 831–841, https://doi.org/10.1080/15563650.2019.1601735.

22. David A. Gorelick et al., "Tolerance to Effects of High-Dose Oral Δ9-Tetrahydrocannabinol and Plasma Cannabinoid Concentrations in Male Daily Cannabis Smokers," *Journal of Analytical Toxicology* 37, no. 1 (February 2013): 11–16, https://doi.org/10.1093/jat/bks081.

23. R. R. Perron, R. L. Tyson, and G. R. Sutherland, "Delta9-Tetrahydrocannabinol Increases Brain Temperature and Inverts Circadian Rhythms," *Neuroreport* 12, no. 17 (December 4, 2001): 3791–3794, https://doi.org/10.1097/00001756-200112040-00038.

24. Kimberly A. Babson, James Sottile, and Danielle Morabito, "Cannabis, Cannabinoids, and Sleep: A Review of the Literature," *Current Psychiatry Reports* 19, no. 4 (April 2017): 23, https://doi.org/10.1007/s11920-017-0775-9.

25. Nadia Montero-Oleas et al., "Therapeutic Use of Cannabis and Cannabinoids: An Evidence Mapping and Appraisal of Systematic Reviews," *BMC Complementary Medicine and Therapies* 20, no. 1 (January 15, 2020): 12, https://doi.org/10.1186/s12906-019-2803-2.

26. Alex Capano, Richard Weaver, and Elisa Burkman, "Evaluation of the Effects of CBD Hemp Extract on Opioid Use and Quality of Life Indicators in Chronic Pain Patients: A Prospective Cohort Study," *Postgraduate Medicine* 132, no. 1 (January 2, 2020): 56–61, https://doi.org/10.1080/00325481.2019.1685298; Philip McGuire et al., "Cannabidiol (CBD) as an Adjunctive Therapy in Schizophrenia: A Multicenter Randomized Controlled Trial," *American Journal of Psychiatry* 175, no. 3 (March 2018): 225–231, https://doi.org/10.1176/appi.ajp.2017.17030325; Franjo Grotenhermen and Ethan Russo, eds., *Cannabis and Cannabinoids: Pharmacology, Toxicology, and Therapeutic Potential* (New York: Haworth Integrative Healing Press, 2002).

27. Kimberly A. Babson, James Sottile, and Danielle Morabito, "Cannabis, Cannabinoids, and Sleep: A Review of the Literature."

28. Anthony N. Nicholson et al., "Effect of Delta-9-Tetrahydrocannabinol and Cannabidiol on Nocturnal Sleep and Early-Morning Behavior in Young Adults," *Journal of Clinical Psychopharmacology* 24, no. 3 (June 2004): 9, https://doi.org/10.1097/01.jcp .0000125688.05091.8f.

29. E. Gouzoulis-Mayfrank et al., "Psychopathological, Neuroendocrine and Autonomic Effects of 3,4-Methylenedioxyethylamphetamine (MDE), Psilocybin and d-Methamphetamine in Healthy Volunteers," *Psychopharmacology* 142, no. 1 (February 18, 1999): 41–50, https://doi.org/10.1007/s002130050860.

30. Daniela Dudysová et al., "The Effects of Daytime Psilocybin Administration on Sleep: Implications for Antidepressant Action," *Frontiers in Pharmacology* 11 (December 3, 2020): 602590, https://doi.org/10.3389/fphar.2020.602590.

31. Manel J. Barbanoj et al., "Daytime Ayahuasca Administration Modulates REM and Slow-Wave Sleep in Healthy Volunteers," *Psychopharmacology* 196, no. 2 (February 2008): 315–326, https://doi.org/10.1007/s00213-007-0963-0.

32. Adam Wichniak et al., "Effects of Antidepressants on Sleep," *Current Psychiatry Reports* 19, no. 9 (September 2017): 63, https://doi.org/10.1007/s11920-017-0816-4.

33. Serena Bauducco, Cele Richardson, and Michael Gradisar, "Chronotype, Circadian Rhythms and Mood," *Current Opinion in Psychology* 34 (August 2020): 77–83, https://doi .org/10.1016/j.copsyc.2019.09.002.

34. Duncan French, author in conversation with, December 21, 2020.

35. Joseph O. C. Coyne et al., "Heart Rate Variability and Direct Current Measurement Characteristics in Professional Mixed Martial Arts Athletes," *Sports* (Basel, Switzerland) 8, no. 8 (July 30, 2020): E109, https://doi.org/10.3390/sports8080109.

## Chapter Ten. Becoming a Downstate Maven

1. Robert Frost, "The Road Not Taken," Poetry Foundation (Poetry Foundation, 1916), https://www.poetryfoundation.org/poems/44272/the-road-not-taken.

2. Michael Pollan, "Six Rules for Eating Wisely," June 4, 2006, https://michaelpollan. com/articles-archive/six-rules-for-eating-wisely/.

3. Christine Runyan, author in conversation with, May 25, 2021.

4. I. Vlaev et al., "Changing Health Behaviors Using Financial Incentives: A Review from Behavioral Economics," *BMC Public Health* 19 (2019): 1059. https://doi.org/10.1186/s12889-019-7407-8; I. Vlaev et al., "Changing Health Behaviors Using Financial Incentives: A Review from Behavioral Economics," BMC Public Health 19 (2019): 1059. https://doi.org/10.1186/s12889-019-7407-8.

5. Llewellyn Vaughan-Lee, *We Are All One: Full Interview from* One the Movie, video recording, fall 2002, https://goldensufi.org/video-single/we-are-all-one-full-interview-from-one-the-movie/.

6. Liv Aanrud, author in conversation with, February 14, 2021.

7. Alessandra Shuster et al., "Sleep and Mood Across the Menstrual Cycle in Young Women," *Sleep* 44, suppl. 2 (May 1, 2021): A39, https://doi.org/10.1093/sleep/zsab072.092.

8. Jonathan S. Emens et al., "Circadian Rhythm in Negative Affect: Implications for Mood Disorders," *Psychiatry Research* 293 (November 2020): 113337, https://doi.org/10.1016/j.psychres.2020.113337.

9. Richard Hammersley, Marie Reid, and Stephen L. Atkin, "How to Measure Mood in Nutrition Research," *Nutrition Research Reviews* 27, no. 2 (December 2014): 284–294, https://doi.org/10.1017/S0954422414000201.

## Epilogue

1. Pema Chödrön, *The Places That Scare You: A Guide to Fearlessness in Difficult Times* (Boulder, CO: Shambhala Publications, 2002).

# Index

# About the Author

**Dr. Sara C. Mednick** is Professor of Psychology at the University of California, Irvine, where she directs the Sleep and Cognition (SaC) lab. Her first book, *Take a Nap! Change Your Life,* put forth the scientific basis for napping to improve productivity, cognition, mood, and health. A world-renowned scientist, Dr. Mednick's lab investigates the mind and body mechanisms that support performance improvement. Her work has been continuously federally funded with grants from the National Institutes of Health, National Science Foundation, Department of Defense Office of Naval Research, and the Defense Advanced Research Projects Agency (DARPA), a United States Department of Defense agency. She has been interviewed by every major magazine and newspaper, including the *New York Times, New Yorker, Los Angeles Times, Washington Post,* and BBC, and has been featured on *Good Morning America*, among others. She resides in San Diego, and with her wife in the Hudson Valley.

AU website: www.saramednick.com
AU social media: @Sara_Mednick (Twitter)